EVALUATION OF
PROTEINS FOR HUMANS

other AVI books

Nutrition and Biochemistry

CARBOHYDRATES AND THEIR ROLES   *Schultz, Cain and Wrolstad*
CHEMISTRY AND PHYSIOLOGY OF FLAVORS   *Schultz, Day and Libbey*
DIETARY NUTRIENT GUIDE   Soft Cover   *Pennington*
DRUG-INDUCED NUTRITIONAL DEFICIENCIES   *Roe*
FOOD ENZYMES   *Schultz*
IMMUNOLOGICAL ASPECTS OF FOODS   *Catsimpoolas*
LIPIDS AND THEIR OXIDATION   *Schultz, Day and Sinnhuber*
NUTRITIONAL EVALUATION OF FOOD PROCESSING, 2ND EDITION   Cloth and Soft Cover   *Harris and Karmas*
PROGRESS IN HUMAN NUTRITION, VOL. 1   *Margen*
PROTEINS AND THEIR REACTIONS   *Schultz*
PROTEINS AS HUMAN FOOD   *Lawrie*
SELENIUM IN BIOMEDICINE   *Muth, Oldfield and Weswig*
SULFUR IN NUTRITION   *Muth and Oldfield*

Food Science

BASIC FOOD CHEMISTRY   Cloth and Soft Cover   *Lee*
BREAD SCIENCE AND TECHNOLOGY   *Pomeranz and Shellenberger*
DAIRY LIPIDS AND LIPID METABOLISM   *Brink and Kritchevsky*
DAIRY TECHNOLOGY AND ENGINEERING   Cloth and Soft Cover   *Harper and Hall*
EGG SCIENCE AND TECHNOLOGY   *Stadelman and Cotterill*
ELEMENTARY FOOD SCIENCE   Cloth and Soft Cover   *Nickerson and Ronsivalli*
ENCYCLOPEDIA OF FOOD ENGINEERING   *Hall, Farrall and Rippen*
ENCYCLOPEDIA OF FOOD TECHNOLOGY   *Johnson and Peterson*
FABRICATED FOODS   *Inglett*
FOOD ANALYSIS LABORATORY EXPERIMENTS   Soft Cover   *Meloan and Pomeranz*
FOOD ANALYSIS: THEORY AND PRACTICE   *Pomeranz and Meloan*
FOOD AND THE CONSUMER   Soft Cover   *Kramer*
FOOD ENGINEERING SYSTEMS, VOL. 1   Cloth and Soft Cover   *Farrall*
FOOD FLAVORINGS, 2ND EDITION   *Merory*
FOOD FOR THOUGHT   Soft Cover   *Labuza*
FOOD PROCESS ENGINEERING   Cloth and Soft Cover   *Heldman*
FOOD PRODUCTS FORMULARY, VOL. 1   *Komarik, Tressler and Long*   VOL. 2   *Tressler and Sultan*   VOL. 3   *Tressler and Woodroof*
FOOD SCIENCE, 2ND EDITION   *Potter*
FREEZING PRESERVATION OF FOODS, 4TH EDITION, VOLS. 1, 2, 3 AND 4   *Tressler, Van Arsdel and Copley*
FUNDAMENTALS OF DAIRY CHEMISTRY, 2ND EDITION   *Webb, Johnson and Alford*
FUNDAMENTALS OF FOOD ENGINEERING, 2ND EDITION   *Charm*
POULTRY PRODUCTS TECHNOLOGY, 2ND EDITION   *Mountney*
SAFETY OF FOODS   *Graham*
SOYBEANS, VOL. 1   *Smith and Circle*
SUGAR CHEMISTRY   *Shallenberger and Birch*

EVALUATION OF
PROTEINS FOR HUMANS

Edited by C. E. BODWELL, Ph.D.
Protein Nutrition Laboratory
Nutrition Institute
USDA, ARS
Beltsville, Maryland

A Volume based on a Symposium held at the 35th Annual Meeting of the Institute of Food Technologists, Chicago, Illinois, June 8–12, 1975; sponsored by the Nutrition Division, IFT.

THE AVI PUBLISHING COMPANY, INC.
WESTPORT, CONNECTICUT

Library of Congress Catalog Card Number: 76-27468
ISBN-0-87055-215-5

Printed in the United States of America
BY THE MACK PRINTING COMPANY

Contributors

L. VAN BEEK, Central Institute for Nutrition and Food Research (CIVO)-TNO, Utrechtseweg 48, Zeist, The Netherlands

C. E. BODWELL, Protein Nutrition Laboratory, Nutrition Institute, USDA, ARS, Beltsville, Maryland

RICARDO BRESSANI, Instituto de Nutrición de Centro América y Panamá (INCAP), Carretera Rossevelt, Zona 11, Guatemala, Central America

ROBERT E. FEENEY, Department of Food Science and Technology, University of California, Davis, California

V. J. FERON, Central Institute for Nutrition and Food Research (CIVO)-TNO, Utrechtseweg 48, Zeist, The Netherlands

A. P. DE GROOT, Central Institute for Nutrition and Food Research (CIVO)-TNO, Utrechtseweg 48, Zeist, The Netherlands

L. ROSS HACKLER, Cornell University, Geneva, New York

D. M. HEGSTED, Department of Nutrition, Harvard School of Public Health, Harvard University, Boston, Massachusetts

G. RICHARD JANSEN, Department of Food Science and Nutrition, Colorado State University, Fort Collins, Colorado

CONSTANCE V. KIES, Department of Food and Nutrition, University of Nebraska, Lincoln, Nebraska

PAUL A. LACHANCE, Department of Food Science, Cook College, Rutgers University, New Brunswick, New Jersey

IRVIN E. LIENER, Department of Biochemistry, College of Biological Sciences, University of Minnesota, St. Paul, Minnesota

WILDA H. MARTINEZ, National Program Staff, USDA, ARS, Beltsville, Maryland

GARY A. MILLER, Department of Food and Nutrition, University of Nebraska, Lincoln, Nebraska

KENNETH W. SAMONDS, Department of Nutrition, School of Public Health, Harvard University, Boston, Massachusetts

NEVIN S. SCRIMSHAW, Department of Nutrition and Food Science, Massachusetts Institute of Technology, Cambridge, Massachusetts

P. SLUMP, Central Institute for Nutrition and Food Research (CIVO)-TNO, Utrechtseweg 48, Zeist, The Netherlands.

DAVID A. VAUGHAN, Protein Nutrition Laboratory, Nutrition Institute, USDA, ARS, Beltsville, Maryland

VERNON R. YOUNG, Department of Nutrition and Food Science, Massachusetts Institute of Technology, Cambridge, Massachusetts

Foreword

This book is the outcome of a symposium sponsored by the Nutrition Division of the "IFT" and is being published because it reflects the most current information available on the use of proteins in human feeding. With the current need for protein in the food supply of the world, it is extremely important that we learn as much about proteins as we possibly can.

We have always been hampered by the need for methods of assaying to determine the real potential of a protein in human feeding and determine the effects of processing on proteins. This book also deals with antinutritional factors found in food that have plagued researchers for many years. This area will be of vital importance in the coming years as more and more sources of proteins are examined. The possibility of many of the anti-nutrients surviving processing is high and the possible deleterious effects on humans could be considerable. Efforts must be made for detection and practical elimination of these factors.

The information in this book does not present easy solutions to difficult problems; however, it does aid the researcher in avoiding pitfalls in the evaluation of proteins and suggests promising leads for additional research that hopefully will culminate in better ways of selection and processing of proteins and in more reliable and less complicated methods for the determination of nutritional quality.

HOWARD E. BAUMAN, Ph.D.
Chairman, Nutrition
Division of the IFT,
1975–1976

May 1976

Preface

Although considerable discussion has evolved recently about whether a lack of protein sources or a lack of dietary energy sources is the primary cause of human malnutrition on a global basis, such discussions do not obviate the central importance of proteins in human nutrition. Likewise, it is not disputed that, in the decades ahead, sources of protein will undoubtedly need to be conserved. One approach for conserving protein sources is to develop methods for more accurately assessing the nutritional value of proteins for human consumption. Such methods would provide a basis for the more efficient utilization of the protein resources which may be available. This is discussed further in the Introductory Chapter which comprises Section I of this book. In Section II, protein and amino acid metabolism and requirements for humans are discussed with particular emphasis on the need for considering these factors in relation to protein quality evaluation. Extant methods for estimating the nutritional value of proteins for humans are critically evaluated (including *in vitro* methods, animal or human bioassays and biochemical indices). Also, techniques used in animal bioassays and human nitrogen balance studies are specifically described. Lastly, in Section III, factors of potential practical importance which may affect nutritional value are considered.

Other books have been published during the past few years which are concerned with the same general subject area. However, for the most part, these have not precisely addressed the problems under consideration in terms of human nutrition *per se*. Accordingly it is hoped that the current volume will be a worthy addition to the existing body of literature.

Contributors from various Federal Agencies are expressing their own opinions and not those of the Federal Government.

All royalties derived from the sale of this volume will be retained by the Nutrition Division of the Institute of Food Technologists for use in sponsoring future programs.

C. E. BODWELL, PH.D.

September 15, 1976

Acknowledgments

Appreciation is expressed to the Institute of Food Technologists and to the IFT Nutrition Division for scheduling and sponsoring the symposium on which this volume is based. Concern is periodically expressed relative to the role of the food industry in, and their contribution to, the nutritional well-being of the national population. The scheduling of two half-day sessions during the annual IFT meeting to the subject of "Proteins for Human Consumption" (as well as numerous other sessions devoted to nutrition) is an expression of a genuine concern to be aware of recent developments in the area of human nutrition as they relate to foods and the food industry.

Appreciation is expressed to the contributors, for without their efforts the symposium and this volume would obviously not have been possible. Those authors who willingly contributed Chapters 1, 7 and 8, on topics not originally included in the symposium, are due a special mention of appreciation. The generous support of the four companies who provided expenses for some of the speakers was essential to the scheduling of the symposium. For their role in making this support available (and to their respective companies), thanks are due to Dr. Howard Bauman (Pillsbury Co.); Dr. Wayne Henry (Far-Mar-Co., Inc); Dr. C. J. O'Donovan (Miles Laboratories, Inc.); and Dr. L. D. Williams (Central Soya Co., Inc.).

The collaboration of the symposium Co-Chairman, Dr. L. D. Williams, in making suggestions for speakers and program topics and for obtaining financial support is gratefully acknowledged. The efforts of Dr. Howard Bauman, Nutrition Division Chairman (1975–1976) and Dr. Miles Sawyer, Nutrition Division Secretary-Treasurer, were particularly helpful in matters related to publication of the symposium. Lastly, appreciation is expressed to Mrs. E. C. Cole for her assistance in preparing some of the manuscripts and the index in a final form for submission to the publishers.

Contents

Introduction

CHAPTER 1

N. S. Scrimshaw
and V. R. Young

Nutritional Evaluation and the Utilization of Protein Resources

At a time when the population of the earth has increased from two billion to four billion people in only 35 yr and is due to add another billion persons in the next 12 yr, problems of maintaining a balance between population and food supplies are becoming ever more serious. Today, disruptions in the world food system, for whatever reason, cause suffering for ever larger numbers of people, and there is increasing concern for the future.

Before 1940, the developing countries of the world were, for the most part, either self-sufficient or food exporters. Of the major regions, only Europe was a net importer of food and food exports from North America were relatively unimportant. However, the pattern of world food exports has undergone a radical change during the last 40 yr, as shown in Table 1.1 for the cereal grains (Brown 1975).

Eastern Europe and the USSR, Africa and Asia, largely Japan, China, and India, have become major importers of grain, whereas North America and Australia have shown dramatic increases in their grain exports. From North America, grain exports have nearly doubled in the last 6 yr, from 56 million metric tons in 1970 to an estimated 100 million tons (approximately) during 1976. A major factor accounting for this shift in the world grain trade is the high rate of world population growth, although other factors are also important. Thus, the fluctuations in the Soviet grain harvest and political decisions to meet the deficit in domestic agricultural production have been largely responsible for the growing imports of grain by the USSR during the past few years.

World food production per caput has maintained a precarious balance with increasing world population. This has not been the case, however, for most developing countries, and in some, periods of unfavorable weather, political upheavals, economic and other factors have precipitated famine.

Less dramatic than famine, but in the aggregate more tragic and important at the national and international levels, is the degradation of immense numbers of human lives, especially those of young children, by

1

TABLE 1.1

CHANGING PATTERN OF WORLD GRAIN TRADE DURING THE PAST 40 YR

Region	Grain Exports (+) and Imports (−) Million Metric Tons				
	1934– 1938	1948– 1952	1960	1970	1976
North America	+5	+23	+39	+56	+94
Latin America	+9	+1	0	+4	−3
Western Europe	−24	−22	−25	−30	−17
Eastern Europe and USSR	+5		0	+1	−25
Africa	+1	0	−2	−5	−10
Asia	+2	−6	−17	−37	−47
Australia and New Zealand	+3	+3	+6	+12	+8

Source: Brown (1975); 1976 values are estimates.

chronic malnutrition (Table 1.2). Estimates of the total number of severely malnourished people in the world today begin at more than 460 million (Natl. Acad. Sci. 1975). Depending upon the criteria, 15–25% of the child populations of developing countries of Asia, Africa, and Latin America are estimated to be seriously malnourished.

NEEDS FOR EXPANDING FOOD AND PROTEIN PRODUCTION

Increasing food production on a global scale is a problem of critical importance and it is exacerbated further by the addition of 200,000 persons per day in the world population. However, the increasing world need for food is due, not only to the growing population, but also to rising affluence. In some developing countries, the average person is sustained by the equivalent of about 400 lb of cereal per year, consumed directly, whereas in the United States, per caput requirement for cereal grain is nearly 2000 lb, most of it fed to animals and consumed ultimately as meat, eggs, and dairy products. It has been estimated that 91% of the cereal, legume, and vegetable protein produced in the United States, and suitable for human use, is fed to livestock (Pimentel *et al.* 1975). Furthermore, the extensive use of grains in livestock and meat production is responsible for the considerable increase which has occurred in the feed-grain imports into Japan during the past decade, making Japan, at present, the world's largest grain importer.

With greater purchasing power, not only are other industrialized countries following this same pattern of increased consumption of animal products, but this is also occurring among upper income populations in developing countries. Thus, available food supplies are not only consumed disproportionately by the more affluent countries, but also by the more prosperous segments of the population within developing countries. Be-

TABLE 1.2

NUMBER OF PEOPLE ESTIMATED BY THE FAO TO HAVE AN INSUFFICIENT
PROTEIN-ENERGY SUPPLY IN 1970, BY REGION

Region	Population (Millions)	Number Below Lower Limit (Millions)
Developed	1,074	28
Developing	1,751	434
Latin America	283	36
Far East	1,020	301
Near East	171	30
Africa	273	67
World	2,825	462

Source: Poleman (1975).

cause of this, estimates of per caput food availability data on either a national or world basis conceal the real extent of undernutrition and malnutrition among those populations that are economically and socially the least privileged. In many developing countries, much of the population is still restricted to diets made up almost entirely of cereal grain, and large numbers do not receive enough for normal health and activity. The urgent need for increasing food production and availability in these countries is apparent.

An adequate supply of protein is a central aspect of the world food problem. Cereal grains are not in themselves nutritionally adequate for man, and do not have the concentration of utilizable protein relative to calories needed for optimum growth and development of young children and the proper nourishment of groups suffering from either physiological or pathological causes of stress. Unless supplemented by legumes, fruits, vegetables, and nuts, and desirably by modest amounts of milk, eggs, meat, or fish, the predominantly cereal diets are inadequate in some of the essential vitamins and minerals, and deficient in protein for growing children, pregnancy, lactation, and disease conditions. Populations, for whom cereals are not sufficiently supplemented by other foods, typically exhibit signs of nutritional deficiency and energy intakes are likely to be inadequate as well.

Because of the high cost of protein of animal origin, the usual cereal diets of low income populations are traditionally supplemented by legumes as a source of more concentrated protein and one whose amino acid pattern complements that of most cereal proteins (see Chapter 10). However, the intensive research on cereal grains has improved the efficiency and profitability to the farmers of cereals compared with legumes. Because of the urgent food needs of the so-called Green Revolution countries with their

TABLE 1.3

RELATIVE IMPORTANCE OF VARIOUS FOOD GROUPS IN AVERAGE WORLD
DAILY PER CAPUT INTAKE

	Calories (Number)	(%)	Proteins (gm)	(%)
Cereals	1,242	52.4	31.1	47.4
Wheat	441	18.6	13.3	20.3
Rice	459	19.3	8.5	13.0
Corn (maize)	147	6.2	3.6	5.5
Millet and sorghum	119	5.0	3.5	5.3
Others	76	3.2	2.1	3.2
Roots and tubers	184	7.8	2.8	4.8
Sugar and sugar products	210	8.8	0.1	0.2
Pulses, nuts and oilseeds	121	5.1	7.9	12.0
Vegetables	36	1.5	2.2	3.4
Fruits	47	2.0	0.6	0.9
Total animal products	322	13.6	20.7	31.5
Meat	168	7.1	9.2	14.0
Eggs	18	0.8	1.4	2.1
Fish	19	0.8	3.0	4.6
Milk	117	4.9	7.1	10.8
Fats and oils	199	8.4	0.1	0.2
Vegetable oils	127	5.3	—	—
Animal fats	72	3.1	0.1	0.2
Total	2,374	100.0	64.6	100.0
Animal origin	396	16.7	20.8	31.7

Source: Univ. of California (1974); based on FAO (1971).

rapidly rising populations, governments have provided special incentives
for cereal grain production. The wheat crop doubled in India within a period
of 6 yr, from 1966–1971, and the country almost reached self-sufficiency
in the early 1970's (Brown 1975). However, a negative effect of this effort
to increase total food production is that there has been a fall in legume
production in many developing countries, shorter supplies of legumes and
higher prices which have led to a further decrease in the adequacy of dietary
protein for the vulnerable groups in these countries.

PRODUCTION AND DISTRIBUTION OF MAJOR FOOD PROTEIN SOURCES

Because this book is devoted to proteins for humans, it is also pertinent
to consider briefly the world availability and distribution of protein foods.
A more detailed assessment of this topic is covered in a number of recent
reviews (e.g., Stillings 1973; Jalil and Tahir 1973; Univ. of California 1974;
Pimentel et al. 1975).

Precise estimates of world protein supplies are difficult to make, for
reasons such as the extensive losses which may occur following harvesting
and because crop yields may be undeclared or subject to large error (Farmer

TABLE 1.4

ENERGY AND PROTEIN SUPPLIES (1963–1965) PER CAPUT PER DAY

Region	Population (1969) (Million)	Energy (kJ)	Animal Protein (Gm)	Total Protein (Gm)
Far East[1]	1966	8580	8.6	54.8
Near and Middle East	166	10080	14.0	71.6
Africa	297	9080	10.9	58.5
Latin America	276	10840	24.1	67.6
Developing Regions	2750	8950	10.7	57.6
Europe[2]	698	12760	42.8	87.6
North America	224	13140	65.3	93.1
Oceania	19	13510	63.9	95.4
Developed Regions	941	12850	48.3	89.1
World	3646	9960	21.0	66.1

Source: Stillings (1973).
[1] Includes Mainland China.
[2] Includes USSR.

1969). However, a recent estimate of the contribution of plant and animal sources to the dietary protein supplies in the world is given in Table 1.3. For the plant sources, cereals (mainly wheat, corn, and rice) provided over $2/3$ of the world plant protein supply and grain legumes under $1/5$. In total, the plant sources provide approximately 70% of the world supply of edible protein, and in the developing countries the contribution is higher.

There is, of course, a marked discrepancy in per caput protein supplies for both animal and plant protein sources between the developed and developing regions of the world, as shown in Table 1.4. Animal products supply about 70% of the protein intake in the U.S. diet, whereas this figure approaches zero for many individuals in rural areas of India and Indonesia.

IMPROVING THE SUPPLY OF PROTEINS AND CHANGE IN PATTERN OF DIETARY PROTEIN

Improving the supply of food protein for man can be approached in a number of ways. In the foreseeable future the bulk of the increase must come from a primary increase in the output of the traditional agricultural sources, as well as through a more efficient use and recovery of protein from these sources. The latter involves, in part, increased utilization of by-products, such as whey and blood in the case of dairy and meat production, and nutritional upgrading of cereal products from low-cost cereal grains. Alternatively, and of significance in the longer-term future, the total supply of protein can be improved by the production of novel primary materials that can be used for food and feed to supplement traditional ones. Single cell protein sources (SCP) offer an example of approaches which depend upon the efficient utilization of nonagricultural materials or agricultural wastes. SCP is a generic term for protein produced through fermentation of petroleum derivatives or organic substrates and wastes by single-cell organisms such as yeasts, bacteria, and microfungi. Some forms of SCP have been used as human food for millennia and new forms have reached the stage of clinical evaluation. Any fermented food will contain significant quantities of cellular organisms as diverse as bacteria, yeast, and fungi. Thus, there should be nothing fundamentally objectionable in the food use of these species, although some will be inadequate for direct human consumption, whereas others will be found to be suitable for this purpose.

In addition to the major problem of national and world protein supplies, the diet of the future is likely to change dramatically from its present form. The introduction of the texturized vegetable proteins from soy and other oilseeds into the diet of the affluent sectors of industrialized nations is a recent example of this. Furthermore, it is anticipated that there will be major changes in the source and physical form of protein-containing foods consumed to meet the physiological and psychological needs for protein, as innovative advances in food production, processing and technology find their application in the market place.

All of these factors, ranging from the planning and improvement in national and world food supplies to the development of new protein sources and introduction of new types of food, require adequate knowledge of human dietary protein and amino acid requirements and the ways in which they can be met effectively. This raises a final problem which must be mentioned and that is the problem of protein requirements and the nutritional evaluation of protein sources.

IMPORTANCE OF NUTRITIONAL EVALUATION

Adequate knowledge of human protein and amino acid requirements is fundamental to the rational development of approaches for improving, and subsequently maintaining, the nutritional adequacy of diets of population groups. During the past 40 yr, changes have occurred among the successive national and international proposals for dietary protein standards, and these changes have important implications with respect to national food and agricultural policies and programs. This point has been emphasized by Whitehead (1973) and it is illustrated in Table 1.5. The interpretation of dietary data for a representative developing country, Uganda, would be quite different, depending upon whether the National Research Council allowances (Natl. Res. Council 1948) were thought to be adequate or if the recent Food and Agriculture Organization/World Health Organization recommendations (FAO/WHO 1973) were considered more appropriate.

TABLE 1.5

THE INTERPRETATION OF DIETARY DATA FROM UGANDA ON THE BASIS OF
NRC (1948) AND FAO/WHO (1973) RECOMMENDED PROTEIN ALLOWANCES

| Nutrient Intake | Ugandan Children (Mean) | NRC (1948) | | | FAO/WHO (1973) | | |
		Recom.	Adequacy (%)	Lim. Factor	Recom.	Adequacy (%)	Lim. Factor
Protein (gm/kg/day)	1.5	4.5	33	+ + +	2.2	68	—
Energy (kJ/kg/day)	280	420	67	—	418	67	+

Source: Modified from and calculated according to Whitehead (1973).
[1] Assuming a 55% nitrogen utilization, relative to egg or milk protein.

In the former case, interpretation of the dietary survey data leads to the conclusion that protein is the major limiting dietary component and the focus of food production programs should be on increasing the availability and consumption of protein foods. However, using the 1973 FAO/WHO guidelines, it would have to be concluded that there was a deficit in the quantity rather than the quality of the diet. Thus, increased production and consumption of the traditional diet should provide for an adequate level of nutritional status for the particular population of concern. Clearly, there is an essential need for sound and adequate data on human protein requirements and dietary protein quality in order to develop satisfactory dietary standards. There are, however, major uncertainties and problems concerned with current estimates of protein requirements and the assessment and practical significance of protein nutritional quality. Although these problems are dealt with in depth in subsequent chapters, it is worth noting in these introductory comments some of the significant limitations in present knowledge as well as to emphasize the need for improved methodological approaches to protein nutritional evaluation.

Firstly, with respect to nutritional requirements, it should be emphasized that a disconcerting fact of the recent international, FAO/WHO (1973) recommendations for protein allowances in adults is that they are based largely on short-term metabolic balance studies carried out in healthy Caucasian university students. Secondly, successive FAO/WHO Expert Committees (FAO/WHO 1965; 1973) have stated that the occurrence of acute and chronic infectious diseases, including intestinal parasites, needs to be taken into account in applying these recommendations to the populations of developing countries. However, such a suggestion is meaningless because no guidelines for doing so have been supplied. In any event, the current recommendations are not adequate for such populations although it is not known, in quantitative terms, how much more protein is required by persons living in these conditions. Furthermore, it is uncertain whether protein nutritional quality has more or less importance under these circumstances than for healthy individuals living in the medically favorable conditions of the industrialized countries. Moreover, additional losses of nitrogen in sweat occasioned by hard physical work under tropical conditions are not taken into account, and the extent to which this is necessary has not been determined. Thirdly, as discussed in Chapter 2, it is now clear that generous energy intakes were supplied in most metabolic nitrogen balance studies, including the ones on which the recommended allowances for protein and the essential amino acid requirements are based. This experimental condition would lower losses of body nitrogen below those occurring at energy intakes appropriate for the maintenance of weight under ordinary conditions. The net result has been an underestimation of the minimum protein and essential amino acid intakes necessary to maintain nutritional status.

Clearly, there is a special need for studies on the determination of protein requirements in various age groups in populations and under conditions relevant to developing countries. For pregnancy and lactation, existing recommendations are based on estimates of the additional protein needs for the fetus and other products of pregnancy and the amount of protein excreted in breast milk, but the data are limited and contradictory. For school-age children, adolescents and the elderly, the data are equally fragmentary. This critical need for improved knowledge of protein requirements in man can only be met through long-term, controlled experiments in different populations and under various conditions, if the human use of food protein supplies is to be planned efficiently without jeopardy to the individual. The lack of a satisfactory and quantitative body of knowledge of human and energy protein requirements is an important reason for the differences in scientific opinion on the extent to which food protein and/or energy supplies limit the nutritional well-being of a large proportion of the world's population.

Even if the human protein requirements, expressed in terms of protein of high quality such as egg or milk, were known with greater precision, current methods of adjusting these figures for differences in dietary quality are not satisfactory. The 1971 FAO/WHO Committee (FAO/WHO 1973) suggests that either amino acid score or bioassay results for net protein utilization (NPU) be used for this purpose, but the amino acid score is unreliable for foods submitted to thermal processing. Moreover, sampling, as well as bioassay procedures, introduce further elements of uncertainty into this method of assessing protein quality and limit its practical significance.

Net protein utilization is usually measured at suboptimal levels of nitrogen intake, and this overestimates protein quality because the degree of efficiency of dietary utilization at these levels of intake is greater than when the intake is just sufficient to maintain nitrogen balance or growth. The FAO/WHO Expert Committee attempted to make an allowance for this effect by adding 30% to their estimate of factorial losses of body nitrogen (obligatory losses in urine, feces, and via the integument under conditions of adequate calories and very low or zero nitrogen intakes). Unfortunately, the available research indicates that the allowance for egg was insufficient and that the inadequacy may be proportionately greater, the poorer the quality of protein. Thus, current recommendations would put the populations of developing countries in multiple jeopardy by underestimating requirements, ignoring adverse environmental factors and by overestimating dietary protein quality.

Finally, a precise method of evaluating protein quality is important, not only to make possible estimation of the amount of a given protein mixture required to meet physiological needs for protein, but also to guide efforts aimed at improving the protein quality of food crops and food mixtures and to monitor the nutritionally adverse effects of food processing procedures. Oilseed meals, for example, are frequently subjected to a thermal processing step in order to remove the oil. Because they are such important potential sources of protein to supplement predominantly cereal diets and provide the protein concentrate of weaning foods, it is essential that adequate approaches be developed for assessing protein nutritional quality in relation to human protein needs.

CONCLUSIONS

This brief introduction has served to emphasize a number of serious problems which have direct relevance to the requirements for proteins and the quantity of various food proteins to meet them. Plant sources, which make the greatest contribution to the world protein supply, are of generally lower quality protein than those of animal origin. Moreover, with the increasing global needs for protein, a proportionate expansion of animal sources of protein will not be as great as that for the plant sources. Furthermore, the production of novel sources of food protein, involving new processing methods, and the development of new food products also are likely to occur at an increasing pace because of pressures on traditional food supplies and their increasing costs. Indeed, an editorial in a recent issue of *Nature* (Vol. 258, p. 373, 1975) stated that Lord Zuckerman suggests that the survival of western civilization is going to depend on a new food revolution.

Improved knowledge of the nutritional value of proteins, including the assessment of human protein requirements, is already of great practical importance. It will be of even greater significance with the continued growth of the world's population, and this book documents the current extent of our knowledge and provides an important stimulus and guide to research needs.

BIBLIOGRAPHY

BROWN, L. R. 1975. The world food prospect. Science *190*, 1053.

FAO. 1971. Agricultural Commodity Projections, 1970–1980, Vol. I and II. Food and Agriculture Organization of the United Nations, Rome, Italy.

FAO/WHO. 1965. Protein Requirements. FAO Nutrition Meetings, Rept. Ser. *37*, Food and Agriculture Organization of the United Nations, Rome, Italy.

FAO/WHO. 1973. Energy and Protein Requirements. World Health Organization, Tech. Rept. Ser. *522*, World Health Organization, Geneva, Switzerland.

FARMER, B. H. 1969. Available food supplies. *In* Population and Food Supply, J. B. Hutchinson (Editor). Cambridge University Press, Cambridge.

JAHIL, M. E., and TAHIR, W. M. 1973. World supplies of plant proteins. *In* Proteins in Human Nutrition, J. W. G. Porter, and B. A. Rolls (Editors). Academic Press, New York.

NATL. ACAD. SCI. 1975. Population and Food. Crucial Issues. National Academy of Sciences, Washington, D.C.

NATL. RES. COUNCIL. 1948. Recommended Dietary Allowances, Revised, 1948. Reprint and Circ. Ser. *129*. Washington, D. C.

PIMENTEL, D., DRITSCHILO, W., KRUMMEL, J., and KUTZMAN, J. 1975. Energy and land constraints in food production. Science *190*, 754.

POLEMAN, T. T. 1975. World Food: A Perspective. Science *188*, 510.

STILLINGS, B. R. 1973. World supplies of animal protein. *In* Proteins in Human Nutrition, J. W. G. Porter, and B. A. Rolls (Editors). Academic Press, New York.

UNIV. OF CALIFORNIA. 1974. A hungry world: The challenge to agriculture. General Report by Univ. of California Food Task Force, Division of Agricultural Sciences, Univ. of California.

WHITEHEAD, R. G. 1973. The protein needs of malnourished children. *In* Proteins in Human Nutrition, J. W. G. Porter, and B. A. Rolls (Editors). Academic Press, New York.

Evaluation

CHAPTER 2

V. R. Young and
N. S. Scrimshaw

Human Protein and Amino Acid Metabolism and Requirements in Relation to Protein Quality[1,2]

Food protein sources differ in their relative capacities to meet human protein requirements. Thus, proteins of plant origin, such as from wheat and oil-seed legumes, are usually required at higher levels of intake than those of animal origin, such as cow's milk and meat, in order to support an adequate protein nutritional status within an individual.

It has generally been concluded that major variations in protein quality are caused by differences in the amino acid composition of food proteins, although other factors may be important in specific cases, as discussed in the subsequent chapters. It is pertinent to consider first the requirements for protein and essential amino acids and the factors which affect them. This will facilitate an evaluation of the nutritional and metabolic significance of dietary protein quality and can potentially lead to a more rational approach to the determination of the nutritive value of food proteins for human consumption.

This review will consider first some general features of protein metabolism in the whole body in order to explore the metabolic basis for protein and amino acid requirements at various stages throughout life. Our purpose is to assess the significance of the changes which occur in body protein and amino acid metabolism during normal growth and development, and later in the aging individual, and their relationships to dietary protein quality. This topic will be followed by an evaluation of the major factors which influence the utilization of dietary protein, giving particular emphasis to the influences of protein and energy intake on adaptive aspects of body protein metabolism and nitrogen retention.

[1] The unpublished results obtained in the authors' laboratories were supported by NIH grants AM15856, AM16654, HD98300, AM16322, a contract with the US Department of Agriculture (No. 12-14-1001-258) and the US National Live Stock and Meat Board.
[2] Publication No. 2675 from the Department of Nutrition and Food Science, Massachusetts Institute of Technology, Cambridge, Massachusetts 02139.

With this background, the approaches taken in arriving at estimations of the quantitative needs for protein and essential amino acids will be discussed to assess the status of current knowledge of human protein and amino acid requirements. The reader is referred also to various reviews and statements concerned with human protein and amino acid requirements (Hegsted 1963; FAO/WHO 1973; Porter and Rolls 1973; Fomon *et al.* 1973; Food and Nutrition Board, 1974A) and nutritional aspects of dietary protein quality (Allison 1964; Campbell and McLaughlan 1971; Bressani and Viteri 1971; White and Fletcher 1974; Young 1975) for more detailed background information in the areas covered in this chapter.

SOME METABOLIC CONSIDERATIONS OF THE DAILY PROTEIN REQUIREMENTS

The quantitatively most important function of dietary protein is to provide the substrate necessary for the maintenance of body protein synthesis in the adult and for a net protein gain in the growing organism. Additional roles played by amino acids include the synthesis of neurotransmitters, nicotinamide, purines and pyrimidines, and other metabolically active products such as creatine, carnosine, anserine, the adrenal medullary, thyroid and peptide hormones, and porphyrins. Although these compounds are of great physiological importance, presumably they do not account for the utilization of a quantitatively significant fraction of the amino acids ingested daily. Therefore, it is worthwhile to explore initially body protein synthesis and how it changes with normal growth and development in the human subject.

It has been recognized for many years that the intensity of protein metabolism in mammalian species is related to the same power of body weight as is basal energy metabolism. Thus, Brody (1945) showed that the variation in obligatory nitrogen losses among nine species, ranging in size from the mouse to the cow, correlated with the 0.72 power of body weight, expressed in kilograms (Fig. 2.1). More recently, Munro (1969) reviewed this aspect of body protein metabolism and computed the power function of body weight which was best correlated among adults of mammalian species with parameters of tissue and whole body protein metabolism, including albumin and ceruloplasmin turnover and liver RNA content.

The estimates of Munro, together with those of Brody (1945) and others (e.g., Smuts 1935; Waterlow 1968), demonstrate clearly the intimate relationships between the intensity of body protein and energy metabolism in the intact organism. Hence, the fall in basal energy expenditure, per unit of body weight in mammalian species, including man, during continued growth and development (see Kleiber 1961) would be expected to reflect a similar decline in the intensity of body protein turnover. Similarly, it would not be surprising to anticipate a fall in dietary protein needs with

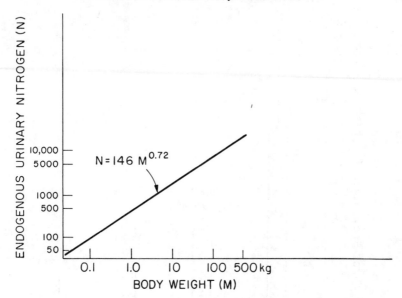

FIG. 2.1.   RELATIONSHIP BETWEEN ENDOGENOUS URINARY NITROGEN AND BODY
SIZE OF MAMMALIAN SPECIES

Schematized from the analysis of Brody (1945).

a decline in the intensity of protein metabolism, in a way analogous to the
reduction in dietary energy needs which accompanies the diminution in
the intensity of energy metabolism with continued development and at-
tainment of maturity.

It is known that the rate of total body protein synthesis, per unit of body
weight, declines with progressive growth and development within a mammalian species (Waterlow and Stephen 1967), again in parallel with the
reduced intensity of body energy metabolism which occurs during the
growth period (Kleiber 1961). A number of separate studies (Nicholson
1970; San Pietro and Rittenberg 1953; Picou and Taylor-Roberts 1969;
Sharp et al. 1957) confirm this for man.

We have recently explored, in man, the quantitative changes in total body
protein synthesis using the same experimental approach at various stages
of life. The isotope method, developed by Picou and Taylor-Roberts (1969)
is based on the continuous administration of ^{15}N-labeled glycine and the
analysis of urinary urea for ^{15}N enrichment after a constant level of isotope
enrichment in the metabolic amino acid pool has been achieved. Details
of the procedures and the subjects have been described (Young et al. 1975;
Steffee et al. 1975; Pencharz 1974; Winterer et al. 1975).

Three age groups have been studied so far: (1) newborn, including six
premature infants and one full-term baby, all of whom were studied during

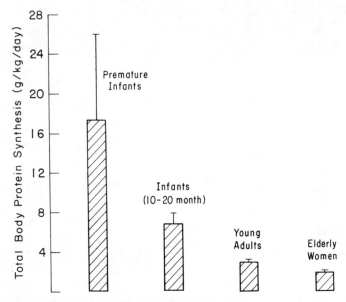

FIG. 2.2. CHANGE IN THE INTENSITY OF TOTAL BODY PROTEIN SYNTHESIS AT VARIOUS TIMES OF LIFE IN HUMAN SUBJECTS

Drawn from the data of Young *et al.* (1975A).

a 30–36 hr ^{15}N tracer period within 1–45 days of life and two babies were studied two or three times; (2) healthy, normal young adults, three male and one female, 20–23 yr old; (3) four healthy, elderly women, 69–91 yr of age. The [15]*N*-glycine was given during a 60-hr tracer period in studies with young adults and the elderly. Diets provided constant intakes of essential nutrients and were judged to be adequate for each age group.

Figure 2.2 portrays results, expressed per unit of body weight, for the three age groups and, for comparative purposes, we have also included the data of Picou and Taylor-Roberts (1969) which were obtained with infants, about 1 yr old. These observations indicate that the intensity of body protein synthesis declines rapidly during the first year of life and in young adults it is about ⅙ of that found in premature babies. Furthermore, the rate of protein synthesis, per unit of body weight, continues to decline, but more gradually, with the value for elderly subjects studied being about ⅔ of that for healthy young adults. Thus, the intensity of protein metabolism, per unit of body weight, in man declines, as in the rat (Waterlow 1968), throughout life.

To examine further the relationship between changes in the intensity of whole body protein synthesis and energy metabolism, we have recalculated the data on the basis of energy expenditure for each of the age groups, as summarized in Table 2.1. Differences in the intensity of protein me-

TABLE 2.1

MEAN TOTAL BODY PROTEIN SYNTHESIS IN RELATION TO BASAL ENERGY
METABOLISM AND DIETARY PROTEIN ALLOWANCES IN PREMATURE BABIES,
INFANTS, YOUNG ADULTS AND ELDERLY WOMEN

Age Group	Dietary Protein Allowance (gm kg^{-1} day^{-1})	Protein Synthesis (gm)	
		per kcal Basal Energy Expenditure	per gm Protein Allowance
Newborn[1]	3.2	0.15 ± 0.09	5.4
Infants (~1 yr)	1.3		5.3
Young Adult	0.57	0.11 ± 0.01	5.2
Elderly	0.42	0.11 ± 0.03	4.5

Source: Taken from Young et al. (1975A). Data for infants from Picou and
Taylor-Roberts (1969).
[1]Premature.

tabolism among the various age groups are essentially eliminated when body
protein synthesis is related to basal energy expenditure. These results in
human subjects confirm the previous observations among and within
mammalian species that the intensity of protein metabolism is closely related to the intensity of energy metabolism (Brody 1945; Waterlow 1968;
Munro 1969).

The lowered rate of body protein synthesis in the elderly age group,
relative to young adults, deserves further consideration, particularly because some investigators have concluded that protein and amino acid requirements change during advanced age (see reviews by Watkin 1957, 1964;
Young et al. 1976). Firstly, the lowered rate of body protein synthesis, per
unit of body weight, may be due to a lower protein mass (Forbes and Reina
1970; Parizkova et al. 1971). Thus, additional ways of comparing the rates
of total body protein synthesis in young adults and elderly subjects are
depicted in Fig. 2.3. Firstly, using creatinine excretion as an index of muscle
mass (Muldowney et al. 1957; Graystone 1968; Alleyne et al. 1970), this
figure shows that total body protein synthesis per gram of creatinine excreted is considerably higher in the aged subject than in the young adult.
Because muscle mass is reduced with advancing age (e.g., Yiengst et al.
1959), the higher turnover of total body protein per unit of creatinine excretion in the elderly may be caused by a relatively greater contribution
by active visceral tissues to whole body protein synthesis in the elderly
subject than in young adults.

This hypothesis can be explored by comparison of urinary N^τ-methyl-
histidine (3-methylhistidine) excretion in young adults and elderly subjects.
This unusual amino acid is present in actin of all muscles and the myosin
of "white" muscle fibers (see Young et al. 1973A and Haverberg et al. 1974
for brief reviews) and the major proportion of protein-bound 3-methyl-

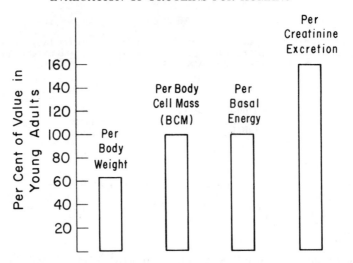

FIG. 2.3.   THE RATE OF TOTAL BODY PROTEIN SYNTHESIS

Expressed per unit body weight, body cell mass, kcal of basal metabolism and creatinine excretion, in elderly women in comparison with
values obtained in young adults. Based on unpublished results of Winterer et al. (1975) and Young et al. (1975B).

histidine is located in skeletal muscle (Haverberg et al. 1975A). In rats
(Young et al. 1972A) and man (Young et al. 1973A; Long et al. 1975) it is
quantitatively excreted in the urine and, unlike the common amino acids
of body proteins, it is not reutilized for purposes of protein synthesis (Young
et al. 1972A) or metabolized via oxidative pathways (Long et al. 1975).
Therefore, we have measured the excretion of 3-methylhistidine as an index
of the rate and extent of muscle protein breakdown in human subjects of
various ages (Havèrberg et al. 1975B).

A summary of our recent measurements on the urinary output of this
amino acid in young adults and elderly women is given in Table 2.2. These
data show that the daily output of 3-methylhistidine is much lower in the
elderly women than in young adults, reflecting the lowered muscle mass
in elderly subjects. However, when normalized for differences in creatinine
excretion, the output of 3-methylhistidine in the elderly women is still below
that for young adults. This observation suggests that, per unit of muscle
mass, the rate of muscle protein breakdown and therefore synthesis declines
with advanced age in man. It is further supported by studies showing reduced muscle protein synthesis (Breuer and Florini 1965; Geary and Florini
1972; Waterlow and Stephen 1968; Britton and Sherman 1975; also reviewed by Young 1974) with increased age in mice and rats. Hence, the
higher rate of body protein synthesis and catabolism per unit creatinine
output in the elderly age group indicates a shift in the distribution of body

TABLE 2.2

A COMPARISON OF MEAN RESULTS FOR URINARY 3-METHYLHISTIDINE
EXCRETION IN YOUNG ADULT MEN AND ELDERLY WOMEN CONSUMING
A FLESH-FREE DIET [1]

Characteristics	Young Adults	Elderly
Body weight (kg)	67.2	56.7
Age (yr)	21	77
3-Methylhistidine (mg)		
per day	33.5	12.7
per kg/day	0.50	0.22
per gm creatinine	21	17

[1] Unpublished results of Haverberg et al. (1975B). The data are based on six subjects in each age group.

protein metabolism. At this later stage in life, the visceral organs, liver, kidney, and intestine, account for a greater proportion of body protein metabolism than during the young adult years. However, as also shown in Fig. 2.3, total body protein synthesis is similar in young adults and elderly women when the data are expressed per unit of body cell mass or basal energy expenditure.

We should point out that our comparisons are based on a cross-sectional comparison and utilize our preliminary results obtained from four elderly *women*. We do not yet know whether quantitatively similar conclusions would apply to data from elderly *men*, but it seems likely, and, therefore, additional studies in aged individuals of both sexes would be highly worthwhile.

The significance of these observations relative to the dynamic aspects of whole body protein metabolism, dietary protein and amino acid needs and the evaluation of protein quality cannot be judged precisely at present. However, when the estimates of whole body protein synthesis rates are compared with the recent Food and Agriculture Organization/World Health Organization allowances (FAO/WHO 1973) for protein (Table 2.1), it is apparent that the fall in protein allowances with age closely parallels the alterations in the intensity of total body protein synthesis. Thus, it appears that the amount of dietary protein required to support body protein synthesis may be similar in all age groups and that protein needs expressed per unit of body weight are related to differences in the amount of protein synthesized per unit time. Furthermore, these observations offer support, as discussed below, for the statement that a major function of the daily protein intake, even in the young child, is associated with the maintenance of tissue protein content (e.g., Hegsted 1971).

Our data also provide a new basis for assessing the marked differences in protein requirements of infants and older children which, hitherto, have

TABLE 2.3

A COMPARISON OF THE RELATIONSHIP OF NET PROTEIN GAIN TO WHOLE BODY
PROTEIN SYNTHESIS IN HUMAN NEONATES AND YOUNG RATS

	Protein Gain	Whole Body Protein Synthesis	Gain, Synthesis (%)
	(gm Protein/kg/Day)		
Human neonate[1]	2.3	17.4	13
Young rat[2]	9.4	40	24

[1] Based on results by Pencharz (1974). Protein gain was estimated from N balance data.
[2] Estimates based on data summarized by Bernhart (1970) and studies of Millward and Garlick (1972) on total body protein synthesis.

not been explained satisfactorily by differences in the absolute amounts of body nitrogen gained daily. Indeed, as shown in Table 2.3, we estimate that the daily protein gain in premature infants accounts for only about 13% of the total amount of protein synthesized per 24 hr (Pencharz 1974). Table 2.3 also provides comparable values for the young rat and shows, in contrast to the human neonate, that protein gain accounts for about 24% of the total body protein synthesis. The implications of this difference for the relevance of rat bioassay procedures of protein quality to human nutrition should be explored.

BODY PROTEIN METABOLISM IN RELATION TO PROTEIN AND ENERGY INTAKES

From the foregoing it is obvious that the rates of whole body protein synthesis and breakdown are considerably greater than the intake of dietary protein estimated to meet the needs for maintenance of N balance or for growth. Thus, there is an extensive reutilization within the body of the amino acids which are liberated during the course of normal protein breakdown. This recycling of amino acids as well as the rates of synthesis and breakdown of body proteins are subject to change in response to various stimuli, including alterations in the level and adequacy of energy, protein and amino acid intakes. This section will review briefly some of the changes in protein and amino acid metabolism which have been observed in human subjects with alterations in dietary protein and energy intake which may be relevant to published estimates of their protein and amino acid needs.

Effects of Reduced Protein and Amino Acid Intakes

It is common knowledge that when a subject is placed on a reduced level of protein intake, urinary nitrogen output decreases until nitrogen equilibrium is again achieved at the new level of protein intake. If the protein intake is reduced below a certain minimum, the subject will not maintain nitrogen equilibrium and there will be a steady depletion of body protein, with associated alterations in cell structure and organ function, and finally death. This reduction in urinary nitrogen excretion is now generally considered to represent adaptive changes in tissue and organ metabolism (Waterlow 1968). A number of mechanisms, which may not be mutually exclusive, could account for the change in N output, such as: (1) a more efficient use of dietary amino acids for purposes of protein synthesis, (2) reduced catabolism of body protein and of the amino acids liberated during the process of tissue protein breakdown.

Although data are limited in human subjects, some observations can be discussed with a view to providing a partial picture of the way in which human protein metabolism adapts to various nutritional states.

Changes in the Metabolism of Amino Acids.—A low-protein diet in adult man leads to a decrease in the concentration of certain essential amino acids in plasma (e.g., Whitehead 1969; Young and Scrimshaw 1968; Young *et al.* 1973B). Based on an extrapolation from studies in experimental animals (see Munro 1970A for review) these plasma amino acid changes may be reflective of reduced levels of amino acids in some tissues such as muscle and liver. Another example of this kind of adaptive response is provided by our studies on the effects of diets devoid of single essential amino acids. When young men consume these diets for 12 days (Young *et al.* 1971; Ozalp *et al.* 1972) their plasma amino acid response varies with the particular amino acid; a phenylalanine-tyrosine devoid diet results in very little change in the level of plasma free phenylalanine whereas a valine-free diet causes a significant decline in its plasma level (Fig. 2.4). These differential effects of specific dietary essential amino acid deficiencies presumably reflect varying differences in the capacity of the metabolic pathways to adjust to alterations in the intake of the specific amino acid.

In addition to the changes in the concentration of the various amino acids in tissues and body fluids in response to inadequate amino acid intakes, there is now evidence that the amino acids are also oxidized less rapidly *in vivo* under these conditions. Indeed, Krebs (1972) has pointed out that because of the high Km (or Michaelis constant) for enzymes of amino acid oxidation and the relatively low tissue concentration of amino acids, they would be *preferentially* catabolized, in comparison with carbohydrate and fat, when consumed in excess of needs. Following this reasoning, if tissue amino acid levels decline in response to lowered amino acid intakes, their rates of oxidation would be expected to fall.

There are now many examples (reviewed by Kaplan and Pitot 1970) which indicate that enzymes of amino acid metabolism adapt with changes in the nutritional environment. A descriptive example is provided by Mauron (1973) who assayed the activities of two model enzymes in the livers of rats fed various levels of protein (Fig. 2.5). The enzymes were serine

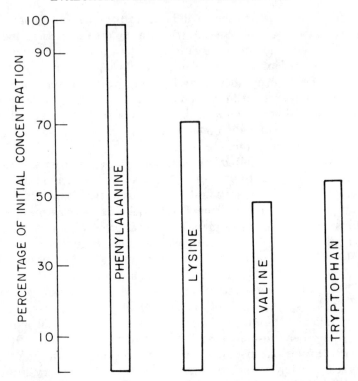

FIG. 2.4.   SCHEMATIC SUMMARY OF CHANGES OBSERVED IN FASTING PLASMA

Amino acid levels in young adults given diets devoid in the single essential amino acid indicated for 12 days. As indicated, each bar represents
plasma changes observed for the test amino acid (lysine, valine or tryptophan) which was omitted; in the case of phenylalanine, both phenylalanine and tyrosine were omitted from the diet. Drawn from the data
of Ozalp *et al.* (1972) and Young *et al.* (1971).

dehydratase (SDH), involved in the conversion of amino acid carbon to
glucose carbon, and 3-phosphoglycerate dehydrogenase (PGDH) involved,
in general terms, with the conversion of carbohydrate carbon to amino acid
carbon. As shown in Fig. 2.5, rats adapted to an increased dietary casein
concentration by *induction* of SDH and reduced PGDH activity. This
suggests, with a high protein or amino acid intake the excess amino acids
are more rapidly catabolized, but that at a low amino acid intake the carbon
from carbohydrate sources must be converted to amino acid carbon to make
the most efficient use of the reduced amounts of available dietary amino
acids. This latter response applies, of course, to the nonessential or dispensable amino acids.

More direct evidence for changes in the extent to which amino acids are
oxidized with varying amino acid intake may be gained from *in vivo* oxi-

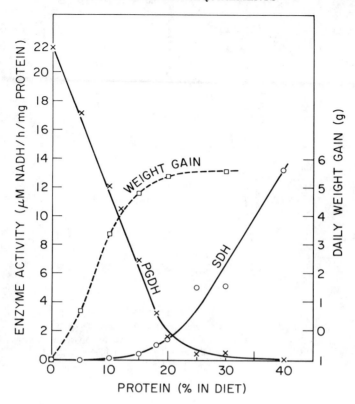

From Mauron (1973)

FIG. 2.5.   WEIGHT GAIN OF RATS GIVEN VARYING DIETARY LEV-
ELS OF CASEIN AND THE ACTIVITIES OF THE LIVER ENZYMES, SER-
INE DEHYDRATASE (SDH) AND 3-PHOSPHOGLYCERATE DEHYDRO-
GENASE (PGDH)

dation studies using ^{14}C-labeled amino acids in experimental animals
(Brookes *et al.* 1972; Sketcher and James 1974; Yamashita and Ashida 1969;
Soliman and Harper 1971; Wang *et al.* 1973). In addition, studies by
Swendseid and Kopple (1973) with ^{14}C-labeled amino acids in adult human
subjects have demonstrated reduced oxidation of histidine and tyrosine
when their dietary supply is low (Fig. 2.6). Information of this type provides
a basis for understanding the mechanisms of adaptation in body protein
metabolism, as well as for evaluating the significance of changes in plasma
amino acid levels, with alterations in amino acid intake, and their relationships to dietary amino acid needs.

From a nutritional, rather than a metabolic, point of view it is important
to consider whether the quantitative extent to which this adaptive decrease
in amino acid oxidation depends upon the relative inadequacy of intake

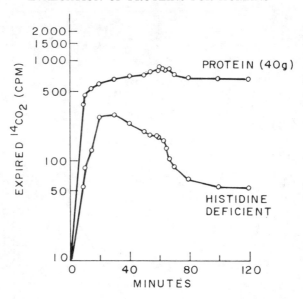

From Swendseid and Kopple (1973)

FIG. 2.6. EFFECT OF A HISTIDINE-FREE DIET ON THE APPEAR-
ANCE OF RADIOACTIVITY IN RESPIRED AIR FOLLWING INJEC-
TION OF ^{14}C-RING LABELED HISTIDINE IN A 53-YR OLD ADULT
MALE SUBJECT

of the amino acid. There is some evidence that it may be geared to nutritional needs (Brookes *et al.* 1972; Young and Munro 1973). For some amino
acids, such as lysine, animal experiments have shown a close relationship
between the dietary intake, the requirement for this amino acid and its
plasma concentration (e.g., Stockland *et al.* 1970). We have explored this
adaptive response in amino acid metabolism as a means of assessing essential amino acid requirements of human subjects of various ages (Young
et al. 1971, 1972B; Tontisirin *et al.* 1972, 1973, 1974).

Total Body N Turnover.—The effects of protein intake on changes in
protein and amino acid metabolism of individual tissues and organs have
been reviewed by others (Munro 1970B; Waterlow and Alleyne 1971) and
will not be discussed here. However, alterations in protein and amino acid
metabolism at the organ level must be finally integrated into the total N
economy of the intact organism. Furthermore, it is the overall total response
of the organism which is of particular interest in reference to the assessment
of protein requirements and dietary protein quality.

This topic may be introduced by pointing out, as shown in Fig. 2.7, that
in addition to the effects of a reduced protein intake in normal subjects,
an adaptive decline in the excretion of urinary N also occurs during star-

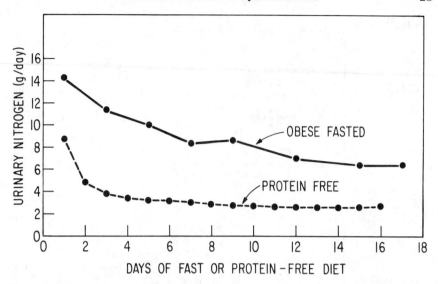

FIG. 2.7. THE EFFECT OF URINARY NITROGEN EXCRETION OF GIVING HEALTHY, NORMAL YOUNG ADULTS A "PROTEIN-FREE" DIET IN COMPARISON WITH THE RESPONSE TO A TOTAL STARVATION IN AN OBESE SUBJECT

These data based on results of Scrimshaw *et al.* (1972) and Young *et al.* (1973A).

vation in obese subjects (Cahill 1970). However, the mechanisms associated with these qualitatively comparable responses to such dietary changes in normal healthy subjects and in obese subjects may be quite different. Evidence that this may be so is suggested by the observation that the changes in plasma amino acid levels differ under these two conditions of dietary protein lack (compare Young and Scrimshaw 1968; Felig *et al.* 1969). Thus, the measurement of N output or N balance does not reveal the ways in which human protein metabolism responds to a given nutritional situation, except in terms of net gain or loss of total body N content. If improved approaches are to be developed for determination of protein and amino acid needs, this must be understood.

Figure 2.8 shows graphically that there are various ways in which whole body protein metabolism may adjust to a new state of nitrogen equilibrium following a change in nitrogen intake. The first possibility shown in the figure is that a reduced rate of body protein breakdown and more efficient retention of dietary N would allow a new equilibrium to be achieved. Here the flux of flow of nitrogen (amino acids) into and out of the metabolic pools is reduced and there is a decline in the intensity of body protein synthesis and breakdown.

The second possibility is that the reduced supply of N or amino acids brings about an enhanced rate of body protein breakdown and that this is

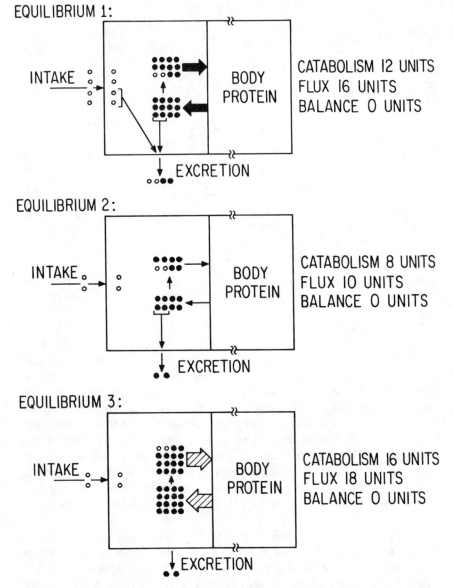

FIG. 2.8. A SCHEMATIC DESCRIPTION OF TWO POSSIBLE WAYS BY WHICH WHOLE BODY PROTEIN TURNOVER RESPONDS TO A REDUCED PROTEIN INTAKE WITH THE ACHIEVEMENT OF A NEW EQUILIBRIUM IN NITROGEN BALANCE

coupled with mechanisms which allow for the overall rate of protein synthesis to increase, the net result of which is a new equilibrium but with an elevation in the rate of turnover of body protein. Clearly, other possibilities

TABLE 2.4

EFFECT OF REDUCED DIETARY PROTEIN INTAKE ON THE FLUX OF NITROGEN
IN THE METABOLIC POOL, WHOLE BODY PROTEIN SYNTHESIS AND PROTEIN
BREAKDOWN IN THE YOUNG ADULT SUBJECTS

Parameter (mg N/kg/hr)	Protein Intake (gm/kg Body wt/Day)		Significance P
	1.5	0.38	
N Flux	28.2	25.7 (−8.8%)	<0.05
Protein synthesis	20.1	23.2 (+15%)	<0.05
Protein breakdown	18.3	23.3 (+27%)	<0.005
$\dfrac{\text{Synthesis}}{\text{N Flux}} \times 100$	71	90 (+27%)	<0.01

Source: Steffee *et al.* (1975). Based on studies in 4 young adult men and 2 young adult women. Dietary periods were 7 days for the 1.5-gm level and 14 days for the 0.38-gm level.

and/or combinations can also be suggested; e.g., the rate of body protein breakdown may not change but the amount of N entering the pool which is excreted may be greatly reduced. Waterlow (1968) has reviewed these aspects of the adaptive nature of body protein metabolism.

There are relatively few studies which allow a distinction to be made among these possibilities. Studies in rats (Waterlow and Stephen 1968) show that *short-term* adaptation to a low-protein diet is not accompanied by a decrease in total body N turnover. A similar conclusion may be drawn from the study of Picou and Taylor-Roberts (1969) with infants given low- and high-protein diets. Using the same approach as in the studies described earlier on the effects of age on body protein synthesis, we have recently investigated the adaptive nature of whole body protein metabolism by measuring total N flux (disposal rate) and total body protein synthesis and breakdown rates in healthy young adult subjects conditioned to differing levels of protein intake. Our findings, summarized in Table 2.4 suggest that, in healthy young adults during short-term adaptation to a low-protein but otherwise adequate diet, there is a small decrease in N flux, a marked increase in the rate of total body protein breakdown and a more efficient utilization of amino acids for protein anabolism with a greater degree of endogenous amino acid utilization.

Hence, total body protein metabolism responds to alterations in the level of protein and amino intake through changes in protein synthesis and breakdown as well as by alterations in the efficiency of amino acid utilization and recycling. These responses account for observed changes in the estimates of biological value (BV) of proteins at different levels of intake within the submaintenance to maintenance range (Bressani and Viteri 1971; Calloway and Margen 1971; Inoue *et al.* 1973, 1975; Scrimshaw and Young

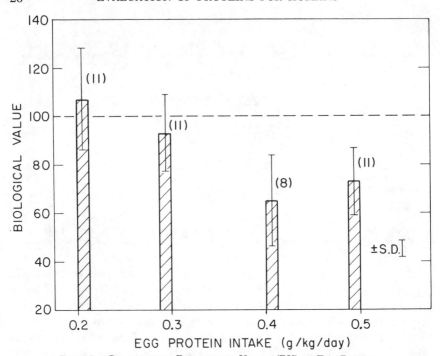

FIG. 2.9.   CALCULATED BIOLOGICAL VALUE (BV) OF EGG PROTEIN

At different levels within the submaintenance to maintenance range of protein intake in young men. Values in parentheses denote the number of subjects studied in each group. Drawn from the results of Young *et al.* (1973B).

1974) (Fig. 2.9). Furthermore, this supports the view that the estimation of protein quality is best approached by measurement of the protein metabolic response to graded levels of protein intake. This subject is considered in more practical terms in the subsequent chapters by Samonds and Hegsted (Chapter 4) and by Bressani (Chapter 5) and we have discussed this previously (Young and Scrimshaw 1974).

Dietary Energy Influences on Nitrogen Metabolism and Protein Utilization.—In addition to the effects of dietary nitrogen or essential amino acid intake on the efficiency of nitrogen utilization, another dietary factor which is important to consider in the assessment of protein quality is the level of energy intake. The topic of protein-calorie interrelationships also has been reviewed extensively (e.g., Munro 1951; Calloway and Spector 1954; Swanson 1959) and only a few points need be made here.

The major evidence, in both experimental animals and man, indicates that dietary caloric restriction leads to a loss of nitrogen from the body and that under these conditions, there is a reduction in the efficiency of dietary nitrogen utilization. However, the extent to which this occurs depends upon the availability of body energy stores as shown by the studies of Cahill

TABLE 2.5

EFFECT OF EXCESS ENERGY INTAKE ON THE UTILIZATION AND
REQUIREMENTS FOR EGG AND RICE PROTEINS IN YOUNG MEN

Protein Source	Energy	Efficiency of N Utilization[1] (%)	Mean Requirement	
			Nitrogen (mg/kg)	Conventional Protein (g/kg)
Egg	Excess	54	67	0.42
	Maintenance	41	90	0.56
Rice	Excess	47	82	0.51
	Maintenance	27	119	0.74

Source: From Inoue *et al.* (1973). Excess energy = 57 ± 2 kcal/kg. Maintenance energy = 45 ± 2 kcal/kg.
[1]Value obtained from slope of regression of N balance on N intake.

(1970) and co-workers on starvation in obese subjects and of Jourdan *et al.* (1974) on nitrogen utilization in obese subjects given different protein and energy intakes. Alternatively, addition of energy, from either carbohydrate or fat sources, to an already adequate diet results in a considerable extra retention of dietary nitrogen. Munro (1964) suggests that for man the magnitude of this effect is about 2 mg N per additional calorie and that the effect may continue for longer than two weeks. However, the quantitative extent of this response to alterations in energy intake depends upon the adequacy of the protein intake and changes in protein intake may also modify the response of body energy metabolism to changes in caloric intake (Calloway and Spector 1954; Munro 1964).

Two aspects of protein-energy relationships are of particular significance in this discussion. Firstly, the effects of excess energy intakes in metabolic N balance experiments concerned with estimating protein or amino acid requirements and dietary protein quality, require consideration. In many previous N balance studies, including our own, experimental dietary regimens have usually been designed to provide generous levels of energy intake so that this factor did not limit the utilization of dietary protein and amino acids. However, it is now beginning to be appreciated more critically that even small excesses of energy intake have important effects on dietary N utilization. This point is well demonstrated by the careful studies of Inoue *et al.* (1973, 1975) which show, as summarized in Table 2.5, that the efficiency of utilization of egg and rice proteins and, therefore, estimated requirements, is markedly affected by changes in the level of energy intake.

In a similar context, Rose and Wixom (1955) maintained two individuals in N balance on a crystalline amino acid diet supplying 3-4 gm N per day.

From their results, these workers concluded that a diet supplying essential amino acids at twice the minimal requirement levels and a total N intake of 3.5 gm per day was adequate for the maintenance of N equilibrium in adult subjects. However, during the 56–60-day experiment, one subject gained more than 5 kg body weight and the other subject gained nearly 2 kg, due to the high energy intake provided by the experimental diet. This not only seriously limits the practical application of the estimated amino acid requirements from the studies of Rose and co-workers (Rose 1957) but also makes it difficult to evaluate the significance of protein quality in adult human protein nutrition.

We (Garza *et al.* 1976A) have also observed, during recent long-term metabolic balance studies, that N balance can be significantly increased in young adult subjects consuming the 1973 FAO/WHO Safe Practical Allowance for protein with increments of 3–9 Kcals per kg body wt per day in energy intake above their estimated requirement level (Fig. 2.10). Because the energy requirement for an individual is difficult to determine precisely, our recent findings serve to underscore further the importance of evaluating the modifying effects of the level of energy intake on the results and interpretation of all metabolic N-balance studies with human subjects.

Secondly, the effects of inadequate or low caloric intakes on the utilization of dietary protein should also be considered here in relation to protein quality. From studies with experimental animals it is apparent that, even when dietary calories are severely limiting, dietary protein is not quantitatively used for meeting the energy deficit. Morrison and Narayana Rao (1967) showed, that, under conditions of restricted caloric intake, dietary proteins are utilized by growing rats for anabolic purposes and that protein sources still differ in their nutritional value, although these differences are less than with *ad libitum* feeding. Similarly, Rosenthal and Allison (1951) showed with well-nourished dogs that the efficiency of dietary nitrogen retention was the same in animals receiving either adequate calories or 50% of their caloric requirements. When caloric intake was reduced to 25%, however, there was a marked reduction in N utilization. Our studies in healthy adults have also demonstrated that the utilization of wheat gluten is significantly improved by lysine fortification even at low energy intakes in subjects undergoing a significant loss of body weight (Scrimshaw *et al.* 1973). Thus, although inadequate intakes of energy reduce overall N utilization, body protein metabolism still responds to changes in the patterns and levels of amino acid intake.

Most human studies concerned with protein requirements, N utilization, and dietary protein quality have probably been carried out at excess energy intakes, leading to enhanced N retention. In view of this fact it is important to reevaluate critically the human requirements for essential amino acids

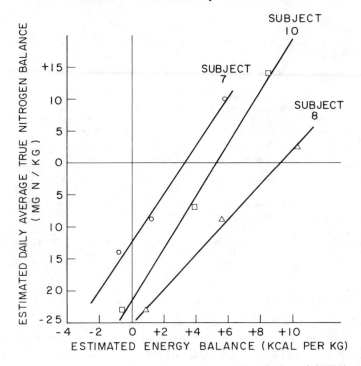

From Garza et al. (1976A)

FIG. 2.10. AN ESTIMATE OF THE EFFECT ON N BALANCE OF IN-
CREMENTS IN ENERGY INTAKE ABOVE ESTIMATED ENERGY NEEDS
IN THREE YOUNG ADULT MEN
Energy balance was estimated by assuming that body weight change, in
excess of that predicted from the N balance results, represented fat deposition equivalent to 7800 kcals per kg body wt. Each subject received
the FAO/WHO (1973) safe practical allowance of egg protein (0.57 g
per kg body wt per day). Results based on diet periods lasting 21–32
days for each energy intake level.

and the nutritive value of food protein sources at levels of energy intake
which are less generous than conventionally given.

METHODS USED FOR ESTIMATING HUMAN PROTEIN AND AMINO ACID NEEDS

With the above background, the metabolic significance of the methods
and approaches which have been used for estimating human protein and
amino acid requirements will not be discussed. The major methods and
approaches, which Table 2.6 summarizes, will be reviewed. Emphasis will
be on their limitations rather than extensive applications.

TABLE 2.6

A LISTING OF MAJOR METHODS AND APPROACHES WHICH HAVE BEEN USED
FOR ESTIMATING PROTEIN AND AMINO ACID REQUIREMENTS IN MAN

Method	Principle	Comment
Factorial method (for total N)	Summation of sources of obligatory N losses plus allowance for growth	Methods involve use of various correction factors. Requires validation
Nitrogen balance response curve	Minimum intake of protein or amino acid for N equilibrium or N retention during growth	Prone to technical errors and other factors. Functional significance of N balance not precisely known
Growth	Minimum protein or amino acid intake for "optimal" growth	Useful only during infancy
Plasma amino acids	Response of plasma amino acid levels to graded amino acid intake	Metabolic significance of plasma amino acid concentrations not known

Nitrogen Balance Measurements

Most of the data available on protein and amino acid requirements are based on results from metabolic N balance studies. Useful information can be gained from N balance determinations when they are carefully conducted, but for application to an assessment of protein and amino acid requirements it is important to appreciate the following limitations.

(1) Maintenance N balance does not necessarily reflect maintenance of a steady state level of organ protein metabolism or of nutritional status because it fails to reveal alterations in the quality and distribution of tissue metabolism and protein content within the body. This point has previously been discussed in relation to the adaptive aspects of body protein metabolism and will be referred to again in a later section.

(2) In addition to the well-recognized cumulative, technical errors, all of the routes of N loss from the body are difficult to quantitate. Furthermore, loss of N via one route may be compensated by changes in the losses of N via another (e.g., Huang et al. 1975). Thus, unless all routes of N are measured, erroneous conclusions may be drawn from apparent N balance values. Most of the N balance data in the literature have involved only measurement of urinary and fecal N losses.

(3) Errors in N balance estimates are larger when the diet is higher in N. Many of the important studies on amino acid requirements of humans have been conducted at relatively high intakes of dietary N (Holt and Snyderman 1965; Rose 1957).

(4) Various factors other than the test nutrient affect the sensitivity and absolute value of the N balances, and these must be considered in an

$$\text{EQUATION: } Q_3 - Q_2 = \frac{f(I_3 - I_2)}{\lambda}(1 - e^{\lambda t}) \quad \ldots\ldots(1)$$

DIFFERENTIATION

$$\text{OF eq. (1): } \frac{dQ}{dt} = f(I_3 - I_2)e^{-\lambda t} \quad \ldots\ldots\ldots(2)$$

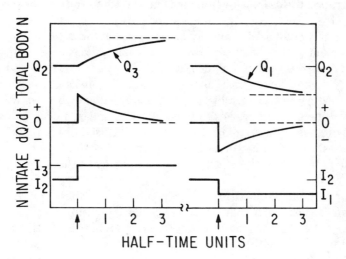

HALF−TIME UNITS

FIG. 2.11. THE MODEL PROPOSED BY FORBES (1973) TO DESCRIBE THE ADJUSTMENT OF N EQUILIBRIUM TO A CHANGE IN N INTAKE IN HUMAN SUBJECTS

Plot of total body N (Q), and daily N balance (dQ/dt). Left hand and right hand portions represent effects of an abrupt increase and decrease in N intake, respectively. Time is in units of half time for N turnover.

evaluation of the conclusions drawn from N balance results. These factors include level of energy intake, as discussed previously, and prior nutritional state of the subject.

Recently, Forbes (1973) has proposed a further limitation of the metabolic N balance method (Fig. 2.11). He has argued that the approach of N balance to a new equilibrium, following a change in dietary N intake, is achieved by metabolic changes which are much slower than hitherto thought. Forbes' argument is based on the description of body protein metabolism by use of the following equation:

$$\frac{dQ}{dt} = \frac{f}{\lambda}(I_3 - I_2)e^{-\lambda t}$$

where f = the percentage of dietary N which is utilized; I_3 and I_2 are the new and previous intakes of N, respectively; λ is the fractional turnover rate of body N; dQ/dt is the instantaneous net change of body N (N balance) per unit of time (t). He assumed a value of about 30% for f and a fractional turnover rate of 0.014 day^{-1}. For adult humans Forbes concludes that with a change in N intake, N balance will approach equilibrium again only after a considerable period of time. This may be as long as 50–150 days, depending upon the assumed value for f and the magnitude of the change in N intake.

There are a number of erroneous assumptions in this assessment. Firstly, the argument that N balance shows an exponential response to altered N intake is based on the N balance data of Deuel *et al.* (1928) and Smith (1926). We consider that the interpretation of Deuel's data is seriously confounded because their subject was receiving a grossly inadequate intake of dietary energy during the experimental period and significantly lost body weight. Similarly, the results of Smith cannot be used as adequate support for Forbes' thesis since the single subject studied by Smith received a variable but generally increasing energy intake throughout a 24-day low-protein period.

A more fundamental criticism is that this model implies that the body's response to a change in N intake is only achieved by altering the size of the body N pool and that values for the efficiency of dietary N utilization and body N turnover are fixed constants, irrespective of the actual level of N intake. We have discussed earlier in this review some of the evidence which shows that neither f nor λ have fixed, constant values but respond to changes in the level and adequacy of dietary N intake. Thus, we consider the model used by Forbes to be invalid.

There is, however, still the problem of determining how long it takes after a change in amino acid or total nitrogen intake, for a new steady state N output to be achieved. In reviewing human studies on the lysine supplementation of wheat proteins, Mickelsen and his colleagues (Vaghefi *et al.* 1974) concluded that, when a diet high in wheat is consumed, the time required for establishing a steady state in N output may be as long as 30 days. This is a much longer balance period than the about 1–2-week balance periods frequently used by investigators working with adult subjects. However, their conclusion was based largely on their own metabolic N balance study (Bolourchi *et al.* 1968) with young adults receiving about 1 gm protein per kg body wt per day (90–95% from wheat flour). Unfortunately, dietary energy intake was increased as the experiment progressed thus seriously confounding the interpretation of the relationship between N balance and the length of time on the diet. There are no definitive published studies which adequately address this important problem and so the design of an N-balance experiment remains largely a matter of the experience of the investigator, coupled with the many constraints imposed in conducting studies with human subjects. It is the responsibility of each investigator to demonstrate that a steady state has been achieved under the conditions of the experiment. A more thorough investigation of this problem in both children and adults is obviously necessary.

Growth

Body weight gain can be used as a measure of dietary protein adequacy in studies with infants. However, except for the very young, it is an insensitive parameter. Furthermore, ethical considerations restrict its use in the younger age groups and an additional problem lies in the uncertainty as to what rate of body weight gain is consistent with optimum long-term maintenance of health and body performance.

Plasma Amino Acids

A new method for assessment of amino acid requirements which we have developed is based on measurements of plasma amino acid concentrations under well-defined experimental conditions (Young et al. 1971, 1972B; Tontisirin et al. 1972, 1973, 1974). Although this method may offer an approach which is independent of the N balance method, few amino acids have been studied so far, and the approach requires refinement. Furthermore, as discussed earlier, the individual essential amino acids do not show the same quantitative plasma response to comparable alterations in their dietary supply. There is, therefore, a need for thorough qualitative and quantitative investigation of the mechanisms associated with the control of plasma amino acid levels before the approach can be adequately evaluated. A similar comment applies to the measurement of plasma amino acid levels for assessing dietary protein quality (see McLaughlan 1974 for a review).

The plasma amino acid method is discussed again, later in this review, in relation to the significance of published studies on the amino acid requirements of children and adults.

APPROACHES IN THE ASSESSMENT OF PROTEIN AND AMINO ACID REQUIREMENTS

Much of the published data has been compiled recently in monograph form by Irwin and Hegsted (1971A, 1971B), and they have pointed out the significant gaps which exist in the available estimates of protein and amino acid needs for the various age groups. These do not need to be repeated here but a brief review will be made of the approaches used in assessing protein and amino acid requirements.

TABLE 2.7

SOME ESTIMATES OF OBLIGATORY NITROGEN LOSSES IN VARIOUS AGE GROUPS

Group	Nitrogen Losses (mg N/kg Body wt/Day)		
	Urine	Feces	Integumental and Miscellaneous
Infants (4–6 months)[1]	42	33	
Children (3–4 yr)[1]	68	31	
Adults			
Men[2]	37.2	8.8	
Women[3]	25.2	8.7	
FAO/WHO (1973)	37	12	5[4]
Elderly Women[5]	24.8	9.8	

[1]Fomon et al. (1965).
[2]Scrimshaw et al. (1972).
[3]Bricker and Smith (1951).
[4]Based, in part, on data of Calloway et al. (1971).
[5]From Perera et al. (1975).

Protein Requirements

Two major approaches have been followed for estimating the minimum physiological needs for total protein: (1) the factorial approach and (2) the determination of the minimum N intake required to support maximum N retention in children or N equilibrium in the adult.

Factorial Approach.—In this approach the losses of "obligatory" N via urine and feces are measured and summated with additional corrections for N losses via the integument and miscellaneous routes. In the case of growth, pregnancy or lactation, further allowances are made for body N gain, the N content of fetus and supporting tissues and the output of milk proteins, respectively. A summary of estimated obligatory N losses in various age groups is given in Table 2.7. A more complete summary of these losses is given in Irwin and Hegsted (1971A) and FAO/WHO (1973).

A major assumption is that losses of N associated with a protein-free intake can be used to estimate the N losses occurring when N intakes just meet the minimum physiological requirement for high-quality protein. In view of the earlier discussion which dealt with the changes in protein and amino acid metabolism with reduced protein intake there is little physiological rationale for this assumption.

It has been demonstrated in both adults (Calloway and Margen 1971; Young et al. 1973B; Inoue et al. 1973) and infants (e.g., Chan and Waterlow 1966; Bressani and Viteri 1971) that it is not possible to achieve adequate N retention in growing children or N equilibrium in adults by providing high quality protein N just to meet the summated obligatory N losses. Additional nitrogen is required because of a fall in the efficiency of N utilization and dietary N retention as N intake approaches the requirement level. A 30% increase in N intake was assumed by the 1973 FAO/WHO Expert Committee to meet this additional need. However, a critical appraisal of the data upon which this estimate was based indicates to us that this value was underestimated by as much as 46% with respect to the additional N required by some individuals. Furthermore, the applicability of the 30% figure to other age groups, particularly children and elderly subjects, has not been tested.

Despite these problems, the method deserves further investigation because, in practice, it offers a convenient means of estimating protein needs of various weight and age groups not all of which cannot be directly studied. For this reason the factorial approach was adopted by FAO/WHO (1973) in arriving at recommendations for dietary protein. However, there are no direct estimates on the obligatory N losses in infants and adolescents, and there are only limited data on children of primary-school age and elderly subjects (Young et al. 1974B). Also, there are no statistically reliable data which provide knowledge of the covariance between obligatory N losses and the minimum protein needs of healthy subjects. Clearly, much further work is needed to establish the relationships between obligatory N losses and the protein needs of individual subjects if the factorial method is to be used for evaluating protein requirements for groups of various ages and physiological states. This can only be done adequately by comparing factorially derived estimates with long-term N balance.

The N Balance Response Curve.—In this approach the N balance response to graded intakes of protein within the region of maintenance N intake is determined. This method is, in theory, the most direct way of estimating protein needs but suffers from the limitations of the N balance method discussed earlier. Only a few studies of this kind have been conducted to provide estimates of the minimum needs for dietary proteins from differing foods or combination of food sources. There is a critical need for studies, with both high- and low-quality proteins, on nitrogen utilization over graded intakes which span the requirement range in human adults. Where feasible, this should also be carried out in younger age groups. Investigations of this kind are necessary to improve our knowledge of human protein requirements and of dietary protein quality. They also provide a direct way of evaluating the factorial approach.

Summary of Protein Allowances.—A number of recent summaries of studies on the estimated requirements for total protein (Hegsted and Irwin 1971A; Natl. Acad. Sci.—Natl. Res. Council 1974A, 1974B; FAO/WHO 1973) have appeared and this makes it unnecessary to provide an additional review of the published data here. Table 2.8 summarizes some of the recent recommendations for protein allowances in various age groups. These values are based on additional considerations of the variability in

TABLE 2.8

A SUMMARY OF SOME RECENT COMMITTEE RECOMMENDATIONS FOR
PRACTICAL PROTEIN ALLOWANCES IN VARIOUS AGE GROUPS

Age Group	Committee Recommendation (gm Protein/kg Body wt/Day)		
	UK 1969[1]	FAO/WHO 1973[2]	US 1974[3]
Infants (1–2 yr)	1.7	1.7	1.8
Teenagers (15 yr, boys)	0.82	1.03	0.89
Adults (~35 yr, males)	0.66	0.82	0.80

[1]U.K. Dept. of Health and Social Security (1969). Assuming an NPU 70%.
[2]FAO/WHO (1973). Assuming a protein score of 70.
[3]Natl. Acad. Sci.–Natl. Res. Council (1974B). Assumes 75% utilization of dietary N.

requirements among apparently similar individuals. Again, the data reveal that reliable estimates of the nature and extent of the variation in the requirements for proteins of differing quality are not available. Indeed, this is true of all nutrients. Thus, if the recommended allowances are to have practical value, there is a critical need to improve our present knowledge of human protein nutrition. A more extensive analysis of the current safe practical allowances, particularly in relation to the 1973 and earlier FAO/WHO recommendations, has appeared elsewhere (Scrimshaw 1976).

Essential Amino Acid Requirements of Various Age Groups

Amino Acid Patterns.—The methods and approaches used in estimating the needs for the individual essential amino acids and their limitations are similar to those for estimating total protein needs. Therefore, this section will be devoted to an appraisal of the current state of knowledge of human essential amino acid requirements.

Some recent estimates of the essential amino acid needs of infants and adults are summarized in Table 2.9. These data do not reveal any clear-cut differences in the pattern of amino acid requirements for the two age groups. Since the estimates for each amino acid are rather imprecise (Hegsted 1963), there is no reason to believe that the essential amino acid pattern differs with developmental age. Furthermore, similar amino acid patterns might be anticipated because it appears, from studies in the rat, that the amino acid composition of the weight gain is similar to that of the whole organism (Bunce and King 1969). This conclusion probably does not apply to the neonate because cystine appears to be an obligatory dietary constituent (Gaull et al. 1972).

Ratio of Essential Amino Acid N to Total Dietary N.—It is generally

TABLE 2.9

PATTERN OF ESSENTIAL AMINO ACID REQUIREMENTS IN INFANTS AND ADULTS

	Relative to			
	Valine		Lysine	
Amino Acid	Infant	Adult	Infant	Adult
Histidine	0.3	—	0.3	—
Isoleucine	0.8	1.0	0.7	0.8
Leucine	1.7	1.4	1.6	1.2
Lysine	1.0	1.2	*1.0*	*1.0*
S-amino acids	0.6	1.3	0.6	1.1
Aromatic amino acids	1.3	1.4	1.2	1.2
Threonine	0.9	0.7	0.8	0.6
Tryptophan	0.2	0.2	0.2	0.3
Valine	*1.0*	*1.0*	0.9	0.8

Source: Calculated from the FAO/WHO (1973) summaries of estimated amino acid requirements in infants and adults.

TABLE 2.10

"PROTEIN QUALITY INDEX" OF COW'S MILK AND CORN PROTEIN
IN RELATION TO AGE

	Cow's Milk	Corn
Infant	100	52
Adult	141	95

Source: Arroyave (1974).

$$\text{Protein Quality Index} = \frac{\text{Protein requirement for age}}{\text{Amount test protein to satisfy requirement for limiting amino acid}} \times 100$$

considered that the requirement for total essential amino acids declines more rapidly with age than does the need for total dietary nitrogen (see FAO/WHO 1973). It has been estimated that the infant requires approximately 37% of total N in the form of an optimal mixture of essential amino acids. In contrast, it is estimated that in the adult only 15% of the total N requirement need be supplied via a balanced essential amino acid pattern. Thus, these estimates indicate that the nitrogen and amino acid requirements vary at different rates with age. On this basis, Arroyave (1974) developed a "Protein Quality Index." A summary of his calculations, based on published estimates of essential amino acid requirements, are given in Table 2.10. From these calculations he concluded that the nutritional quality of a protein will depend upon the age of the individual consuming it. However, the extent to which age affects the quality of a protein source is still, in our opinion, a matter for considerable debate.

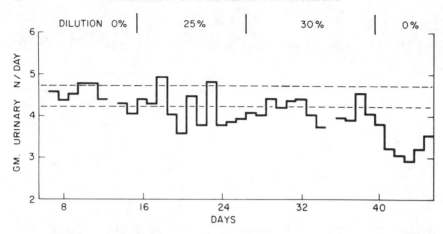

FIG. 2.12. EFFECT OF PARTIAL REPLACEMENT (DILUTION) OF FISH PROTEIN CON-
CENTRATE WITH NONSPECIFIC NITROGEN ON THE URINARY EXCRETION OF TOTAL
NITROGEN IN A SUBJECT DURING CONSECUTIVE DIETARY PERIODS

Total protein intake equivalent (N × 6.25) to 0.4 gm protein per kg per day. From results of
Young and Scrimshaw (1974B).

If changes with age in the proportion of essential amino acid nitrogen
to total nitrogen occur to the extent indicated above, then for adults
high-quality animal protein sources such as eggs, milk, and meat provide
total essential amino acids in considerable excess of the estimate for adult
maintenance. Thus, for adults it should be possible to replace a significant
proportion of the essential amino acids of these protein sources with a
nonspecific N source without influencing their nutritive value, but not to
the same extent in younger individuals.

Although the data of Daniel *et al.* (1970) in girls, aged 10–11 yr, and the
earlier experiments conducted in our laboratories support this premise
(Scrimshaw *et al.* 1966, 1969; Huang *et al.* 1966), a reinterpretation of these
studies and those of others (Kofranyi 1972) is necessary in view of the more
recent observations, discussed above, which show that the efficiency of
dietary N utilization, and presumably that of the essential amino acids,
increases with reductions in protein intake throughout the submaintenance
range. Hence, although we found that the partial replacement of egg, milk,
or meat protein N with nonspecific N did not affect N balance, in the
short-term, the replacement may have resulted in a compensatory increase
in the efficiency of essential amino acid utilization, the net result being no
change in N balance.

Subsequent studies (Young and Scrimshaw 1974B) with fish protein
concentrate (FPC) support this later interpretation; the results obtained
in one subject are shown in Fig. 2.7. N balance was not altered as a result

of the partial replacement of FPC with nonspecific N, but upon reintroduction of the basal FPC diet, there was an immediate and significant decrease in N output and marked increase in N balance. This response suggests the development of an accumulative deficiency of essential amino acids during the "dilution" period and this later resulted in a greater efficiency of dietary N utilization when the richer source of essential amino acid(s) was consumed once again. Thus, the significance of the estimated relationship between the essential amino acid and total N requirements in adults, as given below, remains uncertain.

Our studies on the relationships between intake levels of specific essential amino acids, plasma amino acid levels and the requirement for specific amino acids, discussed earlier, are relevant to this matter. In growing experimental animals (see Young and Scrimshaw 1972 for a brief review) the concentration of a specific essential amino acid in blood plasma remains low and relatively constant until the dietary requirement for that amino acid is met. At about this level of intake, the plasma concentration begins to rise in response to further increases in the intake of the amino acid. We used this response to explore human amino acid requirements, as schematically depicted in Fig. 2.13. The lower "breakpoint," A, in the curve shown in the figure has been interpreted to occur at that intake of the amino acid which just meets the minimum physiological requirement. This operational definition of the plasma amino acid response curve in adult human subjects is based on the broad extrapolation of observations made in experimental animal studies. Our studies have demonstrated that the lower "breakpoint" in the plasma tryptophan (Young et al. 1971), valine (Young et al. 1972B), and threonine (Tontisirin et al. 1974) response curves occur at intakes of the amino acids which correspond to the minimum levels of amino acid intake thought to be sufficient to maintain protein nutritional status.

It might be argued, however, that the physiological requirement for the amino acid is higher than that estimated from the lower "breakpoint" values on the plasma response curve. In fact, it might be postulated that the requirement is met at an intake which corresponds to the upper "breakpoint," B, in the response curve, or at an intake within the range of intakes bounded by these plasma levels. Our studies have not critically examined this upper portion of the response curve but in Table 2.11 we have attempted to identify the minimum levels of intake of the amino acids which would be required to achieve a plasma concentration in the region at the upper plateau value. These levels are compared with the intakes of the amino acids provided by egg protein when consumed at a level of 94 mg N per kg body wt per day. For tryptophan, threonine, and leucine, the upper "breakpoint" occurred at approximately twice the level of intake corresponding to the lower "breakpoint."

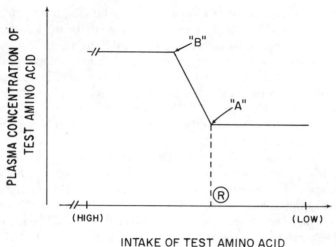

FIG. 2.13. A SCHEMATIC REPRESENTATION OF THE RELATIONSHIP
BETWEEN THE PLASMA CONCENTRATION OF AN ESSENTIAL AMINO
ACID

The intake of the amino acid and the requirement for that amino acid.
This figure is based on the interpretation of studies of the plasma amino
acid response in young men (see text). The "high" level of intake ap-
proximates the level of amino acid which is normally consumed. Point
A represents the lower "breakpoint" and point B corresponds to the upper
"breakpoint."

A further evaluation of N balance studies in children and adults is also
instructive. For example, Table 2.12 shows the results of a study by Rose
et al. (1954). Our estimation suggests that when an estimate of true N
balance is made, assuming 5 mg N body wt per kg for sweat and integu-
mental loss, the subject was not in balance at the level of tryptophan intake
which the authors concluded to be sufficient to meet the minimum requirement. This point is made to emphasize that the criterion used for estimating the minimum requirements for essential amino acids in adults
has neither been precise nor consistent among and within laboratories (see
Hegsted 1963, 1964). The published estimates, therefore, are of doubtful
validity for practical application.

These findings lead to the suggestion that the current estimates (FAO/
WHO 1973) of the quantitative relationship between individual essential
amino acids and total protein requirements may be significantly too low
for adults. The data of Weller et al. (1971) support this view, as do the
earlier studies of Hegsted et al. (1955) who showed that improvements in
N balance occurred following amino acid supplementation of protein even
though the unsupplemented diets apparently already supplied the limiting
amino acid in excess of estimated minimum needs.

TABLE 2.11

INTAKES OF ESSENTIAL AMINO ACIDS ESTIMATED TO BE SUFFICIENT TO
MAINTAIN THEIR PLASMA AMINO ACID LEVELS AT THE LOWER AND UPPER
"BREAKPOINTS" ON THE PLASMA RESPONSE CURVE

| Amino Acid | Intake (mg/kg/day) for | | Intake from 94 mg N/kg/Day from Egg |
	Lower Breakpoint	Upper Breakpoint	
Tryptophan	3	5–6	10
Threonine	7	>18<30	30
Leucine	~22	~40	50
Valine	16	>18<42	42

TABLE 2.12

RESULTS FOR NITROGEN BALANCE WITH SUBJECT R.J.D. STUDIED BY ROSE
ET AL. (1954) FOR MINIMUM TRYPTOPHAN REQUIREMENT

| Period (Days) | Tryptophan Intake[1] | | Apparent Balance gm N/Day | Estimated "True" Balance gm N/Day |
	gm/Day	mg/kg/Day		
5	0.20	3.0	+0.27	−0.06
5	0.10	1.5	−0.37	−0.70
8	0.15	2.25	+0.12	−0.21

Source: From Rose et al. (1954), who concluded from the apparent N balance
data that the minimal tryptophan requirement was 0.15 gm/day. Note, that if
correction of 5 mg N/kg/day for entegumental and miscellaneous losses [FAO/
WHO (1973)] had been made, then a negative "true" balance would have been
observed at 0.15 gm tryptophan per day.
[1]Total N intake, 10 gm/day. Energy intake was 54.5 kcals/kg body wt/day.

Conversely, Fomon et al. (1973) believed that for some amino acids, at
least, previous estimates of requirements in infants are substantially greater
than the true requirements. If so, this would also tend to reduce the apparent differences in the proportion of essential amino acids to total nitrogen required for adequate protein nutrition at various ages.

Some General Comments Concerning Published Estimates.—In
addition to the above observations which indicate the unsatisfactory state
of knowledge of the essential amino acid requirements in man, the practical
significance of published requirements remains highly uncertain for other
reasons.

(1) Studies on requirements for individual essential amino acids have
generally been conducted on a few subjects for each amino acid and the
observations at specified intakes of the amino acid were of short duration.
Some age groups and physiological states (primary school age children,
adolescents, pregnancy, and lactation) have not been studied at all. The
data for elderly subjects are highly contradictory (Young et al. 1976).

(2) Calorie intakes have generally been much higher than normally required by the subjects and this would have a sparing effect on both amino acid and total protein requirements.

(3) The criteria utilized in the various studies have varied and are not precise or even consistent within a given study, making it difficult to evaluate all of the available information on amino acid requirements. Major differences in methodology and experimental protocols occur and the accuracy and reliability of most of the estimates are not known. A statistical appraisal of the published requirements in young women suggests that the mean requirement for some of the available estimates is within no better than 50% (Hegsted 1963).

(4) A wide variation is reported in the requirements for some of the amino acids among individuals. The extent to which methodological and biological factors account for this variation is not known. Considerably more information is required on the variability in essential amino acid requirements among apparently similar individuals.

(5) The major technique followed in the earlier studies was that of N balance, the limitations of which have been referred to earlier.

(6) The dietary amino acid patterns and absolute levels of essential amino acid and total N intake provided by the experimental diets have varied considerably among the various experiments. There has been no systematic attempt to determine the quantitative significance of these dietary differences on estimates of minimum requirements derived from the various studies. In particular, the quantitative significance of metabolic interactions among the essential amino acids and between essential and dispensible amino acids has not been established in the human subject. There is now even uncertainty as to the quantitative relationships between methionine and cystine in relation to the total S-amino acid needs of man (Stegink and DenBesten 1972) and the earlier conclusion that histidine is a nonessential amino acid appears to be no longer tenable (Kofranyi *et al.* 1969; Bergström *et al.* 1970; Fürst 1972; Anderson *et al.* 1975; Kopple and Swendseid 1975).

PROTEIN REQUIREMENTS AND THE EVALUATION OF PROTEIN QUALITY

In estimating the minimum physiological needs for protein by the factorial method a correction is then applied depending upon the quality of protein consumed. However, there is uncertainty with respect to: (1) the importance of protein quality in adults and, perhaps, even in the case of healthy children, (2) the best method to evaluate protein nutritional quality and (3) the significance in human nutrition of results obtained with experimental species in biological assays of protein quality.

The lower utilization by children and young adults of high quality protein, such as egg protein or lactalbumin, compared with the rapidly growing rat, as well as the dog, raises some doubt as to whether rat assays provide valid and quantitatively meaningful information on the potencies of proteins consumed by human subjects. A review of the literature (Young and Scrimshaw 1974A) on the relation of animal to human assays of protein quality shows that the available data are too limited to provide a definitive conclusion. Clinical studies are needed to develop more rapid, sensitive and accurate estimates of dietary protein quality. Appropriate conditions, with adult subjects, should be identified so that the results of such human assays will also have application to younger age groups. Further discussion of the methods and approaches which may be taken in studies with human subjects is the topic of subsequent chapters in this book (Chapters 5, 6, and 8).

The question of protein quality in adult human protein nutrition is worth briefly considering, however, since a correction for protein quality is applied to all age groups in arriving at recommended protein allowances (FAO/WHO 1973; Natl. Acad. Sci.—Natl. Res. Council 1974B). Firstly, it has already been emphasized that uncertainty surrounds the estimated requirements for the essential amino acids in various age groups. Secondly, reliable conclusions cannot be made regarding the proportion of total amino acids that should be provided as a balanced pattern of essential amino acids for any age group because of the necessarily short-term nature of the N balance studies.

A further problem, which arises in relation to the evaluation of dietary protein quality and safe levels of protein intake in adult human subjects, is concerned with the metabolic interactions among amino acids and the effects of the total nitrogen intake in the utilization of essential amino acids. A major assumption still being made in the chemical evaluation of the nutritive value of dietary proteins, by use of the protein score, is that the efficiency of utilization of dietary protein is a simple and direct function of the concentration of the limiting essential amino acid. This implies that the other essential or dispensable amino acids that may be provided in excess of minimum needs do not significantly affect the utilization of the limiting amino acid. However, it has also been frequently emphasized (e.g., Holt and Snyderman 1965; Clark 1965; Clark et al. 1972) that the pattern and level of intake of the essential amino acids play important roles in modifying the utilization of dietary protein. There are a number of practical situations in which the effects of amino acid disproportions have been observed in man and this topic has been reviewed (Harper et al. 1970). These interactions are important to consider in relation to the evaluation of protein quality and the estimation of essential amino acid and protein requirements.

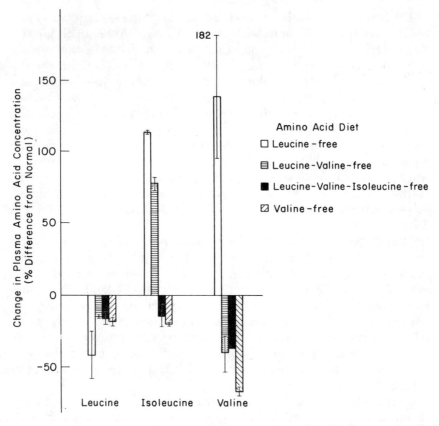

From Hambraeus et al. (1976)

FIG. 2.14.   CHANGES IN THE CONCENTRATIONS OF BRANCHED-CHAIN AMINO ACIDS IN PLASMA OF YOUNG MEN RECEIVING AMINO ACID DIETS DEVOID OF ONE OR MORE BRANCHED-CHAIN AMINO ACIDS FOR FOUR-DAY PERIODS

Values are compared with those obtained after an overnight fast when consuming a normal, free choice diet just prior to the experimental diet period. The bar represents the mean value for the percentage of deviation obtained for the two subjects given each experimental diet. I indicates the range.

The following observations may be used to emphasize and support the possible importance of amino acid interactions in protein utilization: (1) using a basal, egg protein diet Kofranyi (1972) observed that it was possible to reduce the total amount of dietary nitrogen required by about 30% for maintenance in adults by replacing part of the egg protein diet with nitrogen from potato. This optimal balance was associated with an altered ratio of the essential amino acids to each other and to the non-essential amino acid component of the protein mixture. (2) The addition of "nonspecific" nitrogen (i.e., glycine and diammonium citrate or other utilizable nitrogen sources) to a diet may influence the efficiency of utilization of the total nitrogen and essential amino acid intake (Kies *et al.* 1965). (3) The order in which essential amino acids become limiting appears to depend, in part, upon the level of total N intake (Kies and Fox 1970).

Another example of interactions among essential amino acids is shown by our studies (Hambraeus *et al.* 1976) of the response of plasma amino acid levels to changes in the level and pattern of intake of the branched-chain amino acids (Fig. 2.14). Previously we found that with a diet devoid of isoleucine or valine, the concentrations of the branched-chain amino acids are apparently unaffected (Ozalp *et al.* 1972). However, as shown in Fig. 2.14, a diet devoid of leucine results in a significant increase in the concentration of the other two branched-chain amino acids. This suggests that the adequacy and/or level of dietary leucine intake is not only an important factor in the regulation of the plasma levels of all three branched-chain amino acids but that the requirements for isoleucine and valine may be modified by the level of leucine intake.

From these observations it is apparent that the efficiency of utilization of dietary protein cannot be considered simply on the basis of the intake of the limiting essential amino acid. It must include an evaluation of the levels of the other essential amino acids and of the total N intake. It is not possible to do this in terms which have a precise, quantitative, predictive value at this time, but these considerations are meant to emphasize the difficulties which arise in evaluating the significance of protein quality and arriving at recommendations for safe levels of essential amino acid intake in subjects of all ages.

LONG-TERM METABOLIC STUDIES ON HUMAN PROTEIN REQUIREMENTS AND NEEDS FOR RESEARCH

Nitrogen Balance Measurements

Finally, much of the information discussed above is based on short-term experimental diet periods. As discussed earlier, the body responds through complex metabolic changes to a reduction in the intake of specific essential amino acids or of total N intake. For this reason, protein and essential amino acid needs or the assessment of protein quality cannot be measured with confidence solely on the basis of short-term N balance experiments.

Only three relatively long-term studies have been conducted and reported in the literature. Firstly, Bricker *et al.* (1949) attempted to assess the adequacy of estimated protein needs of college women through metabolic studies lasting for 10 weeks. Their subjects received a protein intake of about 31 gm per day from a mixture of beef, bread, cream, oatmeal, and potatoes. They remained in positive balance throughout, although their data suggest a progressive deterioration in the magnitude of N balance as time on the study progressed. A selected number of performance tests gave no indication of change after 10 weeks on the cereal based diet. However, the data of Bricker and co-workers are difficult to evaluate in view of the fact that the 10-week experimental period was preceded by a 5-week period at low, or grossly inadequate, intakes of dietary protein.

The second study is that of Calloway and Margen (1971) who gave two subjects for 88 days a level of N (about 12 gm N per day or about 75 gm high-quality protein) well above apparent minimum requirement levels. These workers observed a marked decline in creatinine excretion, but otherwise the results of this study cannot be used to assess the adequacy of estimated protein needs based on short-term metabolic studies.

The third long-term study is that of Yoshimura (1961, 1971). On the basis of changes in circulating hemoglobin levels and urinary corticosteroid excretion during metabolic balance periods of about 12 weeks, he concluded that the needs for essential amino acids are considerably higher, perhaps two-fold greater, than suggested from short-term studies on the needs for individual essential amino acids. It is also pertinent to point out that positive N balance was maintained in subjects who showed, at the same time, the development of anemia and hypoproteinemia during the long-term experimental balance periods (Yoshimura 1961).

Other Criteria of Dietary Protein Adequacy

N balance alone is not a sufficient criterion for determining the adequacy of protein intakes. It is simply an overall measure which might conceal functional abnormalities related to protein intake. There is an urgent need to develop and utilize as many functional measures as possible in correlation with long-term balance studies in human subjects. For example, as shown in Fig. 2.15, during a pilot long-term study we have recently observed changes in serum glutamic oxaloacetic transaminase activity which suggest that this measurement might prove useful in determining the long-term adequacy of dietary protein.

Those measures which could be followed in long-term studies fall into two categories: (1) the more classical measurements such as N balance, body composition, creatinine and hydroxyproline excretion, total serum proteins, albumin, hematocrit, hemoglobin, other usual hematological indices, blood levels of various serum or blood enzymes, and an assessment of the capacity of the subject to perform physical and mental work; and (2) new parameters which might include, in addition to serum transaminase, measurement of 3-methylhistidine excretion, assessment of changes in the status of the immune system and measurements of other blood constituents, particularly of proteins which turn over rapidly and can be used to assess the function and status of protein metabolism in specific tissues and organs.

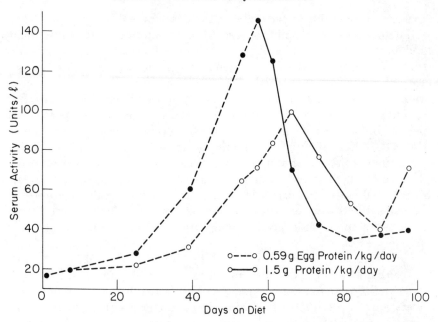

FIG. 2.15.   CHANGES IN SERUM GLUTAMIC OXALOACETIC TRANSAMINASE

Glutamic aspartic aminotransferase activity in two young adult male subjects consuming a diet supplying the FAO/WHO (1973) *Safe Practical Allowance* for egg protein. At the time indicated the protein intake was increased to 1.5 gm protein per kg body wt per day. From results of Garza et al. (1976D).

SUMMARY AND CONCLUSIONS

A major factor in the assessment of protein quality is concerned with the amino acid composition of the different food proteins. Therefore, an adequate knowledge of the needs in man, of all ages, for essential amino acids and total nitrogen and of the quantitative influence of factors which affect these needs is of primary importance in the evaluation of protein quality in human nutrition. In the first portion of this review, changes in human protein and amino acid metabolism with age and in response to alterations in protein and energy intake were discussed. The adaptive nature of body protein metabolism was emphasized. The purpose of this discussion was to provide a metabolic basis for evaluating the approaches taken in the estimation of protein and amino acid requirements and the practical significance of published values for the essential amino acid requirements of man.

The human body responds through complex metabolic changes to alterations in protein, amino acid, and energy intake. For this reason alone, there is considerable uncertainty on the practical value of the published estimates for essential amino acid requirements, particularly in adult man, and on the extent to which the quantitative relationship between the essential amino acid and total nitrogen needs change with age. Further limitations of the data concerned with human protein and amino acid needs were also discussed. Human protein and amino acid requirements cannot be measured with confidence solely on the basis of short-term experimental periods but studies of this type provide most of the current knowledge in this area of human nutrition. Finally, the measurement of N balance as a parameter of protein or amino acid adequacy is not a sufficient criterion. There is an urgent need to explore and apply functional measures of protein nutritional status in correlation with longer-term metabolic studies in human subjects in order to develop a rational and satisfactory basis for the assessment and significance of dietary protein quality in man.

ACKNOWLEDGMENT

We thank all of the members of our research group for their dedicated and careful participation in these studies. We are also grateful for the cooperation of the subjects who volunteered to undertake the demands of the experimental protocols.

BIBLIOGRAPHY

ALLEYNE, G. A. O., VITERI F., and ALVARADO, J. 1970. Indices of body composition in infantile malnutrition: Total body potassium and urinary creatinine. Am. J. Clin. Nutr. 23, 875.

ALLISON, J. B. 1964. The nutritive value of dietary proteins. In Mammalian Protein Metabolism, Vol. II, H. N. Munro, and J. B. Allison (Editors). Academic Press, New York.

ANDERSON, H. L., CHO, E. S., HANSON, K. C., and KRAUSE, G. F. 1975. Effects of low histidine intake on nitrogen utilization of men. Federation Proc. 34, No. 3, 879 (Abstr.).

ARROYAVE, G. 1974. Amino acid requirements by age and sex. In Nutrients in Processed Foods: Proteins, P. L. White, and D. C. Fletcher (Editors). Publishing Sciences Group, Acton, Mass.

BERGSTROM, J., FÜRST, P., JOSEPHSON, B., and NOREE, L-O. 1970. Improvement of nitrogen balance in a uremic patient by addition of histidine to essential amino acid solutions given intravenously. Life. Sci. 9, No. 11, 787.

BERNHART, F. W. 1970. Comparison of the essential amino acid, nitrogen and calorie requirements of the weanling rat and breast-fed infant. J. Nutr. 100, 461.

BOLOURCHI, S., FRIEDEMANN, C. M., and MICKELSEN, O. 1968. Wheat flour as a source of protein for adult human subjects. Am. J. Clin. Nutr. 21, 827.

BRESSANI, R., and VITERI, F. 1971. Metabolic studies in human subjects. Proc. SOS/70., 3rd Intern. Congr. Food Technol., Institute of Food Technologists, Chicago.

BREUER, C. B., and FLORINI, J. R. 1965. Amino acid incorporation into protein by cell-free systems from rat skeletal muscle. IV. Effects of animal age, androgens, and anabolic agents on activity of muscle ribosomes. Biochem. 4, 1544.

BRICKER, M. L., SHIVELY, R. F., SMITH, J. M., MITCHELL, H. H. and HAMILTON, T. S. 1949. The protein requirements of college women on high cereal diets with observations on the adequacy of short balance periods. J. Nutr. 37, 163.

BRICKER, M. L., and SMITH, J. M. 1951. A study of the endogenous nitrogen output of college women, with particular reference to use of the creatinine output in the calculation of the biological values of the protein of egg and of sunflower seed flour. J. Nutr. *44*, 553.

BRITTON, G. W., and SHERMAN, F. G. 1975. Altered regulation of protein synthesis during aging as determined by *in vitro* ribosomal assays. Exptl. Gerontol. *10*, 67.

BRODY, S. 1945. Bioenergetics and Growth. Van Nostrand Reinhold, New York.

BROOKES, J. M., OWENS, F. N., and GARRIGUS, U. S. 1972. Influence of amino acid level in the diet upon amino acid oxidation by the rat. J. Nutr. *102*, 27.

BUNCE, G. E., and KING, K. W. 1969. Amino acid retention and balance in the young rat fed varying levels of lactalbumin. J. Nutr. *98*, 159.

CAHILL, G. F., JR. 1970. Starvation in Man. New Engl. J. Med. *282*, 668.

CALLOWAY, D. H., and MARGEN, S. 1971. Variation in endogenous nitrogen excretion and dietary nitrogen utilization as determinants of human requirements. J. Nutr. *101*, 205.

CALLOWAY, D. H., ODELL, A. C. F., and MARGEN, S. 1971. Sweat and miscellaneous nitrogen losses in human balance studies. J. Nutr. *101*, 775.

CALLOWAY, D. H., and SPECTOR, H. 1954. Nitrogen balance as related to caloric and protein intake in active young men. Am. J. Clin. Nutr. *2*, 405.

CAMPBELL, J. A., and MCLAUGHLAN, J. M. 1971. Applicability of animal assays to humans. Proc. SOS/70, 3rd Intern. Congr. Food Technol. Institute of Food Technologists, Chicago.

CHAN, H., and WATERLOW, J. C. 1966. The protein requirements of infants at the age of about one year. Brit. J. Nutr. *20*, 775.

CLARK, H. E. 1965. Utilization of essential amino acids by men. *In* Newer Methods of Nutritional Biochemistry, Vol. 2, A. A. Albanese (Editor). Academic Press, New York.

CLARK, H. E., HOWE, J. M., MAGEE, J. L., and MALZER, J. L. 1972. Nitrogen balances of adult human subjects who consumed four levels of nitrogen from a combination of rice, milk and wheat. J. Nutr. *102*, 1647.

DANIEL, V. A., DORAISWAMY, T. R., SWAMINATHAN, M., and RAJALAKSHMI, D. 1970. The effect of dilution of milk proteins with nonessential amino acids (L-alanine and L-glutamic acid) on nitrogen retention and biological value of the proteins in children. Brit. J. Nutr. *24*, 741.

DEUEL, J. J., JR., SANDIFORD, I., SANDIFORD, K., and BOOTHBY, W. M. 1928. A study of the nitrogen minimum. The effect of 63 days of a protein-free diet on the nitrogen partition products in the urine and heat production. J. Biol. Chem. *76*, 391.

FAO/WHO. 1973. Energy and Protein Requirements, Report of a Joint FAO/WHO Ad Hoc Expert Committee. World Health Organ., Tech. Rept. Ser. *522*, Geneva, Switzerland.

FELIG, P., OWEN, O. G., WAHREN, J., and CAHILL, G. F., Jr. 1969. Amino acid metabolism during prolonged starvation. J. Clin. Invest. *48*, 584.

FOMON, S. J., DEMAEYER, E. M., and OWEN, G. M. 1965. Urinary and fecal excretion of endogenous nitrogen by infants and children. J. Nutr. *85*, 235.

FOMON, S. J., THOMAS, L. N., FILER, L. J., JR., ANDERSON, T. A. and BERGMANN, K. E. 1973. Requirements for protein and essential amino acids in early infancy. Acta Paediat. Scand. *62*, 33.

FORBES, G. B. 1973. Another source of error in the metabolic balance method. Nutr. Revs. *31*, 297.

FORBES, G. B., and REINA, J. C. 1970. Adult lean body mass declines with age: some longitudinal observations. Metabolism *19*, 653.

FÜRST, P. 1972. ^{15}N-studies in severe renal failure. II. Evidence for the essentiality of histidine. Scand. J. Clin. Lab. Invest. *30*, 307.

GARZA, C., SCRIMSHAW, N. S. and YOUNG, V. R. 1976A. Protein requirements of man: Evaluation of the 1973 FAO/WHO safe level of protein intake for young men at high energy intakes. Brit. J. Nutr. (in press).

GARZA, C., SCRIMSHAW, N. S., and YOUNG, V. R. 1976B. Human protein requirements: the effect of variations in energy intake within the maintenance range. Am. J. Clin. Nutr. *24*, 280.

GAULL, G., STURMAN, J. A., and RÁIHÁ, N. C. R. 1972. Development of mammalian sulphur metabolism: absence of cystathionase in human fetal tissues. Pediat. Res. *6*, 538.

GEARY, S., and FLORINI, J. R. 1972. Effect of age on rate of protein synthesis in isolated perfused mouse hearts. J. Gerontol. *27*, 325.

GRAYSTONE, J. E. 1968. Creatinine excretion during growth. *In* Human Growth, D. B. Cheek (Editor). Lea and Febiger, Philadelphia, Pa.

HAMBRAEUS, L. BILMAZES, C., DIPPEL, C., SCRIMSHAW, N. S., and YOUNG, V. R. 1976. Regulatory role of dietary leucine on plasma branched-chain amino acid levels in young men. J. Nutr. *106*, 230.

HARPER, A. E., BENEVENGA, N. J., and WOHLHEUTER, R. M. 1970. Effects of ingestion of disproportionate amounts of amino acids. Physiol. Rev. *50*, 428.

HAVERBERG, L. N., MUNRO, H. N., and YOUNG, V. R. 1974. Isolation and quantitation of N^τ-methylhistidine in actin and myosin of rat skeletal muscle: use of pyridine elution of protein hydrolysates on ion-exchange resins. Biochim. Biophys. Acta. *371*, 226.

HAVERBERG, L. N., OMSTEDT, P. T., MUNRO, H. N., and YOUNG, V. R. 1975A. N^τ-methylhistidine content of mixed proteins in various rat tissues. Biochim. Biophys. Acta. *405*, 67.

HAVERBERG, L. N. *et al.* 1975B. Unpublished results. Massachusetts Institute of Technology, Cambridge, Mass.

HEGSTED, D. M. 1963. Variation in requirements of nutrients—amino acids. Federation Proc. *22*, 1424.

HEGSTED, D. M. 1964. Protein requirements. *In* Mammalian Metabolism, Vol. II., H. N. Munro, and J. B. Allison (Editors). Academic Press, New York.

HEGSTED, D. M. 1971. Nutritional research on the value of amino acid fortification—Experimental studies in animals. *In* Amino Acid Fortification of Protein Foods, N. S. Scrimshaw, and A. M. Altschul (Editors). MIT Press, Cambridge, Mass.

HEGSTED, D. M., TRULSON, M. F., WHITE, H. S., WHITE, P. L., VINAS, F., ALARISTUR, E., DIAZ, C., VASQUEZ, J., LOO, A., ROCA, A., and COLLAZOS, CH.C. 1955. Lysine and methionine supplementation of all-vegetable diets for human adults. J. Nutr. *56*, 555.

HOLT, L. E., JR., and SNYDERMAN, S. E. 1965. Protein and amino acid requirements of infants and children. Nutr. Abstr. Rev. *35*, 1.

HUANG, P. C., LO, C. C., HO, W. T. 1975. Protein requirements of men in hot climate: decreased urinary nitrogen losses concomitant with increased sweat nitrogen losses during exposure to high environmental temperature. Am. J. Clin. Nutr. *28*, 494.

HUANG, P. C., YOUNG, V. R., CHOLAKOS, B., and SCRIMSHAW, N. S. 1966. Determination of the minimum dietary essential amino acid-to-total nitrogen for beef protein fed to young men. J. Nutr. *90*, 416.

INOUE, G., KISHI, K. MIYATANI, S., and YAMAMOTO, S. 1975. Nitrogen requirement and NPU of egg protein in Japanese young men. *In* Influence of Environmental and Host Factors on Nutritional Requirements, N. Shimazono (Editor). Japanese Panel of Malnutrition, U.S.-Japan Cooperative Medical Sciences Program, Tokyo, Japan.

INOUE, G., FUJITA, Y., and NIIYAMA, Y. 1973. Studies on protein requirements of young med fed egg protein and rice protein with excess and maintenance energy intakes. J. Nutr. *103*, 1673.

IRWIN, M. I., and HEGSTED, D. M. 1971A. A conspectus of research on protein requirements of man. J. Nutr. *101*, 385.

IRWIN, M. I., and HEGSTED, D. M. 1971B. A conspectus of research on amino acid requirements of man. J. Nutr. *101*, 539.

JOURDAN, M., MARGEN, S., and BRADFIELD, R. B. 1974. Protein-sparing effect in obese women fed low calorie diets. Am. J. Clin. Nutr. *27*, 3.

KAPLAN, J. H., and PITOT, H. C. 1970. The regulation of intermediary amino acid metabolism in animal tissues. *In* Mammalian Protein Metabolism, Vol. IV, H. N. Munro (Editor). Academic Press, New York.

KIES, C., and FOX, H. M. 1970. Effect of level of total nitrogen intake on second limiting amino acid in corn for humans. J. Nutr. *100*, 1275.

KIES, C., WILLIAMS, E., and FOX, H. M. 1965. Determination of first limiting nitrogenous factor in corn protein for nitrogen retention in human adults. J. Nutr. *86*, 350.

KLEIBER, M. 1961. The Fire of Life. John Wiley & Sons, New York.

KOFRANYI, E. 1972. Protein and amino acid requirements. A nitrogen balance in adults. *In* Protein and Amino Acid Functions, E. J. Bigwood (Editor). Pergamon Press, New York.

KOFRANYI, E., JEKAT, F., BRAND, E., HACKENBERG, K., and HESS, B. 1969. Die frage der essentialitat von arginin und histidin, Hoppe-Seyler's Z. Physiol. Chem. *350*, 1401.

KOPPLE, J. D., and SWENDSEID, M. E. 1975. Evidence that histidine is an essential amino acid in normal and chronically uremic men. J. Clin. Invest. *55*, 881.

KREBS, H. A. 1972. Some aspects of the regulation of fuel supply in omnivorous animals. *In* Advances in Enzyme Regulation, Vol. 10, G. Weber (Editor). Pergamon Press, New York.

LONG, C. L., HAVERBERG, L. N., KINNEY, J. M., YOUNG, V. R., MUNRO, H. N., and GEIGER, J. W. 1975. Metabolism of 3-methylhistidine in man. Metabolism *24*, 929.

MCLAUGHLAN, J. M. 1974. Nutritional significance of alterations in plasma amino acids and serum proteins. *In* Improvements of Protein Nutriture, Natl. Res. Council—Natl. Acad. Sci., Washington, D.C.

MILLWARD, D. J., and GARLICK, P. J. 1972. The pattern of protein turnover in the whole animal and the effect of dietary variations. Proc. Nutr Soc. (Engl.) *31*, 257.

MORRISON, A. B., and NARAYANA RAO, M. 1967. Some relationships between protein and calories. *In* World Review of Nutrition and Dietetics, Vol. 7, G. H. Bourne (Editor). S. Karger, Basel, Switzerland.

MAURON, J. 1973. Some current problems in protein nutrition. *In* Proteins in Human Nutrition, J. W. G. Porter, and B. A. Rolls (Editors). Academic Press, New York.

MUNRO, H. N. 1951. Carbohydrate and fat as factors in protein utilization and metabolism. Physiol. Rev. *31*, 449.

MUNRO, H. N. 1964. General aspects of the regulation of protein metabolism by diet and by hormones. *In* Mammalian Protein Metabolism, Vol. 1, H. N. Munro, and J. B. Allison (Editors). Academic Press, New York.

MUNRO, H. N. 1969. Evolution of protein metabolism in mammals. *In* Mammalian Protein Metabolism, Vol. III, H. N. Munro (Editor). Academic Press, New York.

MUNRO, H. N. 1970A. Free amino acid pools and their regulation. *In* Mammalian Protein Metabolism, Vol. IV. H. N. Munro (Editor). Academic Press, New York.

MUNRO, H. N. 1970B. A general survey of mechanisms regulating protein metabolism in mammals. *In* Mammalian Protein Metabolism, Vol. IV, H. N. Munro (Editor). Academic Press, New York.

MULDOWNEY, F. P., CROOKS, J., and BLUHM, M. M. 1957. The relationship of total exchangeable potassium and chloride to lean body mass, and creatinine excretion in man. J. Clin. Invest. *36*, 1375.

NATL. ACAD. SCI.-NATL. RES. COUNCIL. 1974A. Improvement of Protein Nutriture. Food and Nutrition Board, Committee on Amino Acids, National Academy of Sciences, Washington, D. C.

NATL. ACAD. SCI.-NATL. RES. COUNCIL. 1974B. Recommended Dietary Allowances. Food and Nutrition Board, Committee on Dietary Allowances, National Academy of Sciences, Washington, D.C.

NICHOLSON, J. F. 1970. The rate of protein synthesis in premature infants. Pediat. Res. *4*, 389.

OZALP, J., YOUNG, V. R., NAGCHAUDHURI, J., TONTISIRIN, K., and SCRIMSHAW, N. S. 1972. Plasma amino acid response in young men given diets devoid of single essential amino acids. J. Nutr. *102*, 1147.

PARIZKOVA, K., EISALT, E., SPRYNAROVA, S., and WACHTLOVA, M. 1971. Body composition, aerobic capacity, and density of muscle capillaries in young and old men. J. Appl. Physiol. *31*, 323.

PENCHARZ, P. B. 1974. Studies in the protein metabolism of human neonates. Ph.D. Thesis, Massachusetts Institute of Technology, Cambridge, Mass.

PERERA, W. D., SCRIMSHAW, N. S., and YOUNG, V. R. 1975. Unpublished data. Massachusetts Institute of Technology, Cambridge, Mass.

PICOU, D., and TAYLOR-ROBERTS, T. 1969. The measurement of total protein synthesis and catabolism and nitrogen turnover in infants in different nutritional states and receiving different amounts of dietary protein. Clin. Sci. *36*, 283.

PORTER, J. W. G., and ROLLS, B. A. 1973. Proteins in Human Nutrition. Academic Press, New York.

ROSE, W. C. 1957. The amino acid requirements of adult man. Nutr. Abstr. Rev. *27*, 631.

ROSE, W. C., LAMBERT, G. F., and COON, M. J. 1954. The amino acid requirements of man. VII. General procedures; the tryptophan requirement. J. Biol. Chem. *211*, 815.

ROSE, W. C., and WIXOM, R. L. 1955. The amino acid requirements of man. XVI. The role of the nitrogen intake. J. Biol. Chem. *217*, 997.

ROSENTHAL, H. L., and ALLISON, J. B. 1951. Some effects of calorie intake on nitrogen balance in dogs. J. Nutr. *44*, 423.

SAN PIETRO, A., and RITTENBERG, D. 1953. A study of the rate of protein synthesis in humans. 2. Measurements of the metabolic pool and the rate of protein synthesis. J. Biol. Chem. *201*, 457.

SCRIMSHAW, N. S. 1976. Strengths and weaknesses of the committee approach—an analysis of past and present recommended dietary allowances for protein in health and in disease. New Engl. J. Med. *294*, 136.

SCRIMSHAW, N. S., HUSSEIN, M. A., MURRAY E., RAND, W. M., and YOUNG, V. R. 1972. Protein requirements of man: variations in obligatory and fecal nitrogen losses in young men. J. Nutr. *102*, 1595.

SCRIMSHAW, N. S., TAYLOR, Y. S. M., and YOUNG, V. R. 1973. Lysine supplementation of wheat gluten at adequate and restricted energy intakes in young men. Am. J. Clin. Nutr. *26*, 965.

SCRIMSHAW, N. S., YOUNG, V. R., SCHWARTZ, R., PICHE, M. L., and DAS, J. B. 1966. Minimum dietary essential amino acid to total nitrogen ratio for whole egg protein fed to young men. J. Nutr. *89*, 9.

SCRIMSHAW, N. S., YOUNG, V. R., HUANG, P. C., THANANGKUL, O., and CHOLAKOS, B. V. 1969. Partial dietary replacement of milk protein by nonspecific nitrogen in young men. J. Nutr. *98*, 9.

SCRIMSHAW, N. S., YOUNG, V. R., SCHWARTZ, R., PICHE, M. L., and DAS, J. B. 1966. Minimum dietary essential amino acid to total nitrogen ratio for whole egg protein fed to young men. J. Nutr. *89*, 9.

SHARP, C. S., LASSON, S., SHANKMAN, S., HAZLET, J. W., and KEDNIS, M. S. 1957. Studies of protein retention and turnover using nitrogen-15 as a tag. J. Nutr. *63*, 15.

SKETCHER, R. D., and JAMES, W. P. T. 1974. Branched-chain amino acid oxidation in relation to catabolic enzyme activities in rats given a protein-free diet at different stages of development. Brit. J. Nutr. *32*, 615.

SMITH, M. 1926. The minimum endogenous nitrogen metabolism. J. Biol. Chem. *68*, 15.

SMUTS, D. B. 1935. The relation between basal metabolism and the endogenous nitrogen metabolism, with particular reference to the estimation of the maintenance requirement of protein. J. Nutr. *9*, 403.

SOLIMAN, A. G., and HARPER, A. E. 1971. Effect of protein content of diet on lysine oxidation by the rat. Biochem. Biophys. Acta. *244*, 146.

STEFFEE, W. P., GOLDSMITH, R. S., PENCHARZ, P. B., SCRIMSHAW, N. S., and YOUNG, V. R. 1976. Dietary protein intake and dynamic aspects of whole body nitrogen metabolism. Metabolism *25*, 281.

STEGINK, L. D., and DEN BESTEN, L. 1972. Synthesis of cysteine from methionine in normal adult subjects: Effect of route of alimentation. Science *178*, 514.

STOCKLAND, W. L., MEADE, R. J., and MELLIERE, A. L. 1970. Lysine requirement of the growing rat; plasma free lysine as a response criterion. J. Nutr. *100*, 925.

SWANSON, P. 1959. Food energy and the metabolism of nitrogen. *In* Protein and Amino Acid Nutrition. A. A. Albanese (Editor). Academic Press, New York.

SWENDSEID, M. E., and KOPPLE, J. D. 1973. Nitrogen balance, plasma amino acid levels and amino acid requirements. Trans. N. Y. Acad. Sci. *35*, 471.

TONTISIRIN, K., YOUNG, V. R., and SCRIMSHAW, N. S. 1972. Plasma tryptophan response curve and tryptophan requirements in children with Down's Syndrome. Am. J. Clin. Nutr. *25*, 976.

TONTISIRIN, K., YOUNG, V. R., MILLER, M., and SCRIMSHAW, N. S. 1973. Plasma tryptophan response curve and tryptophan requirements of elderly people. J. Nutr. *103*, 1220.

TONTISIRIN, K., YOUNG, V. R., RAND, W. M., and SCRIMSHAW, N. S. 1974. Plasma threonine response curve and threonine requirements of young men and elderly women. J. Nutr. *104*, 495.

U. K. DEPT. OF HEALTH AND SOCIAL SECURITY. 1969. Recommended intakes of nutrients for the United Kingdom. Dept. of Health and Social Security. Rept. on Public Health and Med. Subjects. *120*, H. M. Stationery Office, London.

VAGHEFI, S. B., MAKDANI, D. D., and MICKELSEN, O. 1974. Lysine supplementation of wheat proteins. A review. Am. J. Clin. Nutr. *27*, 1231.

WANG, S. H., CROSBY, L. O., and NESHEIM, M. C. 1973. Effect of dietary excesses of lysine and arginine on the degradation of lysine by chick. J. Nutr. *103*, 384.

WATERLOW, J. C. 1968. Observations of the mechanism of adaptation to low protein intakes. Lancet *2*, 1091.

WATERLOW, J. C., and ALLEYNE, G. A. O. 1971. Protein malnutrition in children: Advances in knowledge in the last ten years. *In* Advances in Protein Chemistry, Vol. 25, C. B. Anfinsen Jr., J. T. Edsall, and F. M. Richards (Editors). Academic Press, New York.

WATERLOW, J. C., and STEPHEN, J. M. L. 1967. The assessment of total lysine turnover in the rat by intravenous infusion of L-(U-^{14}C) lysine. Clin. Sci. *33*, 489.

WATERLOW, J. C., and STEPHEN, J. M. L. 1968. The effect of low protein diets on the turnover rates of serum, liver and muscle proteins in the rat, measured by continuous infusion of L-(^{14}C) lysine. Clin. Sci. *35*, 287.

WATKIN, D. M. 1957. The assessment of protein nutrition in aged men. Ann. N. Y. Acad. Sci. *69*, 902.

WATKIN, D. M. 1964. Protein metabolism and requirements in the elderly. *In* Mammalian Protein Metabolism, Vol. 2, H. N. Munro, and J. B. Allison (Editors). Academic Press, New York.

WELLER, L. A., CALLOWAY, D. H., and MARGEN, S. 1971. Nitrogen balance of men fed mixtures based on Rose's requirements, egg white protein and serum free amino acid patterns. J. Nutr. *101*, 1499.

WHITE, P. L., and FLETCHER, D. C. 1974. Nutrients in Processed Foods—Proteins. Publishing Sciences Group, Acton, Mass.

WHITEHEAD, R. G. 1969. The assessment of nutritional status in protein-malnourished children. Proc. Nutr. Soc. (Engl.) *28*, 1.

WINTERER, J. C., SCRIMSHAW, N. S., and YOUNG, V. R. 1975. Unpublished results. Massachusetts Institute of Technology, Cambridge, Mass.

YAMASHITA, K., and ASHIDA, K. 1969. Lysine metabolism in rats fed a lysine-free diet. J. Nutr. *99*, 267.

YIENGST, M. J., BARROWS, C. H., and SHOCK, N. W. 1959. Age changes in the chemical composition of muscle and liver in the rat. J. Gerontol. *14*, 400.

YOSHIMURA, H. 1961. Adult protein requirements. Federation Proc. *20*, No. 1, Part III, Suppl. 7, 103.

YOSHIMURA, H. 1971. Physiological effect of protein deficiency with special reference to evaluation of protein nutrition and protein requirement. *In* World Review of Nutrition and Dietetics, Vol. 14, G. H. Bourne (Editor). S. Karger, Basel, Switzerland.

YOUNG, V. R. 1974. Regulation of protein synthesis and skeletal muscle growth. J. Anim. Sci. *38*, 1054.

YOUNG, V. R. 1975. Recent advances in evaluation of protein quality in adult humans. *In* Proc. 9th Intern. Congr. Nutrition, Vol. 3, A. Chavez, H. Bourges, and S. Basta (Editors). S. Karger, Basel, Switzerland.

YOUNG, V. R., ALEXIS, S. D., BALIGA, B. S., MUNRO, H. N., and MUECKE, W. 1972A. Metabolism of administered 3-methylhistidine: Lack of muscle tRNA charging and quantitative excretion as 3-methylhistidine and its N-acetyl-derivative. J. Biol. Chem. *247*, 3592.

YOUNG, V. R., HAVERBERG, L. N., BILMAZES, C., and MUNRO, H. N. 1973A. Potential use of 3-methylhistidine excretion as an index of progressive reduction in muscle protein catabolism during starvation. Metabolism *22*, 1429.

YOUNG, V. R., HUSSEIN, M. A., MURRAY, E., and SCRIMSHAW, N. S. 1971. Plasma tryptophan response curve and its relation to tryptophan requirements in young adult men. J. Nutr. *101*, 45.

YOUNG, V. R., and MUNRO, H. N. 1973. Plasma and tissue tryptophan levels in relation to tryptophan requirements of weanling and adult rats. J. Nutr. *103*, 1756.

YOUNG, V. R., PERERA, W. D., WINTERER, J. C., and SCRIMSHAW, N. S. 1976. Protein and amino acid requirements of the elderly. *In* Nutrition and Aging, M. Winick (Editor). John Wiley & Sons, New York.

YOUNG, V. R., and SCRIMSHAW, N. S. 1968. Endogenous nitrogen metabolism and plasma free amino acids in young adults given a "protein-free" diet. Brit. J. Nutr. *22*, 9.

YOUNG, V. R., and SCRIMSHAW, N. S. 1972. The nutritional significance of plasma and urinary amino acids. *In* Protein and Amino Acid Functions, E. J. Bigwood (Editors). Pergamon Press, New York.

YOUNG, V. R., and SCRIMSHAW, N. S. 1972. The nutritional significance of plasma and urinary amino acids. *In* Protein and Amino Acid Functions, E. J. Bigwood (Editor). Pergamon Press, New York.

YOUNG, V. R., and SCRIMSHAW, N. S. 1974B. Evaluation of the protein quality of fish protein concentrate for maintenance of adults. *In* The Economics, Marketing and Technology of Fish Protein Concentrate, S. R. Tannenbaum, B. R. Stillings, and N. S. Scrimshaw (Editors). MIT Press, Cambridge, Mass.

YOUNG, V. R. STEFFEE, W. P., PEŃCHARZ, P. B., WINTERER, J. C., and SCRIMSHAW, N. S. 1975. Total human body protein synthesis in relation to protein requirements at various ages. Nature *253*, 192.

YOUNG, V. R., TAYLOR, Y. S. M., RAND, W. M., and SCRIMSHAW, N. S. 1973B. Protein requirements of man: Efficiency of egg protein utilization at maintenance and sub-maintenance levels in young men. J. Nutr. *103*, 1164.

YOUNG, V. R., TONTISIRIN, K., OZALP, I., LAKSHMANAN, F., and SCRIMSHAW, N. S. 1972. Plasma amino acid response curve and amino acid requirements: valine and lysine. J. Nutr. *102*, 1159.

CHAPTER 3

L. Ross Hackler

In Vitro Indices: Relationships to Estimating Protein Value for the Human

Accurate measurements of protein needs, or more specifically amino acid requirements, for humans are crucial to the development of useful *in vitro* indices for evaluating the protein components in human diets.

Mulder (Block and Mitchell 1946) was the first to recognize the importance of proteins to plants and animals. In about 1840 he stated, "In both plants and animals a substance is contained, which is produced within the former, and imparted through their food to the latter. It is unquestionably the most important of all known substances in the organic kingdom. Without it no life appears possible on this planet. Through its means the chief phenomena of life are produced."

Several years elapsed before research on the biological evaluation of proteins attained a sound experimental base in which specific amino acids were recognized as differing in protein-containing foodstuffs. Osborne (1907) concluded his monograph on *The Proteins of the Wheat Kernel* with the following.

The proportion of lysine in wheat gluten is likewise small especially compared with that obtained from the leguminous seeds. The amount of histidine, however, does not differ very greatly from that of the other seed proteins. What significance these differences have in respect to the nutritive value of these different proteins must be determined by future investigation, for it has only very recently been discovered that such differences exist.

It is possible that feeding experiments with proteins of known character in respect to the relative proportions of their decomposition products will throw light on these important questions.

Another period of time elapsed (approximately 30 yr) before Rose's (1938) classic studies on amino acids gave an insight into the body's requirements for specific amino acids. A fact which is often overlooked is that the term "essential amino acid" has significance only when qualified as to species, nutritional or physiological state, and age.

A distinction must be made between protein quality, which is an attribute dependent upon the amino acid composition of proteins, and the efficiency of utilization, which takes into account both protein quality and quantity in the diet. Also, with respect to efficiency of utilization, the adequacy of the total diet to other nutrients, environmental conditions, and the age and physiological state of the recipient must be considered.

AMINO ACID COMPOSITION AND CHEMICAL SCORES

Table 3.1 compares amino acid patterns based on estimates of amino acid requirements as reported by the Food and Agriculture Organization (FAO 1973) and the National Research Council-National Academy of Sciences (Natl. Res. Council–Natl. Acad. Sci. 1974) together with amino acid compositions of human milk, cow's milk and whole egg, and the reference amino acid patterns (FAO 1957, 1973; Natl. Res. Council–Natl. Acad. Sci. 1974). It is readily apparent that chemical indices based on the amino acid composition of egg or milk have a built-in factor of safety. This is also true for the FAO pattern, especially when compared to the values based on estimated requirement levels for the adult. This margin of safety reflects the lack of sufficient information to arrive at firm requirement levels for humans and also recognizes that there is considerable variation between experimental subjects.

A major problem associated with the calculation of scores based on the amino acid compositions of reference proteins and various protein sources is that of obtaining reliable amino acid composition data. Various amino acid compositions of whole egg, which have been used as reference patterns, are listed in Table 3.2. It is obvious that, if these different egg amino acid composition patterns were used for calculating chemical scores of various proteins, different chemical scores would be obtained. Likewise, variation in the analytical estimates of amino acid compositions of various protein sources will be reflected in very different, or even unreliable, chemical scores.

For many years the investigation of the chemical and nutritional attributes of proteins has been hindered by inadequate methods of analysis. The development of automated ion-exchange chromatography procedures for the analysis of amino acids in foods has been of tremendous value to nutrition and food science researchers. However, we have lost sight of some of the problems associated with preparing the sample to be placed on the analyzers. Knipfel et al. (1971) studied the inter- and intra-laboratory variation associated with the analysis of amino acids on automated analyzers and concluded that most of the variation in results was probably due to sample manipulations rather than analysis per se. It has been suggested (Hackler 1974) that more care must be used in preparing samples for amino acid analysis, especially in the removal of air from the hydrolysis tube.

Methionine has been implicated as the amino acid with which the most variation has been observed by ion-exchange chromatography (Knipfel et al. 1971; Derse 1969; Porter et al. 1968). It has been suggested that a shorter hydrolysis of 6 hr will increase the amount of methionine detected (Tamura et al. 1958; Matsuno et al. 1959). On the other hand, Hackler (1971) in a study with pea beans, beef round and gelatin did not observe that a shorter time was desirable (Table 3.3). More uniform results should be obtained

TABLE 3.1

COMPARISON OF AMINO ACID PATTERNS (MG PER GM PROTEIN) BASED ON ESTIMATES OF AMINO ACID REQUIREMENTS, SUGGESTED REFERENCE PATTERNS FOR EVALUATING PROTEINS, AND AMINO ACID COMPOSITIONS OF EGG AND MILK PROTEINS

	Patterns According to Estimated Amino Acid Requirements[1]						Recommended Reference Patterns			Composition		
	Infant (3–6 months)		Children (10–12 yr)		Adult (23–50 yr)		FAO (1957)	FAO (1973)	NAS-NRC (1974)	Human Milk[2]	Cow's Milk[3]	Whole Egg[3]
	a	b	a	b	a	b						
Histidine	14.0	15.0	—	—	—	—			17	26	27	22
Isoleucine	35.0	36.4	37.0	25.9	18.0	15.0	42	40	42	46	47	54
Leucine	80.0	58.2	56.0	38.9	25.0	20.0	48	70	70	93	95	86
Lysine	52.0	44.1	75.0	40.7	22.0	15.0	42	55	50	66	78	70
Methionine + cystine	29.0	20.5	34.0	20.4	24.0	12.5	42	35	26	42	33	57
Phenylalanine + tyrosine	63.0	60.0	34.0	20.4	25.0	20.0	56	60	73	72	102	93
Threonine	44.0	28.6	44.0	25.9	13.0	10.0	28	40	35	43	44	47
Tryptophan	8.5	8.6	4.6	3.7	6.5	3.8	14	10	11	17	14	17
Valine	47.0	40.5	41.0	23.1	18.0	17.5	42	50	48	55	64	66

[1]Values in "a" columns are from FAO (1973); those in "b" columns adapted from Natl. Acad. Sci.—Natl. Res. Council (1974); Body weights of 6, 37, and 70 kg were used in computing the values for infants, children, and adults, respectively; and protein intakes of 2.2, 1.08, and 0.8 gm/kg of body weight for infants, children, and adults, respectively, in the "b" columns.
[2]Composition from FAO (1970); Lindner et al. (1965); and Soupart et al. (1954); also see FAO (1973).
[3]FAO (1970), tryptophan determined microbiologically.
[4]Lunven et al. (1972).

TABLE 3.2

AMINO ACID COMPOSITIONS (MG/GM NITROGEN) OF WHOLE EGG USED AS REFERENCE PATTERNS

	Block and Mitchell (1946)	Oser (1959)	Mitchell (1954)
Isoleucine	500	415	481
Leucine	575	550	575
Lysine	450	400	437
Methionine + cystine	406	342	400
Phenylalanine + tyrosine	675	630	675
Threonine	306	311	268
Tryptophan	93	103	93
Valine	456	464	450
Histidine	131	150	150
Arginine	400	410	

TABLE 3.3

THE EFFECT OF LENGTH OF HYDROLYSIS ON THE METHIONINE COMPOSITION OF PEA BEANS, BEEF ROUND AND GELATIN

Length of Hydrolysis (hr)	Methionine (gm per 16 gm Nitrogen)		
	Pea Beans	Beef Round	Gelatin
5½	0.85	2.16	0.35
11	0.93	2.40	0.61
22	0.96	2.34	0.79
44	0.88	2.44	0.96
66	0.84	2.37	0.98

Source: Hackler (1971); hydrolysis done in 10 ml of 6 N HCl at 110° C (approximately 5 mg nitrogen per sample).

if care is exercised in the removal of oxygen from the hydrolysis flask, removal of acid after hydrolysis, immediately dissolving the dried sample in pH 2.2 buffer and storing in the frozen state. The sample should be thawed just before placing on the ion-exchange column.

Table 3.4 contains information on chemical scores computed from amino acid composition data as measured microbiologically and by column chromatography. Many of the values are in close agreement, however some do not agree (e.g., the values for human milk are very different, 84.1 and 100, when computed from column chromatography and microbiological data, respectively). Other examples of disagreement are the chemical scores for beans and peas. Such variation in amino acid analyses limits the acceptance of *in vitro* indices for estimating protein quality. Also, the specific requirements for amino acids may alter the biological value of protein and this must also be considered in evaluating a chemical or microbiological index of protein quality (see Chapters 2 and 6).

TABLE 3.4

COMPARISON OF CHEMICAL SCORES COMPUTED FROM AMINO ACID
COMPOSITION AS DETERMINED BY COLUMN CHROMATOGRAPHY AND
MICROBIOLOGICALLY

Protein Source	Chemical Score[1]	
	CC[2]	M[2]
Human milk	84.1	100.0
Egg, whole	100.0	100.0
Cow's milk	94.5	94.5
Casein	91.4	92.2
Beef, edible flesh	100.0	100.0
Bean, immature in pod	60.9	63.1
Bean	54.1	39.5
Sesame	50.3	47.0
Coconut	64.7	62.8
Pea	94.8	55.4
Groundnut	65.0	61.8
Rice	66.5	68.2

[1]Chemical scores calculated using FAO (1973) amino acid pattern as the reference pattern.
[2]Scores calculated using amino acid compositions as determined by ion-exchange column chromatography (CC) and microbiologically (M); from FAO (1970).

TABLE 3.5

COMPARISON OF LIMITING AMINO ACIDS IN FOODS CALCULATED BY USING
FAO (1973) PATTERN AS THE REFERENCE PATTERN

Food	Chemical Score[1]	First-limiting Amino Acid	Second-limiting Amino Acid
Whole egg	100.0	—	—
Human milk	84.1	Methionine + cystine	Valine (91.6)[2]
Cow's milk	94.5	Methionine + cystine	—
Casein	91.4	Methionine + cystine	—
Beef, edible flesh	100.0	—	—
Chicken, edible flesh	99.0	Threonine	—
Pork, edible flesh	100.0	—	—
Fish, fresh all types	100.0	—	—
Maize	49.1	Lysine	Tryptophan (73.3)
Millet	62.9	Lysine	Threonine (96.4)
Oats	68.2	Lysine	Threonine (82.8)
Wheat	52.6	Lysine	Threonine (73.2)
Wheat gluten	26.1	Lysine	Threonine (63.6)
Sesame	50.3	Lysine	Threonine (84.2)
Bean, immature pod	60.9	Methionine + cystine	Isoleucine (93.6)
Bean	54.1	Methionine + cystine	Valine (92.6)
Rice, polished	66.5	Lysine	Threonine (82.8)
Yam	75.3	Lysine	Methionine + cystine (78.2)
Groundnut	65.0	Lysine	Threonine (65.2)
Pea	57.7	Methionine + cystine	Tryptophan (93.3)
Coconut	64.7	Lysine	Threonine (84.8)

[1]Scores calculated by using amino acid compositions tabulated by FAO (1970).
[2]Values in parentheses represent scores calculated on the basis of the second most limiting amino acid.

TABLE 3.6

COMPARISON OF SEVERAL METHODS FOR EVALUATING PROTEIN
NUTRITIONAL VALUE

Food	BV[1]	PER[1]	NPU[1]	FAO Score 1970[1]	FAO Score 1973[2]
Maize	59.4	1.12	51.1	41	49.1
Oats	64.9	2.25	65.7	57	68.2
Rice	64.0	2.18	57.2	56	66.5
Wheat	64.7	1.53	40.3	44	52.6
Beans	58.0	1.48	38.4	34	54.1
Groundnuts	54.5	1.65	42.7	43	65.0
Peas	63.7	1.57	46.7	37	57.7
Sesame	62.0	1.77	53.4	42	50.3
Beef	74.3	2.30	66.9	69	100.0
Egg	93.7	3.92	93.5	100	100.0
Fish	76.0	3.55	79.5	70	100.0
Milk, cow's	84.5	3.09	81.6	60	94.5
Casein, cow's	79.7	2.86	72.1	58	91.4

[1]Data for biological value (BV), protein efficiency ratio (PER), net protein utilization (NPU) and FAO score (1970) compiled from FAO (1970).
[2]FAO score, based on FAO (1973) recommended amino acid pattern.

The chemical scores obtained using the FAO suggested pattern of amino acid needs are based on the chemical score for the first-limiting amino acid. This utilizes the approach described in the classic paper of Block and Mitchell (1946). Table 3.5 compares the limiting amino acids in foods as determined by the FAO pattern of 1973. The chemical score for a wide variety of foods shows lysine to be first-limiting in approximately 50% of the foods and methionine + cystine first-limiting in approximately 30%. Threonine was first-limiting in one of the foods, but it was the second-limiting amino acid in 38% of the foods. Tryptophan and valine were second-limiting in two of the foods, while methionine + cystine and isoleucine were each second-limiting in one food. This suggests that we may need to concern ourselves with only three or four amino acids in arriving at an estimate of protein quality for humans.

Although it is not the intent of this paper to discuss the various bioassay methods for evaluating protein quality, it is desirable to compare bioassay data with chemical scores (Tables 3.6 and 3.7). All of the simple correlation coefficients are higher than the required value of 0.684, which indicates significance at the 1% level of probability. Thus, each protein index has a strong linear association with any of the others. Although the bioassay data are from rat studies, these high correlation coefficients suggest that chemical indices based on the amino acid composition of proteins foods in a diet should be useful in estimating the nutritional value of human diets.

TABLE 3.7

SIMPLE CORRELATIONS[1] FOR DATA IN TABLE 3.5 ("COMPARISON OF SEVERAL METHODS FOR EVALUATING THE PROTEIN NUTRITIONAL VALUE")

	BV[2]	PER[2]	NPU[2]	FAO Score 1970[2]	FAO Score 1973[3]
BV	1.0000				
PER	0.9039	1.0000			
NPU	0.9216	0.9420	1.0000		
FAO score, 1970	0.8668	0.8930	0.9882	1.0000	
FAO score, 1973	0.8521	0.8938	0.8734	0.8379	1.0000

[1]$P < 0.01$ requires a coefficient of 0.684 for significance.
[2]Data compiled from FAO (1970); see Table 3.5 for definitions.
[3]Based on the FAO (1973) amino acid pattern.

TABLE 3.8

COMPARISON OF THE ESSENTIAL AMINO ACID INDEX (EAAI), EXPERIMENTALLY DETERMINED BIOLOGICAL VALUES, AND BIOLOGICAL VALUES PREDICTED FROM EAAI VALUES

Protein Source	EAAI	Biological Value Predicted	Biological Value Observed
Milk, cow	88	84	90
Casein	88	84	72
Lactalbumin	89	85	84
Egg, whole	100	97	96
Beef	84	80	76
Fish	80	76	85
Gelatin	25	16	25[1]
Peanuts	69	64	57
Soybeans	83	78	75
Sesame	73	68	71
Oats	72	67	65
Wheat	64	58	67

Source: Data from Oser (1959).
[1]Bender *et al.* (1953) have stated that the often-quoted biological value of 25 for gelatin is incorrect, and they reported duplicate values of 4 and 1.

ESSENTIAL AMINO ACID INDEXES

Oser (1951) pointed out that it would be more reasonable to base a protein rating on the contribution a protein makes in respect to all the essential amino acids rather than simply on the one in greatest deficit, and he proposed an essential amino acid index (EAAI) based on 11 amino acids.

Mitchell (1954) proposed a modified essential amino acid index (MEAAI). In the MEAAI, arginine was omitted as being nonessential and tyrosine was included, in addition to phenylalanine because of its partial replacement value for phenylalanine. Oser (1959) considered the arginine modification as inconsequential and concluded that omitting it from consideration had little, if any, effect upon the EAAI value. For practical purposes, except for infants, arginine and histidine can both be eliminated from consideration in evaluating protein quality for humans.

Table 3.8 compares the EAAI with the biological value for several foods. Oser (1951), Mitchell (1954), Stillings and Hackler (1966) and Hackler *et al.* (1967) have pointed out that the correlation between the EAAI (or MEAAI) and various biological procedures is consistently high under well-controlled conditions. Thus, estimates of biological quality may be made from essential amino acid analyses with at least an equal degree of accuracy as can be obtained from the usual bioassays. It should be emphasized, of course, that such a system as the EAAI (or MEAAI) makes no allowance for the availability of amino acids to the body and is based on the amino acid composition of the test protein in relation to egg amino acids. This may or may not be representative of the amino acids needed by the body. Furthermore, it was mentioned earlier that the literature values for the amino acid composition of the reference protein (egg) varies among laboratories.

AVAILABLE LYSINE (CHEMICAL) AND HEAT PROCESSING

Carpenter's available lysine method is the most widely used chemical procedure for determining chemically available lysine (Carpenter 1960; Carpenter and Booth 1973). This procedure will yield useful information about food proteins that contain lysine as the first-limiting essential amino acid. However, chemical estimates of available lysine are not always related to nutritive value (e.g., Hackler *et al.* 1967; Boctor and Harper 1968; Atkinson and Carpenter 1970). Serious analytical problems exist in applying the method to high carbohydrate protein sources (see Bodwell 1976).

The procedure may also be useful in monitoring the effect of heat processing on protein quality (Hackler *et al.* 1965). The effect of heat processing on available lysine is shown in Table 3.9. It is readily apparent from the data presented that it is necessary to inactivate antinutritional substances in legume products in order for available lysine to be useful in monitoring the effect of heat processing on products such as soy milk. Once the antinutritional factors are inactivated in legumes then Carpenter's available lysine procedure is useful in monitoring products for over heat-processing, even though lysine may not be the first-limiting essential amino acid in the product.

The usual acid hydrolysis procedure will release the biologically unavailable lysine; thus Carpenter's method is also useful in extending our knowledge about a product for which only amino acid data are available. Unfortunately, no single chemical procedure is adequate by itself for predicting protein quality for all proteins.

TABLE 3.9

THE EFFECT OF HEAT PROCESSING ON PROTEIN UTILIZATION OF SOY MILK AS
MEASURED BY PROTEIN EFFICIENCY RATIO (PER) AND AVAILABLE
LYSINE PROCEDURE

min at 121°C	PER	Available Lysine (gm per 16 gm Nitrogen)
0	0.65 ± 0.11	6.0
5	2.24 ± 0.05	6.0
10	2.20 ± 0.08	6.0
20	2.00 ± 0.08	5.9
40	1.83 ± 0.10	5.7
60	1.74 ± 0.04	5.5
120	1.37 ± 0.06	5.0

Source: Hackler *et al.* (1965).

TABLE 3.10

COMPARISON OF AVAILABLE LYSINE VALUES ESTIMATED BY USING
TETRAHYMENA ASSAYS, THE FDNB CHEMICAL METHOD, AND RAT
GROWTH ASSAYS

Protein Source	Available Lysine (gm per 16 gm Nitrogen)			
	Tetrahymena[1] —	+	FDNB	Rat Growth Assays
Fish meal	4.8	7.0	6.1	6.9
Meat meal	1.1	3.1	4.1	4.3
Groundnut meal, 101	2.4	3.5	2.6	3.5
Groundnut meal	2.1	3.0	3.0	3.2
Groundnut meal, heated	0.6	1.7	1.3	1.0
Soybean meal	4.2	4.4	5.4	5.0
Soybean meal, heated	1.0	2.4	2.4	1.3
Cod muscle	6.4	8.6	8.5	10.9
Cod muscle, heated	1.0	5.0	5.6	4.3
Casein	8.1	—	8.4	8.6

Source: Data presented by Shorrock and Ford (1973).
[1]Samples in the *Tetrahymena* column (—) received no predigestion, those in (+)
column were predigested with papain.

MICROBIOLOGICAL METHODS

Where a single amino acid analysis is suitable for monitoring or estimating protein quality, a microbiological procedure may be useful. Lawrie
(1937) observed that *Tetrahymena pyriformis* W. were strongly proteolytic
and efforts to use them for measuring amino acids have been sporadic.
Shorrock and Ford (1973) have compared available lysine values determined with *Tetrahymena,* 1-fluoro-2,4-dinitrobenzene (FDNB), and in
growth tests with rats (Table 3.10). The data obtained with *Tetrahymena*
(samples predigested with papain), FDNB and rat growth are in general

agreement. This suggests that *Tetrahymena,* as well as the chemically available lysine method, may be useful for the evaluation of protein quality for humans. However, it should be noted that the microbiological procedures have not gained wide acceptance because of the unfamiliarity of many nutritionists with microbiological techniques. Also, Shorrock and Ford (1973) observed that the *Tetrahymena* assay still needs further development, especially a faster method (or an alternative procedure) for counting cells needs to be resolved, and a further problem stems from the lack of fundamental information on the nutritional needs of the organism.

Microbiologically available methionine has been used for assessing the nutritional value of proteins by Ford (1960, 1962, 1964). Boyne *et al.* (1967), as a result of collaborative studies with *Streptococcus zymogenes,* proposed an assay procedure for available methionine. Kelly (1971) eliminated the predigestion of the sample with papain, consequently digestion depended on the proteolytic action of *Streptococcus zymogenes.* Kelly also used only a 24-hr incubation. Leleji *et al.* (1972) found it necessary to increase the incubation period to 72 hr before satisfactory results could be obtained with Kelly's procedure. Thus, microbiological procedures may be useful in predicting protein quality where only one or two amino acids need to be determined.

ENZYME DIGESTION

Sheffner *et al.* (1956) attempted to overcome the limitations associated with a chemical determination of amino acids, which employed an acid for hydrolysis of the protein, by using an enzymatic digestion to release the amino acids. This procedure has been referred to as the PDR index (Pepsin Digest Residue index). It is questionable whether the added labor involved in obtaining data for calculating PDR indexes is worthwhile. However, where the history of the product is not known, especially where excessive heat processing may have occurred in the presence of reducing compounds, it may be more useful than total amino acid composition as determined by an acid hydrolysis procedure. Also, Akeson and Stahmann (1964) suggested a pepsin-pancreatin-digest index for the evaluation of protein quality. As with the earlier work of Sheffner *et al.* (1956), Akeson and Stahmann (1964) wanted to overcome the limitations associated with the acid hydrolysis of protein to amino acids and arrive at a value which would more readily define the availability of the amino acids in an intact animal.

The enzyme digestion procedures yield data which will correlate with biological data (Table 3.11; also Mauron, 1973), but these methods are more laborious. Also, there are limitations with the enzymatic digestion procedures, because they do not duplicate the conditions in the gastrointestinal tract. The enzyme digestion procedures do yield information on the amino acids released which is valid for the conditions employed. Szmelcman and

TABLE 3.11

COMPARISON OF PEPSIN PANCREATIN DIGEST INDEX (PPDI) WITH BIOLOGICAL
VALUE (BV) IN THE RAT, AND THE ESSENTIAL AMINO ACID INDEX (EAAI)

Protein Source	BV[1]	PPDI[2]	EAAI[3]
Whole egg	96	100	100
Cow's milk	90	86	88
Lactalbumin	85	87	89
Beef	76	78	84
Casein	69	79	88
Wheat flour	52	52	61

[1]Data of Block and Mitchell (1946).
[2]Data of Akeson and Stahmann (1964).
[3]Data of Oser (1959).

Guggenheim (1967) reviewed a number of *in vitro* digestion techniques and concluded that such techniques can at best serve only as guides to the amounts of amino acids which may be released by enzymatic digestion in the intestine.

DYE BINDING

Dye-binding procedures for the evaluation of protein quality have potential value under well-defined conditions. Several researchers have used the disulfonic acid dye, orange G, to monitor protein content and quality. Fraenkel-Conrat and Cooper (1944) demonstrated that the basic groups on the protein molecule form a protein–dye complex. Lakin (1973) has reviewed various dye-binding procedures and concluded that the empirical measurement of the total content of the basic amino acids in proteins is influenced by two factors: the total protein content and the amino acid composition. Thus, it is necessary for the protein quantities to remain relatively constant in a group of samples for meaningful comparisons to be obtained.

CONCLUSIONS

There is very little information concerning the relationship of *in vitro* protein quality indexes with protein nutritive value for the human. Furthermore, most of our biological testing of proteins has been with laboratory animals fed a single source of protein, whereas humans consume a mixture of proteins which varies from meal to meal and day to day. Lastly, protein is really not a limiting factor in the United States, but with recent nutritional labeling regulations, we do need a simple method (or methods) for monitoring protein quality for humans. Although, a major problem associated with scores based on amino acids is obtaining reliable amino acid composition data, amino acid analyses should be a logical technique for monitoring protein quality.

BIBLIOGRAPHY

AKESON, W. R., and STAHMANN, M. A. 1964. A pepsin pancreatin digest index of protein quality evaluation. J. Nutr. *83*, 257.

ATKINSON, J., and CARPENTER, K. J. 1970. Nutritive value of meat meals II. Influence of raw materials and processing on protein quality. J. Sci. Food. Agr. *21*, 366.

BENDER, A. E., MILLER, D. S., and TUNNAH, E. J. 1953. The biological value of gelatin. Chem. Ind. *1953*, 799.

BLOCK, R. J., and MITCHELL, H. H. 1946. The correlation of the amino acid composition of proteins with their nutritive value. Nutr. Abstr. Rev. *16*, 249.

BOCTOR, A. M., and HARPER, A. E. 1968. Measurement of available lysine in heated and unheated foodstuffs by chemical and biological methods. J. Nutr. *94*, 289.

BODWELL, C. E. 1976. Status of chemical methods to determine biologically available lysine in wheat proteins. 9th National Conference on Wheat Utilization, Seattle, Wash., Oct. 8–10, 1975. Publ. *ARS-NC40*, U.S. Dept. Agr., Washington, D.C.

BOYNE, A. W., PRICE, S. A., ROSEN, G. D., and STOTT, J. A. 1967. Protein quality of feeding-stuffs. 4. Progress report on collaborative studies on the microbiological assay of available amino acids. Brit. J. Nutr. *21*, 181.

CARPENTER, K. J. 1960. The estimation of the available lysine in animal-protein foods. Biochem. J. *77*, 604.

CARPENTER, K. J., and BOOTH, V. H. 1973. Damage to lysine in food processing: Its measurement and its significance. Nutr. Abstr. Rev. *43*, 423.

DERSE, P. H. 1969. Amino acid analysis employing microbiological assays and automated analyzers. Feedstuffs *41*, No. 6, 42.

FAO. 1957. Human protein requirements and their fulfilment in practice. *In* Proceedings of a Conference in Princeton, United States (1955), J. C. Waterlow, and J. M. L. Stephen (Editors). John Wright & Sons Ltd., Stonebridge Press, Bath Road, Bristol, of England.

FAO. 1970. Amino Acid Content of Foods and Biological Data on Proteins. FAO, Rome, Italy.

FAO. 1973. Energy and protein requirements. Report of a joint FAO/WHO ad hoc expert committee, Rome, 22 March–2 April 1971, FAO, Rome, Italy.

FORD, J. E. 1960. A microbiological method for assessing the nutritional value of proteins. Brit. J. Nutr. *14*, 485.

FORD, J. E. 1962. A microbiological method for assessing the nutritional value of proteins. 2. The measurement of available methionine, leucine, isoleucine, arginine, histidine, tryptophan, and valine. Brit. J. Nutr. *16*, 409.

FORD, J. E. 1964. A microbiological method for assessing the nutritional value of proteins. 3. Further studies on the measurement of available amino acids. Brit. J. Nutr. *18*, 449.

FRAENKEL-CONRAT, H., and COOPER, M. 1944. The use of dyes for the determination of acid and basic groups in proteins. J. Biol. Chem. *154*, 239.

HACKLER, L. R. 1971. Methods of analyses for the sulfur amino acids. Feedstuffs *43*, No. 9, 18.

HACKLER, L. R. 1974. Amino acid analysis of foods with emphasis on cystine and methionine. Presented at the 34th Annual IFT Meeting, New Orleans.

HACKLER, L. R., STILLINGS, B. R., and POLIMENI, R. J., Jr. 1967. Correlation of amino acid indexes with nutritional quality of several soybean fractions. Cereal Chem. *44*, 638.

HACKLER, L. R., VAN BUREN, J. P., STEINKRAUS, K. H., EL RAWI, I., and HAND , D. B. 1965. Effect of heat treatment on nutritive value of soy milk protein fed to weanling rats. J. Food Sci. *30*, 723.

KNIPFEL, J. E., AITKEN, J. R., HILL, D. C., MCDONALD, B. E., and OWEN, B. D. 1971. Amino acid composition of food proteins: Inter- and intralaboratory variation. J. Assoc. Offic. Agr. Chem. *54*, 777.

LAKIN, A. L. 1973. Evaluation of protein quality by dye-binding procedures. *In* Proteins in Human Nutrition, J. W. G. Porter, and B. A. Rolls (Editors). Academic Press, New York.

LAWRIE, N. R. 1937. Studies in the metabolism of protozoa. III. Some properties of a proteolytic extract obtained from *Glaucoma piriformis.* Biochem. J. *31,* 789.

LELEJI, O. I., DICKSON, M. H., and HACKLER, L. R. 1972. Effect of genotype on microbiologically available methionine content of bean seeds. Hort. Sci. *30,* 277.

LINDNER, K., TAYAN, R., KRAMER, M., and SZOKE, K. 1965. Pr. Mater. nauk. Inst. Matki Dziecka, *6,* 337, as reported in FAO (1973).

LUNVEN, P., LeCLEMENT DE ST. MARCQ, C., CARNOVALE, E., and FRATONI, A. 1972. Unpublished data, Nutr. Div. of FAO and Natl. Nutr. Inst., Rome, Italy as reported in FAO (1973).

MATSUNO, N., NISHIBARA, A., and ISOBE, S. 1959. Studies on the determination of amino acids (Report 2) on the effect of hydrolysis time of protein on the determination of amino acids. *In* Annual Report of the National Institute of Nutrition, Toyanako, Tokyo.

MAURON, J. 1973. The analyses of food proteins, amino acid composition and nutritive value. *In* Proteins in Human Nutrition, J. W. G. Porter and B. A. Rolls (Editors). Academic Press, New York.

MITCHELL, H. H. 1954. The dependence of the biological value of food proteins upon their content of essential amino acids. Wiss. Abhandl. Deut. Akad. Landwirtschaftwiss. Berlin. Band V/2, 279.

MULDER, G. J. 1840. The chemistry of animal and vegetable physiology. As reported by R. J. Block, and H. H. Mitchell, The correlation of the amino-acid composition of proteins with their nutritive value, 1946. Nutr. Abstr. Rev. *16,* 249.

NATL. ACAD. SCI.–NATL. RES. COUNCIL. 1974. Improvement of Protein Nutriture. Committee on Amino Acids, Food and Nutrition Board. National Academy of Sciences, Washington, D.C.

OSBORNE, T. B. 1907. The proteins of the wheat kernel. Carnegie Inst., Washington, Publ. *84.*

OSER, B. L. 1951. Method for integrating essential amino acid content in the nutritional evaluation of protein. J. Am. Dietet. Assoc. *27,* 396.

OSER, B. L. 1959. An integrated essential amino acid index for predicting the biological value of proteins. *In* Protein and Amino Acid Nutrition, A. A. Albanese (Editor). Academic Press, New York.

PORTER, J. W. G., WESTGARTH, D. R., and WILLIAMS, A. P. 1968. A collaborative test of ion-exchange chromatographic methods for determining amino acids. Brit. J. Nutr. *22,* 437.

ROSE, W. C. 1938. The nutritive significance of the amino acids. Physiol. Rev. *18,* 109.

SHEFFNER, A. L., ADACKI, R., and SPECTOR, H. 1956. Measurement of the net utilization of heat processed proteins by means of the pepsin digest-residue (PDR) amino acid index. J. Nutr. *60,* 507.

SHORROCK, C., and FORD, J. E. 1973. An improved procedure for the determination of available lysine and methionine with *Tetrahymena. In* Proteins in Human Nutrition, J. W. G. Porter, and B. A. Rolls (Editors). Academic Press, New York.

SOUPART, P., MOORE, S., and BIGWOOD, E. J. 1954. Amino acid composition of human milk. J. Biol. Chem. *206,* 699.

STILLINGS, B. R., and HACKLER, L. R. 1966. Amino acids studies on the effect of fermentation time and heat-processing of tempeh. J. Food Sci. *30,* 1043.

SZELCMAN, S., and GUGGENHEIM, K. 1967. Availability of amino acids in processed plant protein food stuffs. J. Sci. Food Agr. *18,* 347.

TAMURA, E., NISHIHARA, A., ISOBE, S., and MATSUNO, N. 1958. Studies on the determination of amino acids (Report 1) on the hydrolysis-time of protein and the effect of carbohydrate and changes of the hydrolysate during storage. *In* Annual Report of the National Institute of Nutrition, Toyanako, Tokyo.

CHAPTER 4

K. W. Samonds
and D. M. Hegsted

Animal Bioassays: A Critical Evaluation with Specific Reference to Assessing Nutritive Value for the Human[1]

There is abundant evidence from animal experiments that proteins differ in their abilities to promote growth and meet maintenance needs. Poor quality proteins, however, presumably can suffice, unless they are extremely low or void of an essential amino acid, if they are fed at sufficiently high levels. Consumption of a protein with 50% of the nutritive value of the best quality proteins would double the amount of that protein needed. The requirement will be quadrupled if nutritive value falls to 25%.

The need for a simple, inexpensive, and reproducible method for measuring protein quality seems self-evident, but these factors should not override other factors which affect the utility of the results. The selected method should have sufficient precision to discriminate between proteins of different quality, should provide an internal test of its own validity to determine whether the results are relatively independent (of the amount of protein fed, the amount of food consumed, the kind of subject used, etc.), should give a result which is proportional to the true potency of the material tested, and, hopefully, would give a result which would be applicable to measures of human protein requirements. Clearly, no single method combines all the desired criteria, and the selection of a method involves a trade-off of one characteristic versus another.

Since all animal assays for measuring protein quality are derived from the same relationship between the change in body nitrogen (or some correlate of body nitrogen) and nitrogen intake, it is worthwhile to begin with this relationship in comparing the similarities and differences, and the shortcomings, of the various methods.

ASSAY METHODS

Figure 4.1 shows some sample data resulting from the feeding of various levels of lactalbumin to young, growing rats and the measuring of weight

[1]Supported in part by a grant-in-aid from the National Institutes of Health (AM-09520) and the Fund for Research and Teaching, Department of Nutrition, Harvard School of Public Health.

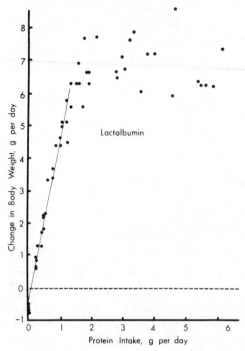

FIG. 4.1. THE GROWTH RESPONSE OF YOUNG RATS TO VARIOUS
LEVELS OF DIETARY LACTALBUMIN

Protein is the limiting factor up to an intake of approximately 1.5 gm
per day.

gain as an indicator of nitrogen gain or loss. The response is generally linear
up to an intake at which protein is no longer the limiting factor. Above this
level, energy intake or the animal's inability to grow any faster presumably
becomes the limiting factor. Now, if we superimpose upon these data the
conditions of a protein quality assay, the qualities and limitations of the
various methods should become evident.

Protein Efficiency Ratio

[In the determination of protein efficiency ratio (PER), a single level of
protein is fed, usually 9% of the diet, and the ratio of the weight gain over
a four-week period to the protein intake is calculated.] As can be seen from
Fig. 4.2, PER is, in fact, the average of the slopes of the lines connecting the
weight gains of these animals to the origin. Variations in food intake, and
therefore in protein intake, increase the variability between the individual
PER lines which decreases the precision of the method particularly for poor
quality proteins. The measurement of PER is dose-dependent, rising as

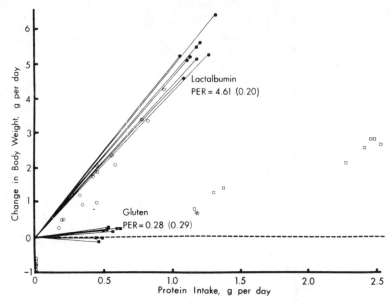

FIG. 4.2.   A GRAPHIC REPRESENTATION OF THE CALCULATION OF PER FROM
THE GROWTH RESPONSE AND PROTEIN INTAKE OF YOUNG RATS

In this and subsequent figures, filled symbols represent data used in the calculation
of the protein quality estimator, while open symbols represent data at other levels
of intake; values given in parentheses are standard errors of the estimate.

intake increases (Fig. 4.3), plateauing as the growth rate reaches the maximum, and then falling slowly at higher intakes. As an estimate of protein
quality, PER consistently underestimates the true slope of the dose-response curve, and, although it tends to roughly rank the proteins according
to their quality, the estimate is not proportional to true protein quality.

Net Protein Ratio, Net Protein Utilization, Biological Value

Other methods attempt to correct for the major flaw in the PER method
by including a second group of animals fed a diet containing no protein and
calculating a new "slope" which takes into account the loss of body weight
or body nitrogen by this group. Net protein ratio (NPR) uses weight change
as the dependent variable and, in fact, uses the same data points as PER
but calculates the slope through the new intercept (Fig. 4.4). Net protein
utilization (NPU) measures the change in body nitrogen between the two
dietary groups and a group of animals sacrificed at the beginning of the
feeding period, and biological value (BV) uses the estimate of retained nitrogen derived from the difference between ingested nitrogen and that
accounted for in urine and feces. In all three of these methods, variations

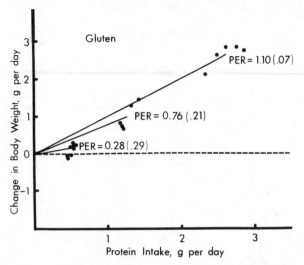

FIG. 4.3.   THE ESTIMATE OF PER IS DOSE DEPENDENT

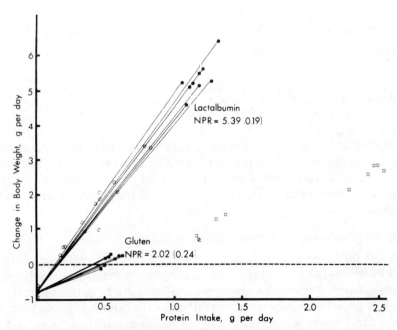

FIG. 4.4.   A GRAPHIC REPRESENTATION OF THE CALCULATION OF NPR FROM
THE GROWTH RESPONSE AND PROTEIN INTAKE OF YOUNG RATS

For a description of symbols, see legend of Fig. 4.2.

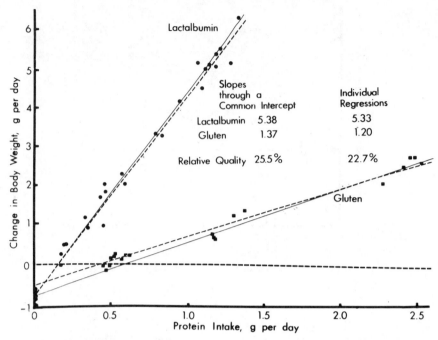

FIG. 4.5. REGRESSION LINES FOR LACTALBUMIN AND GLUTEN

Solid lines were fitted using the multiple regression analysis of the slope ratio assay with the assumption that the lines had a common intercept. Broken lines were fitted individually for the two proteins, omitting the data for the group fed zero protein and without the assumption of a common intercept. Calculated from the slopes through a common intercept, equals the relative nutritive value (RNV) for gluten; relative quality value for gluten calculated from individual regression equations equals relative protein value (RPV).

in food intake tend to make the animals fall along the dose-response line which is an improvement in precision over PER. All the methods, however, are essentially "two point" assays with only the tacit assumption that the response is linear between the zero intercept and the points for animals fed 9% protein.

Slope Ratio Assay: Relative Nutritive Value

A test for linearity is provided by the slope ratio assay (Hegsted *et al.* 1968) which is based upon the assay for relative potency commonly used to evaluate drugs or vitamin supplements (Finney 1964). In this assay, three levels of protein are selected which fall along the relatively linear portion of the curve where protein is limiting. In addition, a zero-protein group is included. Regression lines (relating changes in body weight or body water to nitrogen intake) are fit to the data for individual proteins by Least Squares analysis, and all lines are fit either through the zero protein in-

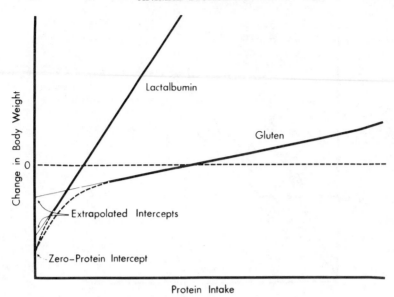

FIG. 4.6.   RELATIVE QUALITY VALUES FOR GLUTEN

Dose-response relationship (see text for discussion).

tercept or through the best fitting common intercept for the various lines
(Fig. 4.5, solid lines). A measure of protein quality, relative nutritive value
(RNV), is then calculated by dividing the slope of a test protein by the slope
of the reference protein, lactalbumin. This method offers a high degree of
precision and an internal test of its own validity, but requires some advance
knowledge of a protein's quality so that appropriate levels can be selected.

Modified Slope Ratio Assay: Relative Protein Value

After several years it has become increasingly clear that all of these
methods suffer from the common misconception that the dose-response
relationship is linear from zero intake up to some preselected level which
varies with the method and with the investigator's interpretation. The relationship for most, if not all, proteins is now known to be as shown in Fig.
4.6. There is curvature at very low intakes. The degree of curvature depends
upon which essential amino acid is most limiting in the protein being
studied and is particularly large with proteins limiting in lysine and to a
lesser degree with proteins limiting in methionine or total sulfur amino
acids. The reason for this curvature is now reasonably clear, although the
biochemical basis has not been explained. The rate of catabolism of some
amino acids, particularly lysine, seems to be dependent upon the availability
of that amino acid (Yamashita and Ashida 1969, 1971). When lysine intake

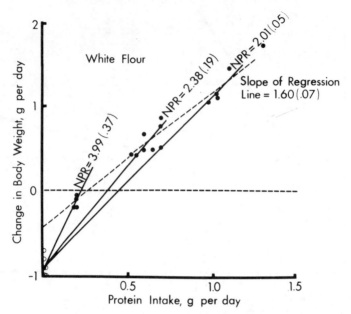

FIG. 4.7. THE CALCULATION OF NPRS FOR THREE LEVELS OF
WHITE FLOUR DEMONSTRATES THAT NPR IS DOSE DEPENDENT FOR
LYSINE-LIMITING PROTEINS

is low, catabolism of lysine is retarded, resulting in the conservation and reutilization of this amino acid. Threonine, on the other hand, appears to have no conservation mechanism. These differences are particularly apparent in long-term feeding studies in which adult rats are fed diets void of one of these amino acids. Lysine-deficient animals survive for months, whereas threonine-deficient animals are moribund within a few weeks (Said and Hegsted 1970; Said *et al.* 1974). Therefore, as one lowers the intake of a lysine-limiting protein, one eventually reaches a level near maintenance at which lysine is no longer limiting because it is conserved. Presumably, another amino acid or total nitrogen for the synthesis of dispensable amino acids becomes the limiting factor and the response line plunges to a lower intercept (Said and Hegsted 1969).

Since BV, NPU, and NPR all utilize the response at zero protein intake to calculate the slope of a regression line, these values will be dose-dependent falling as the level of intake is raised (Fig. 4.7). This dose dependency has led to vigorous disagreement about whether the response line is curvilinear throughout its entire range or essentially linear with curvature at the lower end. Statistical tests for curvature fail to show deviations from linearity over a very wide range of intakes for proteins such as gluten, indicating to us that the latter model is the correct one. The resulting error and dose dependency in the slope ratio assay are less than in BV or NPU since it is based upon multiple points and the slope is not totally dependent upon the zero intercept. Nevertheless, the RNV assay technique can be considered to be valid only if the dose-response lines have a common intercept, and it must therefore be abandoned. In each of these methods the aberration from the expected zero protein intercept often results in a rather gross overestimate of the qualities of lysine-limiting poor quality proteins. The best solution, though not ideal, is the measurement of the slope of the dose-response relationship for individual proteins in the region of intake where it is essentially linear, from approximately the maintenance level to the level at which protein is no longer limiting eliminating the feeding of zero protein diets entirely (Fig. 4.5, broken lines). As in the slope ratio assay, the ratio of the slope of the test protein to the slope of lactalbumin gives an estimate of the relative quality (Fig. 4.5). Appropriate estimates of the confidence interval can be calculated taking into account the variability in both the numerator and denominator of the ratio. This modification has been labeled relative protein value (RPV) to distinguish it from relative nutritive value (RNV).

INTERLABORATORY COMPARISONS OF METHODS

RPV has been compared to PER and NPR in a collaborative assay by eight laboratories experienced in measuring protein quality (Samonds and Hegsted, 1976). Seven proteins were compared: lactalbumin, casein, defatted meat, soy flour, a soy protein isolate, wheat gluten and white flour. The results of this study were, at the same time, disconcerting and enlightening. Not only was there a considerable difference in the precision of the various laboratories, there was also considerable disagreement between the laboratories when the same proteins were evaluated using the same methods. In each laboratory with each test, lactalbumin was judged to be of the highest quality while gluten or white flour was found to be the poorest. Intermediate quality proteins, however, could not be consistently differentiated by PER or NPR, or even ranked in the same order by the laboratories. RPV resulted in consistent ranking of proteins, but frequently could not distinguish between their qualities with an acceptable degree of statistical significance. Only RPV resulted in a significant reduction in the laboratory-to-laboratory variability inherent in the other methods, presumably by reducing or eliminating the effects of different strains of animals, different environmental conditions, etc., by expressing the protein quality relative to an internal standard, lactalbumin (Table 4.1). The laboratory X protein interaction, however, remained significant. It is of interest to note that this kind of correction is relatively more successful than a similar correction of PER values to a common PER for casein of 2.50 (Samonds and Hegsted, 1976). This is probably due to the inherent variation

TABLE 4.1

ANALYSES OF VARIANCE OF PER, NPR AND RPV FROM THE COLLABORATIVE ASSAY

Source	df	Sum of Squares	Mean Square	F
Protein Efficiency Ratio (PER)				
Laboratories	6	6.5936	1.09893[1]	6.666[3]
Proteins	6	68.0700	11.34500[1]	68.816[3]
Laboratory × protein interaction	36	5.9350	0.16486[2]	9.753[3]
Total	48	80.5986		
Method variance	474		0.01690	
Net Protein Ratio (NPR)				
Laboratories	6	3.4132	0.56886[2]	5.5499[3]
Proteins	6	40.2953	6.71588[2]	65.5208[3]
Laboratory × protein interaction	36	3.6900	0.10250[3]	7.4116[3]
Total	48			
Method variance	474		0.01383	
Relative Protein Value (RPV)				
Laboratories	6	0.05786	0.009643[2]	2.3276 (N.S.)
Proteins	5	2.25580	0.451160[2]	108.8970[3]
Laboratory × protein interaction	30	0.12429	0.004143[3]	2.1020[3]
Total	41	2.43795		
Method variance	727		0.00197	

Source: Samonds and Hegsted, 1976.
[1] Tested versus the laboratory × protein interaction in the F test.
[2] Tested versus the method variance in the F test.
[3] $P < 0.001$

in the PER method caused by changes in food intake, which was discussed earlier, and to the lack of reliability or consistency evident in the PER estimates for casein in these laboratories. This study has led to the recommendation that a first-action collaborative study be carried out according to the protocols of the Association of Official Analytical Chemists in order to replace the currently accepted PER method by a multiple-dose, slope estimate method.

When proteins are compared in this manner, some rather striking differences in quality are found when the new estimates are compared to commonly assumed qualities. Wheat gluten, which in textbooks is presented as having a quality of roughly 40% that of egg or lactalbumin, has a RPV of only 23%. As indicated earlier, such differences in quality estimates would almost double the estimated protein requirement.

DISCUSSION

It should be emphasized that RPV measures the ability of a protein to support growth. Because of the ability of the animal to conserve lysine, and other amino acids to some extent when the supply is limited, a protein may

TABLE 4.2

THE COMPARISON OF THE RELATIVE QUALITIES (RELATIVE PROTEIN VALUE)
OF THREE PROTEINS FOR THE GROWTH OF YOUNG RATS AND YOUNG
CEBUS MONKEYS

	Quality, Relative to Lactalbumin (%)	
Protein	Rats	Cebus Monkeys
Soy	56.7 (8.5)[1]	43.1 (4.3)
Wheat gluten	27.8 (1.9)	15.5 (2.4)
Wheat gluten + lysine	56.8 (3.6)	51.5 (3.6)

[1] Numbers in parentheses represent standard errors.

have widely divergent qualities depending upon whether it is to be used
for the synthesis of new tissue in the infant or to meet maintenance needs
of an adult. This difference in quality has been demonstrated in young
(Hegsted and Chang 1965) and adult (Said and Hegsted 1969) rats and in
infant (Samonds and Hegsted 1973) and adult (unpublished data) cebus
monkeys. These data also give us some idea about the ability to extrapolate
from rat-assessed protein requirements to species farther up the evolutionary ladder. In young monkeys, gluten has a RPV relative to lactalbumin
of only 16%, while lactalbumin itself has an efficiency of utilization of approximately 70% compared to the almost 100% efficiency of this protein
in young rats. Identical samples of soy protein and gluten supplemented
with lysine (supplying 6% of the total nitrogen) demonstrated relatively
poorer quality for the support of growth when fed to monkeys than when
fed to rats (Table 4.2). In the adult monkey, however, wheat protein supplied as a mixture of gluten and bread was able to meet maintenance needs
when fed at only 1.7 times the lactalbumin requirement, for a relative
quality of approximately 60%—very close to the estimate of 54% derived
from adult rats.

The role of amino acid conservation in human nutrition and its implications upon the estimates of amino acid requirements is worthy of consideration. As emphasized by the Food and Agriculture Organization/World
Health Organization report on "Energy and Protein Requirements" (WHO
1973), estimates of amino acid needs are limited to infants and adults except
for the studies of Nakagawa et al. (1960, 1961A, 1961B, 1962, 1965) on 10–12
yr old school children. The amino acid requirements of the infant are high,
both in terms of body weight or per unit of protein, with a daily requirement
on the order of 2 gm per kg per day with 35–40% of the nitrogen supplied
as essential amino acids. From infancy to adulthood the total nitrogen requirement per kg falls to about 1/4, while the total essential amino acid

requirement appears to fall to about 10%. The most rational explanation of this would appear to be the differences in the amino acid requirements for maintenance and growth. However, if this were true and if the requirements were cumulative, one would expect the 10–12 yr olds to have requirements more similar to adults than to infants since their growth rate is small relative to their maintenance needs. The data of Nakagawa *et al.*, however, indicate that the amino acid requirements of these children are more similar to infants than to adults. One may, of course, speculate about the accuracy of the estimates of amino acid requirements which are generally quite variable. Also, the criteria upon which the requirements are based differ among investigators.

Another explanation is possible, however. The amino acid requirements of adults are, by necessity, measured at low intakes in which case the adaptive response to conserve the amino acid would presumably be fully operative. On the contrary, if children are to be allowed to grow, the amino acid intake must be above the maintenance requirement and probably the adaptive response cannot be called into play. Thus, the protein needs of children might better be approximated by the needs of infants even though children are growing substantially slower. If this is true, then the theoretical estimate of needs arrived at by the summation of maintenance needs (estimated from adults) and the amount of an amino acid needed to form new tissue (Hegsted 1957; WHO 1973) would certainly be too low.

We conclude that the technical problems associated with the assessment of protein quality in young rats have been examined and that a reasonably satisfactory and practical assay method is now available. The major feature of this assay is the comparison of the slope of the dose-response line of a test protein with that of a high quality standard protein over the range of intakes within which the dose-response relationships are essentially linear. The rat assay is probably a severe test of protein quality, and there is every reason to believe that proteins which are of high quality by this test will also be of maximal quality for man, although the relative efficiency of utilization may be lower in man. Previous methods such as BV and NPR tend to overestimate the quality of poor quality proteins, resulting in an underestimate of the needs for these proteins for growth. Even RPV tends to overestimate the quality of proteins when compared to similarly assessed qualities in young monkeys. On the other hand such data as are available on the amino acid requirements and BV of proteins in adult animals, including man, indicate that protein quality is probably of less significance in adults than in growing animals, and that the rat assay may well underestimate the quality of many dietary proteins for adult man. How well these estimates apply to human infants and slow-growing children is unknown. The development of appropriate animal assays for these conditions is a matter for the future.

SUMMARY

The commonly used animal assay procedures—PER and NPR—as well as other methods based upon similar assumptions, fail to meet several of the basic criteria for a suitable assay. They are dose-dependent, of limited statistical validity (being either one- or two-point assays), and are not reproducible in different laboratories. BV and NPR tend to overestimate the qualities of poor quality proteins resulting in an underestimate of the needs of these proteins. A suitable alternative method has been proposed which compares the slope of a test protein to that of a high quality standard protein over ranges of intake within which the dose-response relationships are relatively linear. The resulting quality estimate reflects a protein's ability to support growth only, and may well underestimate the quality of many dietary proteins for maintenance of adults. How well these estimates reflect human needs awaits the evaluation of the utilities of a variety of proteins in human subjects.

BIBLIOGRAPHY

FINNEY, D. J.   1964.   Statistical Method in Biological Assay.   Hafner Publishing Co., New York.

HEGSTED, D. M.   1957.   Theoretical estimates of the protein requirements of children.   J. Am. Dietet. Assoc. *33*, 225.

HEGSTED, D. M., and CHANG, Y.   1965.   Protein utilization in growing rats at different levels of intake.   J. Nutr. *87*, 19.

HEGSTED, D. M., NEFF, R., and WORCESTER, J.   1968.   Determination of the relative nutritive value of proteins.   Factors affecting precision and validity.   J. Ag. Food Chem. *16*, 190.

NAKAGAWA, I., TAKAHASHI, T., and SUZUKI, T.   1960.   Amino acid requirements of children.   J. Nutr. *71*, 176.

NAKAGAWA, I., TAKAHASHI, T., and SUZUKI, T.   1961A.   Amino acid requirements of children: Isoleucine and leucine.   J. Nutr. *73*, 186.

NAKAGAWA, I., TAKAHASHI, T., and SUZUKI, T.   1961B.   Amino acid requirements of children: Minimal needs of lysine and methionine based on nitrogen balance method.   J. Nutr. *74*, 401.

NAKAGAWA, I., TAKAHASHI, T., SUZUKI, T., and KOBAYASHI, K.   1962.   Amino acid requirements of children: Minimal needs of threonine, valine, and phenylalanine based on nitrogen balance method.   J. Nutr. *77*, 61.

NAKAGAWA, I., TAKAHASHI, T., SUZUKI, T., and KOBAYASHI, K.   1965.   Amino acid requirements of children: Quantitative amino acid requirements of girls based on nitrogen balance method.   J. Nutr. *86*, 333.

SAID, A. K., and HEGSTED, D. M.   1969.   Evaluation of protein quality in adult rats.   J. Nutr. *99*, 474.

SAID, A. K., and HEGSTED, D. M.   1970.   Response of adult rats to low dietary levels of essential amino acids.   J. Nutr. *100*, 1363.

SAID, A. K., HEGSTED, D. M., and HAYES, K. C.   1974.   Response of adult rats to deficiencies of different essential amino acids.   Brit. J. Nutr. *31*, 47.

SAMONDS, K. W., and HEGSTED, D. M.   1973.   Protein requirements of young cebus monkeys (*Cebus albifrons* and *appella*).   Am. J. Clin. Nutr. *26*, 30.

SAMONDS, K. W., and HEGSTED, D. M.   1976.   A collaborative study to evaluate four methods of estimating protein quality: Protein efficiency ratio, net protein ratio, protein value and relative protein value.   *In* Evaluation of Protein Foods (revision of Publ. *1100*), National Academy of Sciences, Washington, D.C.

WHO. 1973. Energy and Protein Requirements. World Health Organization Tech. Rept. Ser. *522*, Geneva.

YAMASHITA, K., and ASHIDA, K. 1969. Lysine metabolism in rats fed lysine-free diets. J. Nutr. *99*, 267.

YAMASHITA, K., and ASHIDA, K. 1971. Effect of excessive levels of lysine and threonine on the metabolism of these amino acids in rats. J. Nutr. *101*, 1607.

CHAPTER 5

R. Bressani

Human Assays and Applications

A primary function of dietary protein is to supply the organism with a mixture of amino acids in an adequate balance for the synthesis and maintenance of tissue proteins. Since the role of dietary protein is to provide the organism with sufficient amounts of the essential amino acids and nitrogen, the quality of the protein depends on how closely it can supply these amino acids in accordance with the specific needs of the organism. The specific needs for these essential amino acids may change according to age and physiological function, implying, therefore, that the quality of the protein is dependent upon such different physiological states. The relative adequacy of a protein to supply the amino acid pattern required by a given organism and its physiological condition is the determining factor of the magnitude of the observed biological responses. Therefore, from the practical point of view, all methods used for evaluating the nutritive quality of proteins are directly or indirectly related to the relative efficiency of the different proteins in satisfying the essential amino acid requirements of the test organism.

In general, all methods commonly used to evaluate the nutritive quality of proteins measure the biological response obtained under controlled experimental conditions. The efficiency and usefulness of any method depend critically on the complete control of the experimental conditions so that the dietary protein becomes the only limiting factor responsible for the response obtained.

It is important to point out that the biological value and the nutritive value of dietary protein are not to be taken as synonyms. The first concept evaluates exclusively, at a specific intake level of protein, the amount and balance of essential amino acids available to the organism to satisfy the requirements for its particular physiological state. The second concept, on the other hand, may be defined as the effectiveness of a protein in terms of both protein quality (biological value) and quantity, together with other nutrients, in inducing an adequate nutritional status.

The objective of this work is to discuss, in a summarized way, the several methods commonly used to evaluate the efficiency of utilization or the biological value of proteins, to comment on the factors affecting the results obtained, and to present some practical applications.

TABLE 5.1

INTAKE OF ESSENTIAL AMINO ACIDS FROM A QUANTITY OF CORN PROTEIN
CALCULATED TO SATISFY ADULT AMINO ACID REQUIREMENTS

	Amino Acids		Daily Intake of Corn Protein to Satisfy Amino Acid Requirement (gm/kg Body wt)	Amino Acids in a Daily Protein Intake of 0.59 gm Corn Protein/kg Body Weight (mg/kg Body wt)
	In 0.55 gm of Ideal Protein[1] (mg)	In Corn Protein (mg/gm Protein)		
Isoleucine	9.9	37.0	0.27	21.8
Leucine	13.8	125.0	0.11	73.7
Lysine	12.1	27.0	0.45	15.9
T.S.A.A.[2]	13.2	35.0	0.38	20.6
T.A.A.A.[3]	13.8	87.0	0.16	51.3
Threonine	7.2	36.0	0.20	21.2
Tryptophan	3.6	6.1	0.59	3.6
Valine	9.9	48.0	0.21	28.3

[1] According to FAO/WHO (1973).
[2] Total sulfur-containing amino acids (methionine + cysteine + cystine).
[3] Total aromatic amino acids (tyrosine + phenylalanine).

THE CONCEPT OF EFFICIENCY OF PROTEIN UTILIZATION

Most of the biological methods used to determine the quality of proteins specify the need to have protein as the only variable in relation to other dietary nutrients, and to reduce the protein content of the diet or the intake of protein to levels below those needed for optimum growth and performance by the test organism. The reason for the first condition is obvious since limitations of other nutrients in the diet will affect the utilization of the protein. The reason for the second condition lies in the attempt to induce a stress condition between the needs of the organism and the capacity of the protein to meet those needs. Evidence supporting this condition has been provided quite often (Allison 1955).

The above implies that only quantities of amino acids are important; however, the quality of the protein also depends on how closely the protein under study can supply the amino acid pattern needed by the organism. This characteristic has given rise to the concept of amino acid balance. Therefore, both conditions, the quantities and balance of the essential amino acids, determine the efficiency of protein utilization. Protein quality assays measure both conditions.

To clarify the concept of amino acid balance, and of efficiency of utilization of the amino acid pattern ingested, use will be made of a common calculation made to indicate that most proteins when consumed in ample amounts can meet amino acid needs. The example is shown in Table 5.1. In this table, the quantities of essential amino acids in 0.55 gm of ideal protein are listed (first column) which, according to FAO/WHO (1973), supposedly satisfy the adult amino acid requirement (when the intake level is 0.55 gm per kg body wt per day). In the next column, the essential amino acid content of corn, expressed as mg per gm of protein, is shown. From these two sets of figures, the intake of corn protein necessary to satisfy the amino acid requirements of adults was calculated and expressed as gm of protein per kg body wt per day, as shown in the third column. The calculation shows that 0.59 gm of corn protein (per kg body wt per day) are needed to meet the need of 3.6 mg of tryptophan (per kg body wt per day) which is the requirement figure for the adult. In the fourth column, calculations were made on the amounts (per kg body wt per day) of other amino acids supplied by 0.59 gm of corn protein (per kg body wt per day). The values in this column show that, with the exception of tryptophan, all of the essential amino acids are present in 0.59 gm of corn protein (per kg body wt per day) at levels up to six times the adult requirement. Since the quality of the protein is controlled by the amino acid present in the lowest amount (relative to requirements), those present in excess will be wasted. This results, therefore, in a low efficiency of utilization of the ingested amino acids present in the pattern shown.

Since in the example, 0.59 gm of corn protein per kg body wt per day meets the needs of all the essential amino acids, it has been suggested that, according to such calculations, the quality of corn proteins is high. This has led to the suggestion that the experimentally determined biological value of corn proteins for the adult is meaningless. The biological value of corn proteins, assayed in adult human subjects, is of the order of 52% (Bressani 1975B). The rationale of the above calculation is not difficult to follow and, in general, it can be accepted. However, as noted, it contradicts the numerical figures obtained from experimental work. Therefore, this contradiction raises a number of questions. Are the methods used for protein quality evaluation poor? Or are the requirements for amino acids underestimated? The answer to both questions is "no." Even though they need improvement, both the methods used and the requirement estimates reflect the best conditions or estimates according to the information available. The problems lie in the fact that allowances are not made in the mathematical calculations for the effects of amino acid excesses or imbalances on protein quality. Furthermore, the excessive use at the desk level of the results of the great number of biological methods available (NPU, ND_p Cal%, PER, etc.) has led to conclusions which eventually may have a negative impact on the population. At one time, protein was the subject of tremendous amounts of research all over the world. Now, the nutrient receiving the most attention is calories (energy). The real need is for attention to be focused on groups of foods with different protein quality and energy content (and

TABLE 5.2

"PROTEIN" LOSSES AT NITROGEN EQUILIBRIUM IN ADULTS FED COMMON AND OPAQUE-2 CORN PROTEINS[1]

	Common Corn (gm/Day)	Opaque-2 Corn (gm/Day)
Corn intake for nitrogen equilibrium	620.0	250.0
Protein intake	43.8	29.0
Apparent coefficient of digestibility	76.5	76.5
"Protein" absorbed	33.3	22.2
Biological value (%)	57.0	82.0
"Protein" retained	19.0	18.0
"Protein" lost in feces	10.5	6.8
"Protein" lost in urine	14.3	4.2

Source: From Kies *et al.* (1965); Clark *et al.* (1967); Truswell and Brock (1962); Young *et al.* (1971).
[1] Protein = protein equivalents as calculated from nitrogen balance data; i.e., "protein" = 6.25 × nitrogen absorbed, retained, lost in feces, or lost in urine.

a variety of other nutrients as well) which, when consumed together in a balanced diet, provide good nutrition.

The effect of amino acid balance on the efficiency of protein utilization can also be seen in the following example, shown in Table 5.2. In this case, corn is also used as the protein under discussion, providing in one case the normal protein associated with common corn and, in the second, the improved quality protein found in Opaque-2 corn.

The results from experimental work in humans have shown that nitrogen equilibrium is obtained with an intake of 250 gm of Opaque-2 corn or 620 gm common corn (Kies *et al.* 1965; Clark *et al.* 1967). With these intakes of grain, an adult therefore is not losing or gaining nitrogen. These figures, in terms of protein, are equivalent to intakes of 29.0 and 43.8 gm of protein from Opaque-2 and common corn, respectively. The "protein" ($N \times 6.25$) absorbed was then calculated by multiplying the ingested protein by the apparent protein digestibility. The biological values of the two corns have been obtained from human studies, being 82% for Opaque-2 and 46.5% for common corn (Bressani 1975; Young *et al.* 1971). Since biological value is defined as the amount of nitrogen retained from that which is absorbed, then the product of "protein" absorbed, times the biological value, gives the amount of "protein" retained. This calculation gives 18 gm of "protein" retained for Opaque-2 and 19 gm for common corn protein. It should be pointed out at this time that since the calculations are based at the nitrogen equilibrium point, the "protein" really is not retained; it rather represents the amount used for anabolic processes. From the protein intake figure and that used for anabolism, nitrogen equivalent to 11 gm of protein is not used in the case of Opaque-2 corn while nitrogen equivalent to 25 gm of protein is lost from common corn. These results indicate, therefore, that because of an improved essential amino acid balance in Opaque-2 corn over common corn, lower quantities of protein, and thus of grain, are needed to attain the same condition. Furthermore, the superior amino acid balance in Opaque-2 corn increases the efficiency of utilization which significantly reduces the amounts of wasted nitrogen. The amount of wasted nitrogen is greater in urine than in feces (Bressani 1974). Taken into consideration the relatively large increases in world population and the low availability of foods, it is of great importance to achieve the best amino acid balance possible to maximize efficiency of utilization of protein.

The FAO/WHO (1973) report indicates that a distinction has to be made between protein quality, depending mainly on its amino acid pattern, and the efficiency of utilization, which depends on both the quality and the quantity of protein in the diet and the completeness of the total diet in terms of all nutrients.

The concept of efficiency of utilization expressed in the present paper differs from that of the FAO/WHO in that the amino acid balance or pattern itself determines to a very high degree the extent of utilization independent of protein content. In the FAO/WHO description of the concept, consideration is not clearly given to the influence that excess amino acids, in relation to the limiting one, may have in the overall utilization of the protein. The fact is that a deficient protein may be properly supplemented with the limiting amino acids resulting in an increase in protein quality; however, the quality values obtained in most cases do not reach the values of the high quality proteins.

HUMAN ASSAYS OF PROTEIN QUALITY

The quality or efficiency of utilization of dietary protein and its nutritive value depend on three broad factors: the intake of protein, its breakdown in the gastrointestinal tract and the metabolic utilization of the digestion products. This process is represented in a simplified manner in Fig. 5.1. It is rather obvious that if the carrier of protein (i.e., the food) is not readily ingested, its amino acid pattern is of little value in terms of practical applications. The second factor, which has a more specific effect on protein quality (and one which deserves more attention), is the efficiency with which the protein molecule is broken down to simpler units at the gastrointestinal level, giving rise to a fraction called fecal nitrogen and one which is called the absorbed nitrogen. This implies that the nitrogen fraction which is absorbed may or may not have the same pattern of amino acids as that present in the nitrogen source ingested. Once the amino acids are absorbed, they are utilized through anabolic and catabolic enzymatic processes which give rise to the nitrogen in urine and a fraction of retained nitrogen which is used for growth, maintenance and production. The quality

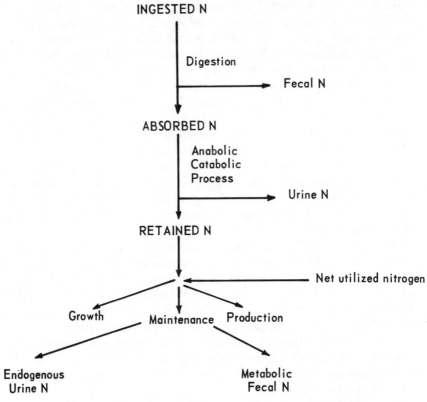

FIG. 5.1.   FOOD PROTEIN NITROGEN UTILIZATION SCHEME

or nutritive value of this retained protein depends almost entirely on the efficiency with which the amino acids (in the retained protein) are utilized for the metabolic processes previously mentioned (growth, maintenance and production). It should be pointed out at this time, that two other nitrogen fractions, the endogenous urinary nitrogen and the metabolic fecal nitrogen, play a role in the numerical calculation of some protein quality assay techniques.

Based on the scheme shown in Fig. 5.1, of the subjects to be discussed in the present paper, protein digestibility will be considered first.

Digestibility of Proteins

The first factor that affects the efficiency of utilization of dietary protein is the degree to which this protein can be hydrolized in the digestive tract. This aspect of utilization of protein is measured by determining the digestibility of the ingested protein. The digestibility of a protein is defined as the fraction of ingested nitrogen which is absorbed.

TABLE 5.3

APPARENT AND TRUE PROTEIN DIGESTIBILITY

$$(1) \quad A_D \ (\%) = \frac{Ni - Fn}{Ni} \times 100$$

$$(2) \quad T_D \ (\%) = \frac{Ni - (Fn - Mn)}{Ni} \times 100$$

A_D = Apparent protein digestibility
T_D = True protein digestibility
Ni = Nitrogen intake
Fn = Fecal nitrogen
Mn = Metabolic fecal nitrogen

Apparent digestibility can be calculated by the first formula shown in Table 5.3. Fecal nitrogen in the equation represents the total sum of nitrogen in fecal matter which includes the nitrogen from any food which is not hydrolyzed plus the nitrogen from the intestinal flora, the intestinal tissue, the digestive enzymes and possibly other sources. The sum of all these sources, with the exception of the nitrogen from any unhydrolyzed food, is called metabolic fecal nitrogen. Therefore, apparent protein digestibility is calculated from a figure for fecal nitrogen which has not been corrected for metabolic fecal nitrogen. When this correction is included in the formula (Allison 1955), the result is true protein digestibility which can be represented by the second equation shown in Table 5.3.

Fecal metabolic nitrogen has been estimated in experimental animals and in humans by feeding the experimental subjects a nitrogen-free diet for up to 16 days. This system, however, has been criticized because the absence of nitrogen from the digestive tract can modify the intestinal flora as well as other metabolic sources of fecal nitrogen. Therefore, some workers have proposed the use of proteins with a 100% digestibility so as to obtain a more representative value for metabolic nitrogen. Table 5.4 summarizes results on metabolic fecal nitrogen in human subjects of various ages. For adults, the values vary from 9 to 17 mg per kg body wt per day after 10–16 days on a nitrogen-free diet. In children, the values are higher, varying from 20–25 mg per kg body wt per day.

The percentage of digestibility of the protein is determined by feeding it to the experimental subject for several days in a known, low and constant amount. The length of protein feeding after metabolic adjustment is around 6–9 days. It is necessary to make quantitative fecal collections which are then analyzed for their nitrogen content. The same procedure is carried out with a nitrogen-free diet in order to measure metabolic nitrogen. To separate feces from the different periods, a marker such as carmine is used.

TABLE 5.4

ENDOGENOUS NITROGEN EXCRETION IN HUMAN SUBJECTS

Subjects	Endogenous Urinary Nitrogen (mg/kg Body wt/Day)	Metabolic Fecal Nitrogen (mg/kg Body wt/Day)
Adult	39	17
Adult	35	9
Adult	37	9
Adult	39	12
Adult	38	14
Adult	39	9
Adult	33	13
Adult	44	14
Children	57	24
Children	48	25
Infants	37	20

Source: Bressani et al. (1972B); Viteri and Bressani (1972); Calloway and Margen (1971); Scrimshaw et al. (1972); Murlin et al. (1946); Young and Scrimshaw (1968); Huang et al. (1972).

TABLE 5.5

RELATIONSHIP BETWEEN NITROGEN INTAKE AND APPARENT AND TRUE PROTEIN DIGESTIBILITY

Corn-Soybean-Cottonseed Protein Mixture			Milk Protein		
Nitrogen Intake (mg/kg Body wt/Day)	Digestibility Apparent (%)	True (%)	Nitrogen Intake (mg/kg Body wt/Day)	Digestibility Apparent (%)	True (%)
473	77.6	83.7	477	86.4	91.2
398	77.6	84.9	386	88.3	94.3
311	75.9	85.2	303	84.1	91.7
234	76.9	89.3	225	81.3	91.5
168	71.4	88.7	164	78.0	92.1
103	63.1	91.3	95	69.5	93.7

Source: Bressani et al. (1972B).

The true protein digestibility tends to increase with a decrease in protein intake, especially with proteins of vegetable origin, and values may be over 100% when protein intake is below 0.4 gm per kg body wt per day. Table 5.5 summarizes the apparent and true protein digestibility from metabolic studies with children fed decreasing levels of milk and a vegetable protein mixture based on corn, soybean and cottonseed (Bressani et al. 1972). The figures show increases in the true digestibility as the protein intake was decreased, for both protein sources. On the other hand, apparent digestibility decreased as protein intake decreased for both sources. This observation was attributed to the metabolic fecal nitrogen values which were increasingly higher, relative to the total fecal nitrogen, as the protein intake decreased.

The true protein digestibility of animal proteins is superior, at the same protein intake, to that of proteins of vegetable origin. For example, true protein digestibility values for egg and milk of 92.8 and 91.0%, respectively, at intakes of 432 and 473 mg per kg body wt per day, have been reported. For mixtures of three vegetable proteins at similar protein intakes (435–473 mg per kg body wt per day), the true protein digestibility varied from 77.4 to 84.6% (Bressani et al. 1972B). The reason for the lower digestibility of vegetable proteins has not been completely explained; possibly there are several factors involved. The fact in itself is important, but it becomes of even greater significance with the currently increasing use of vegetable proteins in foods for human feeding.

Nitrogen Balance

Definition.—The principle on which nutritional balance studies is based is no different from that in other sciences, since its purpose is to measure the net gain or loss occurring in the utilization of the several substances needed by the organism. A living organism consumes nitrogen in the food and eliminates it constantly; therefore, the determination of nitrogen in the food and excreta affords a quantitative measure of protein metabolism. Besides, it also indicates whether the organism is losing or gaining protein under the prevailing conditions at the time the measurements were taken.

As shown in Fig. 5.2, nitrogen balance can be defined as the quantity of nitrogen intake that has been retained in the body. In the formula, Nb stands for nitrogen balance, Ni for nitrogen intake, Fn for fecal nitrogen, and Un for urinary nitrogen.

The apparent nitrogen absorbed is equal to the difference between nitrogen intake and fecal nitrogen. The nitrogen absorbed minus the nitrogen in the urine gives nitrogen balance. According to this formula, nitrogen balance is positive when intake is higher than the sum of urinary and fecal nitrogen, and in this case there is a net body gain of nitrogen. All growing animals are, under normal conditions, in positive nitrogen balance. If nitrogen intake is equal to the sum of urinary and fecal nitrogen, nitrogen balance is zero, in which case the individual is in nitrogen equilibrium. Adult animals, under normal conditions, are in nitrogen equilibrium. If on the contrary, the sum of fecal and urinary nitrogen is higher than nitrogen intake, nitrogen balance is negative.

It is possible, however, to obtain a positive nitrogen balance when there is a simultaneous loss of nitrogen by some tissues. Allison (1955), for example, demonstrated that under stress conditions some tissues are main-

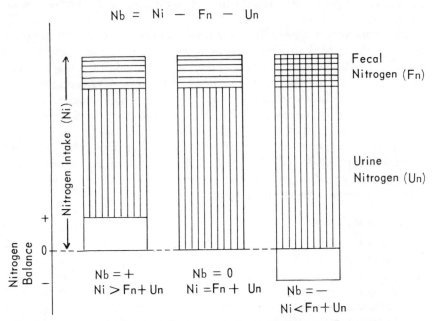

$$Nb = Ni - Fn - Un$$

FIG. 5.2.   SCHEMATIC REPRESENTATION OF NITROGEN BALANCE

(See text for definitions.)

tained at the expense of others and that in spite of this fact, it is possible to obtain a positive nitrogen balance. Similarly, maintaining nitrogen equilibrium does not mean that all tissues are in this state. Neither does the fact that nitrogen intake may be enough to maintain nitrogen equilibrium in an adult necessarily mean that all nitrogen requirements are being satisfied. Nitrogen equilibrium can be adjusted at different levels of intake through metabolic adaptations in such a way that it is possible to maintain an individual in a protein depletion state and still maintain nitrogen equilibrium.

In spite of the fact that for practical purposes, nitrogen balance is equal to nitrogen intake minus the sum of fecal and urinary nitrogen, some results obtained recently indicate that the original formula

$$Nb = Ni - (Fn + Un)$$

is not altogether correct. Several investigators (Calloway and Margen 1971; Young and Scrimshaw 1968; Huang *et al.* 1972; Sirbu *et al.* 1967) have demonstrated that besides fecal and urinary nitrogen, which represent the highest losses of nitrogen, there are other losses of this element that, under special situations, can have a practical significance. In human subjects, for

TABLE 5.6

EFFECT OF NITROGEN INTAKE (SKIM MILK) ON NITROGEN BALANCE
IN CHILDREN (MG N/KG BODY WT/DAY)

Nitrogen Intake	Fecal Nitrogen	Urinary Nitrogen	Nitrogen Absorbed	Nitrogen Retained
477	65	313	412	99
386	45	258	342	83
305	48	185	255	69
225	42	132	184	52
164	36	74	128	54
95	29	50	66	15

Source: Bressani *et al.* (1972B).

example, it has been demonstrated that significant amounts of nitrogen are eliminated in sweat. In long-term studies, losses of nitrogen from skin and hair can be also significant. In view of all these findings, it is considered that a better way to estimate nitrogen balance is to take into account all these losses, which could be called insensible nitrogen losses or Ns; in other words, the original formula would be modified thus:

$$Nb = Ni - (Fn + Un + Ns)$$

This modification, however, is necessary only when nitrogen requirements are being estimated. It is not required for establishing comparative measures of nitrogen balance between several proteins in treatments of short duration and under controlled experimental conditions, in which case an apparent nitrogen balance is adequate.

Factors Affecting Nitrogen Balance.—There are several factors affecting nitrogen balance. Table 5.6 shows the effect of decreasing nitrogen intake on nitrogen balance in children fed skim milk (Bressani *et al.* 1972B). Decreasing intake from 477 to 95 mg per kg body wt per day decreased nitrogen balance from 99 to 15 mg per kg body wt per day.

The values in the table also show that, upon decreasing nitrogen intake, urinary nitrogen losses have a greater influence on nitrogen balance than fecal nitrogen losses. These results imply that when various protein sources are to be compared, in terms of protein quality evaluated by the nitrogen balance method, it is necessary to compare them at a fixed level of protein intake.

As with other techniques of evaluating protein quality, applied either to experimental animals or to man, nitrogen balance is not capable of detecting small differences in quality, as suggested by essential amino acid content, when total nitrogen intake is high. An example is shown in Table 5.7. In this case, children were fed the same amount of various proteins at intakes of around 2.0 gm of protein per kg body wt per day, at equal intakes

EVALUATION OF PROTEINS FOR HUMANS

TABLE 5.7

NITROGEN BALANCE OF VARIOUS PROTEINS FED AT RELATIVELY
HIGH LEVELS OF INTAKE[1]

Protein	(mg/kg Body wt)				
	Ni	Fn	Un	Na	Nr
Skim milk	386	45	258	342	83
Egg	385	42	262	343	80
Corn/cottonseed flour mixture	398	89	216	309	93
Corn/cottonseed/soy mixture	388	110	201	277	77

Source: From Bressani et al. (1972B).
[1] Caloric intake: 90—100 kcal/kg body wt/day; Ni = nitrogen intake, Fn = fecal nitrogen, Un = urinary nitrogen, Na = nitrogen absorbed, and Nr = nitrogen retained.

of calories of 100 per kg body wt per day (Bressani et al. 1972B). In the examples shown, nitrogen balance was essentially the same for all proteins tested, whether of animal or vegetable origin (mixtures based on cottonseed, soybean, and corn flour, or on cottonseed and corn flour). The results also show that the ingestion of vegetable proteins resulted in higher amounts of fecal nitrogen, suggesting a lower digestibility than that for the animal proteins. What is of interest is that, of the nitrogen absorbed, similar amounts of retained nitrogen were obtained from all proteins, suggesting that the amino acid balance of this fraction from the vegetable protein mixtures was as good as that from the proteins of animal origin.

Therefore, when the nitrogen balance method is utilized to evaluate protein quality, not only is it essential to keep nitrogen intake constant but it is also necessary to carry out the tests at nitrogen intakes which will maximize the differences in quality. In animal testing, 10% protein diets are used since it was found that, at this level, quality differences become more evident. Little work has been done on this point in children; however, results of some relevant studies (Bressani et al. 1972B) are shown in Table 5.8. To determine the level of nitrogen intake at which significant differences in nitrogen balance can be obtained, the nitrogen balance values observed at intakes between 360 and 81 mg of nitrogen were grouped (as shown in the table) and evaluated statistically. The analysis indicated that highly significant differences in nitrogen balance values can be detected among different proteins in children at intakes between 156 and 251 mg of nitrogen per kg of body wt per day.

An example of the importance of calories on nitrogen balance is shown in Fig. 5.3 (Clark et al. 1960). The subject in this study received 1500 mg of lysine and 9 gm of nitrogen per day. There was no apparent difference in nitrogen retention as calories decreased from 4350 to 3550 kcal per day,

TABLE 5.8

AVERAGE NITROGEN BALANCE IN CHILDREN AT VARIOUS LEVELS OF
NITROGEN INTAKE

	Nitrogen Balance at Nitrogen Intake Range (mg/kg Body wt/Day)			
Protein Foods Tested	310–360	230–251	156–174	81–114
Milk	62	50	54	8
Cottonseed/corn mix	64	40	26	−4
Soybean/corn mix	86	65	38	0
CSF/SBF/corn mix	59	51	24	−5
Soybean tex. food	82	49	9	−10
Whole egg	80	80	49	—
F value	1.51	5.85[2]	11.06[2]	1.84
LSD (0.01)[1]	45	22	21	20
No. observations	31	31	32	22

Source: From Bressani et al. (1972B).
[1] Least significant difference.
[2] Highly significant.

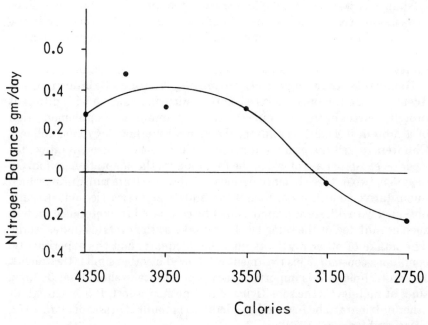

From Clark et al. (1960)

FIG. 5.3. EFFECT OF CALORIC INTAKE ON NITROGEN BALANCE AT CONSTANT NITRO-
GEN AND LYSINE INTAKE (HUMAN SUBJECTS)

TABLE 5.9

EFFECT OF CHANGES IN WATER INTAKE ON NITROGEN BALANCE
AT CONSTANT NITROGEN INTAKE

Water Intake (ml/Day)	Nitrogen Balance (mg/kg Body wt/Day)			
	Intake	Fecal	Urinary	Retained
400	692	41	374	277
1000	701	57	517	127
400	703	51	443	204
1000	665	28	450	187
400	668	36	388	244
1000	673	42	464	167

Source: Bressani and Braham (1964); dogs were used as the experimental animal.

but further restriction caused a downward trend, reaching a negative balance when the subject received 2750 kcal per day.

The effect of changes in water intake on nitrogen balance is shown in Table 5.9. The results of these studies demonstrate that quite independent from the nitrogen intake, low water intake results in lower nitrogen retention figures. It could very well be that the excess in water intake has a flushing effect on the catabolic nitrogen from protein metabolism, since it was found that, with high intakes of water, most of the nitrogen in the urine was in the form of ammonia rather than urea. In any case, results indicate that when using nitrogen balance as a protein evaluation method, intake of water must be kept constant (Bressani and Braham 1964).

General Methodology for Determining Nitrogen Balance in Children.—When the purpose is to compare nitrogen balance with different protein sources or to determine the effect of amino acid supplementation of a protein in healthy children, the general methodology is as follows. Children are fed the protein under study at a constant level of intake for a period of 10–13 days of which the first four are the adaptation period. On days 6–9, two or three balance periods of 3 days each are run, during which quantitative collections of food, feces and urine are carried out. Results obtained with different proteins must be compared to a reference protein such as milk fed at the same levels of intake as the proteins under study. The intake of other nutrients must be adequate, and the experimental conditions constant. This treatment is followed by other similar treatments. In this technique it is important that protein intake should not be high, since at high levels the sensitivity of the method is lost. It is essential for other nutrients to be ingested in adequate amounts (Bressani et al. 1972; Viteri and Bressani 1972).

General Methodology for Determining Nitrogen Balance in Adults.—The application of the nitrogen balance method in young adults must include a period of protein depletion to sensitize the subject to the protein under study. The method generally used is the following. The subjects are depleted for a day by feeding a nitrogen-free diet which helps in adapting the individual more rapidly to the protein intake. The second period, that of adaptation, consists in feeding the subject for 5 days the protein under study at an intake level that will compensate the losses in feces and urine. The adaptation period is followed by two consecutive periods of 5 days each, at the same level of intake, for quantitative collection of feces and urine. Again, results must be compared with those obtained with a reference protein fed at the same intake levels of protein and calories. The reference protein in this case is whole egg protein (Kies *et al.* 1965; Clark *et al.* 1967; Young *et al.* 1971; Scrimshaw *et al.* 1972; Young and Scrimshaw 1968).

Applications.—Using the technique described in a general way in the previous section, the nitrogen balance method has been extremely useful in studying problems related to protein metabolism in at least two major areas, namely, in the evaluation of protein quality and in determining protein and amino acid requirements.

In the area of evaluating protein quality, the application of the method under well-controlled and standardized conditions has been very useful in classifying food proteins according to their nutritive value.

With respect to the use of nitrogen balance as a method to study the effect of amino acid supplementation, some relevant results are presented in Table 5.10 (Bressani 1971). In this example, children were fed wheat flour alone or supplemented with the amino acids shown. Each dietary treatment lasted 13 days, of which the first 4 days were used as an adaptation period and the other 9 days as balance periods (nine periods, each of 3 days duration). Examination of the nitrogen retention values, obtained at a relatively constant level of nitrogen intake, shows a definite response to the addition of only lysine. There was also a further improvement (in addition to that obtained with lysine supplementation alone) in wheat flour protein quality when it was supplemented with lysine plus tryptophan or lysine plus tryptophan and methionine. The effect of tryptophan, however, is questionable.

These results, as well as others using corn, rice, and oats, have confirmed results with experimental animals. The sensitivity of children was such that it was possible to detect effects of amino acid imbalances and interrelationships between amino acids (Bressani 1971).

The supplementary effect of proteins can also be detected by means of nitrogen balance. An example is shown in Table 5.11 for young adults fed rice and rice supplemented with chicken meat (Lee *et al.* 1971). Nitrogen retention on rice was 0.18 gm per day on an intake of 6.31 gm. Replacement of 15% of this intake by chicken meat nitrogen caused an increase in ni-

TABLE 5.10

AMINO ACID SUPPLEMENTATION OF WHEAT FLOUR[1]

	Nitrogen Balance (mg/kg Body wt/Day)				
Diet	*Ni*	*Fn*	*Un*	*Na*	*Nr*
Milk	307	61	172	246	74
Basal (B)	326	47	252	279	27
B + Lysine	335	47	228	288	60
B + Lysine + Tryptophan	330	41	222	289	67

B + Lysine
  + Tryptophan
  + Methionine
	337	38	225	299	74

B + Lysine
  + Tryptophan
  + Methionine
  + Threonine
	338	37	223	301	78

B + Lysine
  + Tryptophan
  + Methionine
  + Threonine
  + Isoleucine
  + Valine
	336	49	204	281	83

Source: Summary of results from Bressani (1971); see Table 5.7 for definitions of abbreviations used.
[1] Amino acids added, as indicated, to give (per gm nitrogen in the diet) 270 mg lysine, 90 mg tryptophan, 270 mg methionine, 270 mg isoleucine, 270 mg valine, and 180 mg threonine.

TABLE 5.11

SUPPLEMENTARY EFFECT OF CHICKEN MEAT TO RICE

	Nitrogen Balance (gm/Day)			
Diet	Intake	Urine	Feces	Retained
100% Rice	6.31	4.82	1.32	0.18
85% Rice, 15% Chicken	6.31	4.79	1.15	0.39
70% Rice, 30% Chicken	6.31	4.88	1.14	0.30

Source: Lee *et al.* (1971).

trogen balance to 0.39 gm per day. The results were not statistically significant because intake of protein was higher than needed for sufficient sensitivity; however, even at this level of protein intake, some increased response was observed.

A further application is the use of the method to distinguish between the nutritive value of proteins. An example is shown in Table 5.12. In this case a high-protein rice and common rice were each fed at an equal intake of 480

TABLE 5.12

NUTRITIVE VALUE OF THE PROTEIN OF RICE

	High-Protein Rice		Common Rice
Intake, gm/day	480	480	480
Total N intake, gm/day	12.06	6.72	12.06[1]
Nitrogen balance, gm/day	1.41	0.24	0.48
Lysine in rice, mg/gm N	193	235	235
Threonine, mg/gm N	262	278	278
Total S amino acids, mg/gm N	222	362	362

Source: Clark et al. (1971).
[1] Nonprotein nitrogen added (consisting of glycine, glutamic acid, and diammonium citrate).

TABLE 5.13

NUTRITIVE VALUE OF THE PROTEIN IN FOUR DIETS BASED ON WHEAT BREAD

	Diet Intake (gm/Day)			
Wheat bread	492	393	393	393
Pinto beans	—	108.6	—	—
Rice	—	—	273	—
Peanut butter	—	—	—	26.1
N balance, gm/day	1.07	1.20	1.22	1.23
Lysine in diet, gm/day	1.87	2.32	1.89	1.87

Source: Edwards et al. (1971).

gm of grain per person per day. Because of differences in protein content between the two types of rice, intakes of nitrogen were 12.06 and 6.72 gm per day (high-protein and common rice, respectively). In order to remove the nitrogen intake variability, the common rice was supplemented with nonprotein nitrogen to give an intake of 12.06 gm per day. The nitrogen balance results show higher nitrogen retention values for the high-protein rice over the common rice with or without nonprotein nitrogen supplementation. The authors explained these results on the basis of a higher intake of essential amino acids from the high-protein rice than from common rice (Clark et al. 1971). It should be indicated that if protein quality differences were intended to be shown, the high-protein rice should have been fed at an intake equal to that of common rice, that is at a nitrogen intake of 6.72 gm. ·

A final example is the use of nitrogen balance to assess the quality of diets. An example is shown in Table 5.13 for young adult students consuming diets based on wheat; the ingredient compositions of the diets are also partially indicated in the table (Edwards et al. 1971). The nitrogen balance results show that from the wheat diet a nitrogen retention of 1.07 gm per day was obtained, which increased slightly when the diet contained beans, rice or peanut butter to values of 1.20, 1.22, and 1.23 gm per day, respectively. Protein intake was 46 gm per day, of which wheat provided 35 gm and other foods 11 gm. When either beans, rice or peanut butter was used to replace 20% of the protein supplied by wheat, the nitrogen balances obtained were no different than that from wheat alone. Actually, on the basis of amino acid content, an improvement should have been obtained from the wheat and bean diet, since bean protein is a rich source of lysine while wheat protein is deficient in this amino acid. The conclusion was reached that no supplementary effect was observed, which is true due to the fact that the study was carried out at relatively high protein intakes, reducing therefore, the sensitivity of the method. In this case, the nitrogen balance method was used to determine the nutritive value of the protein at the levels fed, but not its quality *per se.*

Other useful applications include the interrelationships between several nutrients and protein metabolism. In the area of establishing protein requirements for physiological purposes, the nitrogen balance method has been indeed useful. For this purpose, it has been necessary to determine not only the usual losses of nitrogen in the feces and urine, but also other losses such as through sweat, breathing and intestinal gas (Young *et al.* 1971; Calloway and Margen 1971; Scrimshaw *et al.* 1972; Young and Scrimshaw 1968; Inoue *et al.* 1973; Inoue *et al.* 1974).

Finally, the introduction of several modifications to the described method of nitrogen balance has permitted the development of other approaches for determining protein quality, such as the biological value and nitrogen balance index methods.

Biological Value

The information derived from nitrogen balance studies has been used for over 60 yr in the calculation of the biological value of proteins (Thomas 1909). Biological value is defined as the percentage of absorbed nitrogen which is retained by the organism. This value can be expressed mathematically as shown in Table 5.14. The method has been extensively studied, modified and applied to the study of the biological value of many proteins (Mitchell 1923–1924; Mitchell 1924). By using the method, estimates are obtained, not only of the biological value, but also of the true digestibility of the protein.

For the determination of biological value, it is necessary to take into account the contribution of endogenous fecal and urinary nitrogen to total fecal and urinary nitrogen excretion. Therefore, in the equation in Table 5.14, Ni is equal to nitrogen intake, Fn to fecal nitrogen, Mn to metabolic fecal nitrogen, Un to urinary nitrogen and En to endogenous urinary ni-

TABLE 5.14

BIOLOGICAL VALUE

$$BV = \frac{Ni - (Fn - Mn) - (Un - En)}{Ni - (Fn - Mn)} \times 100$$

$NPU = BV (\% D)$

Ni = N intake
Mn = Metabolic fecal nitrogen
Un = Urinary nitrogen
En = Endogenous urinary nitrogen
Fn = Fecal nitrogen
NPU = Net Protein Utilization
D = Protein digestibility

trogen. In theory, all the figures in the equation should be measured at the same time and in each study. Nevertheless this is not possible in practice, and the endogenous fractions of nitrogen metabolism are measured in separate trials where the animals (or subjects) are fed a nitrogen-free diet. In any case, the calorie intake as well as the intake of other nutrients must be kept constant during the feeding of the nitrogen-free diet as well as in the periods where the proteins under study are being evaluated. The nitrogen intake must be low but yet high enough to permit growth, if the experimental animals used are young, or nitrogen equilibrium, if adult animals are used.

Several investigators have studied the factors affecting the values obtained in studies conducted to estimate the biological value. One of these factors is the protein concentration in the diet or the protein intake. Representative results from metabolic studies in children fed various kinds of proteins are shown in Fig. 5.4. The results show an inverse relationship between protein intake and biological value.

The biological value of these proteins is dependent on protein intake; however, the quantitative relations among proteins depend on the protein level at which comparisons are made (Bressani et al. 1972).

In recent reports, the biological value of wheat gluten and egg in relation to protein intake was studied in young men (Inoue et al. 1974; Young et al. 1973). The results are shown in Table 5.15. In the studies with wheat gluten, it was found that there was not a rectilinear relationship between nitrogen absorbed and nitrogen balance at intakes of wheat gluten protein below 0.29 gm per kg body wt per day. Actually the relationship was curvilinear. Therefore, in order to express the inverse relationship between protein intake and biological value, it was expressed as a fractional equation. In any case, as with children, the biological value of wheat gluten protein decreased as protein intake increased.

Age as a variable affecting biological value has not been studied with human subjects. It is assumed on the basis of amino acid requirements that,

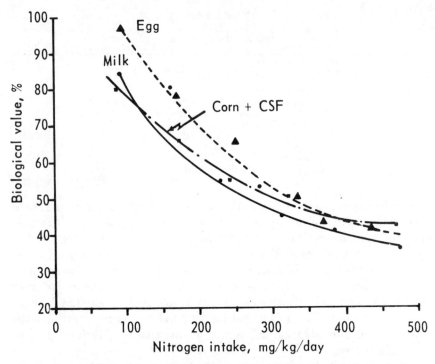

FIG. 5.4.   EFFECT OF PROTEIN INTAKE ON BIOLOGICAL VALUE (CHILDREN)

TABLE 5.15

BIOLOGICAL VALUES OBTAINED IN STUDIES WITH YOUNG MEN GIVEN VARIOUS
LEVELS OF EGG AND WHEAT GLUTEN

| Protein Level | Biological Value | |
(g/kg Body wt/Day)	Wheat Gluten[1]	Egg Protein[2]
0.1	106 ± 2	—
0.2	85 ± 9	103 ± 19
0.3	—	89 ± 14
0.4	45 ± 3	61 ± 18
0.5	—	71 ± 13
0.6	37 ± 1	—
1.0	24 ± 2	—

[1] From Inoue *et al.* (1974).
[2] From Young *et al.* (1973).

for a given protein, its biological value for adults is higher than for growing children. Limited results with experimental animals suggest this to be the case (Forbes *et al.* 1958; Henry and Kon 1957).

However, a brief compilation of biological value figures, as shown in Table

TABLE 5.16

EFFECT OF AGE ON BIOLOGICAL VALUE OF PROTEINS

Protein	Subject	Protein Intake (gm/kg Body wt/Day)	Biological Value (%)	Reference
Milk	Children	0.6	84	Bressani and Viteri (1971)
Milk	Adult	0.4	74	Bricker et al. (1945)
Egg	Children	0.6	97	Bressani and Viteri (1971)
Egg	Adult	0.3	89–96	Young et al. (1969)
Egg	Adult	0.2	94	Hawley et al. (1948)
Opaque-2 corn	Children	0.6	87	Bressani et al. (1969)
Opaque-2 corn	Adult	0.3	80	Young et al. (1971)
Common corn	Children	2.2	32	Bressani (1972)
Common corn	Adult	—	57	Truswell and Brock (1962)
Common corn	Adult	0.6	46	Kies et al. (1965)

5.16, suggests that there is not a clear tendency in regard to age. In general, the figures tend to be similar, particularly for the better quality proteins (Kies et al. 1965; Young et al. 1971; Bressani et al. 1969; Bressani 1973; Truswell and Brock 1962; Bricker et al. 1945; Hawley et al. 1948). The difference between laboratory findings and expected figures may be due to an unsatisfactory application of the method in children; likewise, it could be due to the possibility that the proportionality pattern of essential amino acids is similar for both children and adults, even though present proposed requirements do not indicate this to be true (FAO/WHO 1973). Finally on the basis of endogenous nitrogen excretion values and with the same intake levels of protein, the biological value of a protein should be higher in children than in adults. Therefore, more information regarding this point should be obtained.

Another factor which affects the biological value of proteins is caloric intake. This effect is to be expected since, as indicated previously, energy intake influences nitrogen metabolism. Recent studies (Inoue et al. 1973) have suggested that the NPU values of egg and rice proteins were 44 and 33, respectively, with an energy intake fixed at the maintenance level. On the other hand, the NPU values were 63 and 50 for egg and rice proteins, respectively, with an excess energy intake. It is reasonable to indicate that, from various points of view, the values obtained with intake of energy at the maintenance level are more realistic.

There are other factors that can also interfere with the determination of the biological value of proteins. Among these, perhaps the most important is the state of protein depletion of the animal organism; the more depleted the organism, the higher the biological value obtained. Therefore, when the biological values of several proteins are to be determined or compared, it is essential to standardize the method as much as possible.

General Technique for Determining Biological Value.—Few investigators in recent times have used the biological value technique for determining protein quality. During the last few years, however, some authors have been using it in studies with adult humans as subjects (Young *et al.* 1971; Inoue *et al.* 1973; Inoue *et al.* 1974; Young *et al.* 1973). In these studies, the authors have used the following sequence of diets with good results. The experimental subjects are fed a protein-free diet for 3 days; this propitiates a rapid adaptation to a reduced protein intake. After the nitrogen-free diet period, subjects are fed the protein under study for a 10-day period, of which the first 5 days are considered as the adaptation period and the other 5 days as the balance period. This treatment is followed by another 10-day period with another protein or with the reference protein which, in most cases, is whole egg protein. During the protein feeding period, its intake is generally set at 0.3–0.4 gm per kg body wt per day for the higher quality proteins with an adequate caloric intake for each subject. For poorer quality proteins, the intake is higher. In any case, however, the protein intake should be close to the point of nitrogen equilibrium. The standardization of the individuals in terms of degree of protein depletion is of importance as well.

Applications.—The principal application of the method is obviously in obtaining the true value of the efficiency of utilization of a given protein. Since in obtaining a figure for biological value, it is necessary to determine the digestibility of the protein, the two figures can be used to calculate other parameters of protein quality and the economic effectiveness of one protein over another. Even though this last exercise can be performed with other measures of protein quality, it is easier to do and to understand by using biological value figures. An example is shown in Table 5.17.

This information was obtained from the results of trials carried out with human adults fed normal and Opaque-2 corn (Kies *et al.* 1965; Clark *et al.* 1967). The same can be demonstrated with other foods or food mixtures. It has been found that an individual can cover his protein requirements by consuming 547 gm of normal corn, in comparison to only 250 gm of Opaque-2 corn; the difference shows the efficiency of one type of corn over the other. Speaking of land and production, one hectare of common corn yields enough corn protein to feed 5484 individuals, while one hectare of Opaque-2 corn yields enough corn protein to feed 10,800 individuals. The efficiency, however, does not end there. Applying experimental figures of protein utilization, in the example, it was calculated that 23 out of the 44 gm of protein ingested from common corn were lost by lack of utilization, while only 5 gm of the same protein were lost when Opaque-2 corn was consumed on the basis of an intake of 28 gm. When these data are converted

TABLE 5.17

EFFICIENCY OF LAND UTILIZATION THROUGH THE CULTIVATION OF
HIGH-LYSINE CORN FOR HUMAN NUTRITION

	Normal	Opaque-2
Intake of corn needed for nitrogen equilibrium (gm/day)	547	250
Corn yield (kg/ha)[1]	3000	2700
No. of individuals in nitrogen equilibrium from 1 ha of corn	5484	10800
Protein intake (gm/day)	44	28
Biological value of corn (%)	46.5	82
Protein retained (gm)	21	23
Protein loss (feces + urine) (gm)	23	5
Amount of corn equivalent to protein loss (gm)	255	55
Total amount of corn × No. of individuals (kg)	1398	594
Ha of land	0.47	0.22
Nutritional production (efficiency of land) (%)	53	78

Source: Kies *et al.* (1965); Clark *et al.* (1967).
[1] One hectare (ha) = 2.47 acres.

into cultivated land, it is found that when common corn is grown, 53% of the hectare is efficiently utilized, while 78% is utilized when Opaque-2 corn is cultivated.

Various groups (Calloway and Margen 1971; Murlin *et al.* 1946; Huang *et al.* 1972; Inoue *et al.* 1973; Inoue *et al.* 1974; Young *et al.* 1973; Bricker *et al.* 1945; Hawley *et al.* 1948) have used biological value figures as a means to estimate minimum protein requirements.

Nitrogen Balance Index

Allison (1955), using adult dogs as experimental animals under adequate conditions, found that a straight line relationship could be demonstrated between absorbed nitrogen (Na) and nitrogen balance (Nb). The relationship between nitrogen absorbed and nitrogen retained is linear in the region of negative nitrogen balance; this linearity extends somewhat to the positive side and then becomes frankly curvilinear in the region of high positive nitrogen balance. The empirical equation of the linear region of the relationship between Na and Nb is shown in Fig. 5.5. In equation No. 1, Nb equals nitrogen balance, Na absorbed nitrogen, and NEo the sum of fecal and urinary nitrogen obtained in the animals fed a nitrogen-free diet. Using the other equations it can be demonstrated that K is the slope of the line or the rate of change of nitrogen balance in relation to absorbed nitrogen (the nitrogen balance index), which is equal to the biological value (Allison 1955).

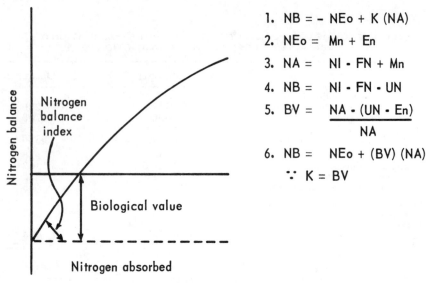

1. $NB = -NEo + K\,(NA)$
2. $NEo = Mn + En$
3. $NA = NI - FN + Mn$
4. $NB = NI - FN - UN$
5. $BV = \dfrac{NA - (UN - En)}{NA}$
6. $NB = NEo + (BV)\,(NA)$

$\therefore K = BV$

FIG. 5.5.   NITROGEN BALANCE INDEX

This method of protein quality assay has been tested in both experimental animals and in young and adult humans with good results. The main difference between this method and nitrogen balance and biological value is that it is a multiple point assay, that is, it requires feeding of the protein under study at different intake levels. Furthermore, there is no essential need to feed protein-free diets, since total endogenous nitrogen excretion can be calculated from the regression equation which relates nitrogen absorbed to nitrogen balance. Since the method is based on nitrogen balance, the values calculated from the use of the method are affected by those conditions which affect nitrogen balance. However, protein level of intake is not a variable if the protein levels fall within the area of a linear or straight line relationship between nitrogen absorbed and nitrogen balance. Since a highly significant straight line relationship has also been demonstrated between nitrogen balance and nitrogen intake, the nitrogen balance index can also be calculated from these values.

Representative results from two laboratories, one using children, and one young adults, fed whole egg protein, have been included in Fig. 5.6. Also shown are the two regression equations of nitrogen balance on nitrogen intake (Bressani et al. 1972B; Young et al. 1973). The figure shows several points of interest. First of all, the coefficients of regression are quite similar between children and young adults, with a value of 0.59 for the children and a value of 0.65 for the adults. As indicated before, the coefficient of regression is a dynamic index of biological value, which is slightly higher for

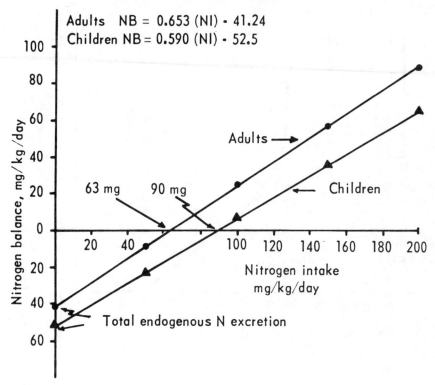

FIG. 5.6. NITROGEN BALANCE INDEX OF CHILDREN (BRESSANI ET AL. 1972B) AND ADULTS (YOUNG ET AL. 1973) FED EGG

adult subjects than for children. This confirms to some extent a relationship between age and protein quality. A second point of interest is that total endogenous nitrogen excretion is higher for children than for adults, confirming again results presented in a previous section of this paper. Of interest also is that the two regression lines spread apart as nitrogen intake increases and thus intercept the zero balance at different points, about 63 mg per kg body wt for young adults and around 90 mg per kg body wt for children. These figures represent the apparent minimum protein requirements for adults and children. Likewise, they represent the minimum needs of essential amino acids which obviously are ingested in greater quantities by children, than by young adults; however, the balance or proportions between them are quite similar.

The information, therefore, obtained from a nitrogen balance index assay is quite complete, making this method one of the best for protein quality determinations. However, it is important to calculate the regression coefficient or the nitrogen balance index from nitrogen balance values obtained

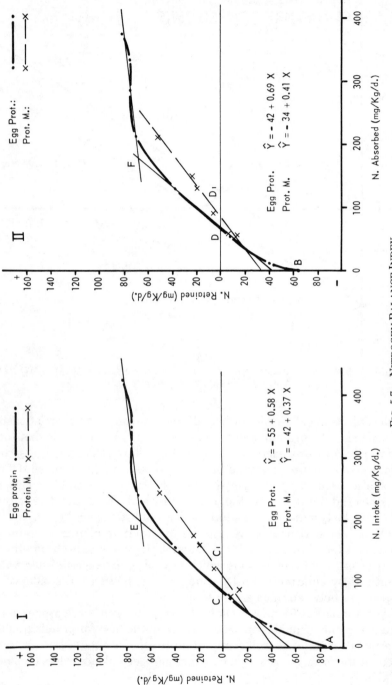

FIG. 5.7. NITROGEN BALANCE INDEX

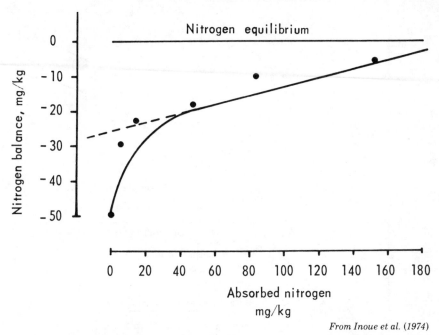

From Inoue et al. (1974)

FIG. 5.8. NONRECTILINEAR RELATIONSHIP BETWEEN ABSORBED N AND N BALANCE
IN YOUNG MEN FED VARIOUS LEVELS OF WHEAT GLUTEN

at nitrogen intakes slightly above and below the nitrogen equilibrium line.
The reason for this is that the relationship between nitrogen intake or absorbed nitrogen and nitrogen balance, much below or above the nitrogen
equilibrium line, is no longer a straight line. The curvilinear relationship
at high intakes is easy to understand; however, the curvilinear relationship
at very low intakes has no apparent explanation. These observations have
been made in both children and young adults. An example for results with
children is shown in Fig. 5.7. The curve representing changes in nitrogen
balance relative to nitrogen intake is made of three segments (Bressani *et
al.* 1972B; Viteri and Bressani 1972; Bressani and Viteri 1971). One corresponds to intakes from approximately 0 to 50 mg nitrogen intake per kg
body wt per day, the second segment is enclosed between nitrogen intakes
of 50–200 mg per kg body wt per day, and the last segment (where curvili-
nearity starts again), at intakes above 200 mg. If the figures for nitrogen
intake from 0 to 50 are used, the quality of the protein is overestimated,
and if the figures above 200 are used, the quality is underestimated.
Therefore, as indicated above, the nitrogen balance index should be calculated from nitrogen intake values from the second segment. Apparently,
intakes between 50 and 200 mg will magnify differences between proteins
as it was previously indicated in the section on nitrogen balance (Table
5.8).

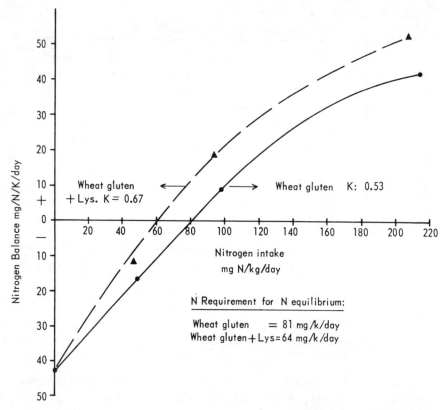

From Hoffman and McNeil (1949)

FIG. 5.9.   NITROGEN BALANCE INDEX OF WHEAT GLUTEN AND OF WHEAT GLUTEN +
LYSINE IN ADULT HUMAN SUBJECTS

The same type of response is obtained in adults as shown in Fig. 5.8. In this case, the point of inflection is at about 0.2 gm of protein intake (per kg body wt) for wheat gluten (Inoue *et al.* 1974). If the nitrogen balance index is calculated at protein intakes from 0 to 0.2 gm per kg body wt, the quality of wheat gluten is overestimated, approaching the quality value for egg protein. The reason for this type of response has not been explained. As it can be seen, total endogenous nitrogen excretion is higher than that resulting from regression analysis. Results from animal work (Bressani *et al.* 1972A) suggest that such an effect may be due to an energy deficiency, or to the way the levels of protein were fed (whether in a descending or ascending order) or even to the state of protein depletion of the experimental subjects. In this last case, it is probable that if the subjects are protein depleted, such curvature may not be found. In this respect, it is of interest to study the results shown in Fig. 5.9, obtained with protein-depleted adult human subjects (Hoffman and McNeil 1949). As can be seen, in the region of negative nitrogen balance the relation between nitrogen absorbed and nitrogen balance is linear, but for intakes higher than 100 mg per kg body wt per day the response is curvilinear. The nitrogen balance index for wheat gluten is 0.53 and for gluten supplemented with lysine, 0.67. The nitrogen requirement to attain equilibrium is 81 and 64 mg per kg body wt per day, respectively.

General Technique for Determining Nitrogen Balance Index in Humans.—The nitrogen balance index represents possibly one of the best systems to evaluate protein quality. In the first place, it does not require (as the estimation of biological value does) feeding a nitrogen-free diet to estimate metabolic fecal nitrogen and endogenous urinary nitrogen. In the second place, it is a dynamic method since several protein intakes are fed to the experimental subjects as opposed to the low nitrogen intake close to the nitrogen equilibrium point used in the static biological value method. Nitrogen balance index (NBI), however, requires that intakes should be in that region where the relationship between absorbed nitrogen and nitrogen balance is linear, and this region falls between intakes of 50–200 mg per kg body wt per day in children, and in a lower range in adults.

When using adults as experimental subjects, the method is carried out by feeding a nitrogen-free diet for 3 days in order to adapt the individual to low levels of protein intake. Then three or four levels of protein intake are fed for three to four periods, each of 7 days duration. One of the levels of protein intake should be below the region of nitrogen equilibrium, another in the region of nitrogen equilibrium and one or two levels above the region of nitrogen equilibrium. Of the 7 days, three are an adaptation period and the last four the balance period. At each level of intake, nitrogen balance is calculated. With increasing levels of intake, nitrogen balance changes from negative to frankly positive. The relationship between absorbed nitrogen and nitrogen balance is then plotted and the coefficient of regression is the nitrogen balance index.

The method, when carried out in children or growing animals, is used in a similar way but there is no need to feed them a nitrogen-free diet to adjust them to low levels of nitrogen intake. It is necessary, however, to run a 12-day adaptation period to a low protein diet. After this period they are fed three or four levels of nitrogen intake including a level of about 1 gm protein per kg body wt per day, one level above this intake and one below. Again, the coefficient of regression between absorbed nitrogen and nitrogen balance is the nitrogen balance index or protein quality of the protein under test. In these studies, it is convenient to determine the index of a reference protein which can be whole egg for adults, milk for children, and casein for animals. Likewise, it is necessary that energy and the intake of other nutrients be provided at constant and adequate levels.

TABLE 5.18

COMPARISON OF NITROGEN BALANCE INDICES FOR EGG FED TO
YOUNG HUMANS

Protein	Method	Regression Equation[1]	Correlation Coefficient	Reference
Fresh egg	Short term	$-59.45 + 0.678\ X$	0.79	INCAP[2]
Fresh egg	Short term	$-53.93 + 1.072\ X$	0.89	INCAP
Egg powder	Short term	$-46.08 + 0.481\ X$	0.72	INCAP
Fresh egg	Conventional	$-39.65 + 0.577\ X$	0.82	INCAP
Egg	Conventional	$-36.20 + 0.538\ X$	0.95	Inoue et al. (1974)
Egg	Conventional	$-33.87 + 0.633\ X$	0.94	Young et al. (1973)

[1] Regression equations of nitrogen absorbed on nitrogen balance.
[2] Instituto de Nutrición de Centro América y Panamá, unpublished data.

TABLE 5.19

REQUIRED NITROGEN ABSORBED TO MAINTAIN NITROGEN EQUILIBRIUM IN
ADULTS FED VARIOUS PROTEIN SOURCES

Protein	Reference	Nitrogen Absorbed (mg/kg Body wt/Day)
Egg	Calloway and Margen (1971)	68
Egg	Young et al. (1973)	73
Egg	Inoue et al. (1973)	100
Egg	INCAP[1] (Short term)	77
Egg	INCAP (Conventional)	83
Egg	INCAP (Short term)	92
Casein	INCAP (Short term)	103
Milk	Bricker et al. (1945)	60
Milk	INCAP (Short term)	73
Milk	INCAP (Short term)	77

[1] Instituto de Nutrición de Centro América y Panamá, unpublished data.

Short-term Nitrogen Balance Index Method.—Based on a large series
of studies with growing dogs, the results of which suggested that the NBI
method could be shortened with respect to the experimental time used
(Navarrete et al. 1975), attempts are being made to apply such a modification to human subjects. In the shortened method, subjects are fed a
protein-free diet for 3 days, followed by daily increasing intakes of the
protein under study. Such intakes go as high as 0.6 gm or 0.7 gm protein
per kg body wt per day. Table 5.18 summarizes the results of various assays
with egg protein with the above modifications in comparison with results
using the conventional technique. The results suggest that the modified
method offers good possibilities for rapid protein quality assays in humans,
particularly if conditions are controlled and standardized. In all cases, the

TABLE 5.20

NITROGEN BALANCE INDICES OF VARIOUS PROTEIN
SOURCES FED TO CHILDREN

| Protein Source | Regression Coefficient Between N Balance and | | Nitrogen Equilibrium Attained with | |
| | N Intake | N Absorbed | N Intake | N Absorbed |
	(mg/kg Body wt/Day)		(mg/kg Body wt/Day)	
Whole milk	0.64	0.73	84	56
Whole egg	0.58	0.69	90	70
CSM	0.37	0.41	115	82
ARL	0.40	0.51	88	55
TRL	0.47	0.58	80	48
IRL	0.48	0.58	90	53
INCAP 9	0.35	0.49	100	60
INCAP 14	0.59	0.62	92	60
INCAP 15	0.43	0.47	113	78

Source: Viteri and Bressani (1972).

subjects were protein depleted for 3 days, except in the results shown in the second line, where the regression coefficient is 1.072. In this case, the subjects were fed decreasing levels of protein from 0.7 to "0" gm per kg body wt per day, held on "0" for 3 days and then fed daily increments of protein back to 0.7 gm per kg. The regression coefficient value was higher than the others because the subjects were probably protein depleted. Allison (1955) indicated that NBI values around or above 1 resulted when the experimental subjects were protein depleted. These results thus suggest that the quality of proteins can be determined in human subjects in a short time. The point which is essential is to standardize the degree of protein depletion prior to feeding either the reference or experimental proteins. Other proteins tested so far are confirming the above statements. Additional evidence is presented in Table 5.19, where nitrogen absorbed values, at nitrogen equilibrium, are presented. The values shown for the short-time NBI method fall within the range of values obtained with the conventional NBI method by other workers.

Applications.—The nitrogen balance index is a very useful method in evaluating protein quality. Results obtained in children fed various proteins are shown in Table 5.20. As with other methods, NBI also classifies the various proteins according to their quality (Bressani *et al.* 1972; Viteri and Bressani 1972). Since these figures are based on data obtained from feeding various levels of protein intake, it is felt that they represent true estimates of the nutritive value of the proteins. Such values are also estimates of the true protein quality, independent of protein intake level. The NBI method can be used, however, for other practical purposes due to the system used

TABLE 5.21

ESSENTIAL AMINO ACIDS ABSORBED AND UTILIZED BY CHILDREN FED COMMON CORN, COMMON CORN SUPPLEMENTED WITH LYSINE AND TRYPTOPHAN, AND OPAQUE-2 CORN

	Common Corn	Common Corn + Lysine + Tryptophan	Opaque-2 Corn
N intake at N equilibrium[1]	360	176	135
N absorbed at N equilibrium[1]	272	158	99
Biological value (%)	31	53	72
N utilized at N equilibrium[1]	84	84	71

Amount of Amino Acids in N Utilized[1]

Amino Acids	Common Corn Absorbed	Common Corn Utilized	Common Corn + Lysine + Tryptophan Absorbed	Common Corn + Lysine + Tryptophan Utilized	Opaque-2 Corn Absorbed	Opaque-2 Corn Utilized	FAO/WHO Estimated Amino Acid Requirement
Arginine	52	16	30	16	41	29	—
Histidine	41	13	24	13	19	13	—
Isoleucine	74	23	43	23	24	17	30
Leucine	203	63	118	63	61	43	45
Lysine	47	14	43	23	29	21	60
Total S.A.A.	59	18	34	18	21	15	27
Total aromatic A.A.	150	46	87	46	52	37	27
Threonine	65	20	38	20	24	17	35
Tryptophan	4.9	1.5	14	7.6	9	6.6	4
Valine	76	23	44	23	34	24	33

[1] Mg/kg body wt/day.

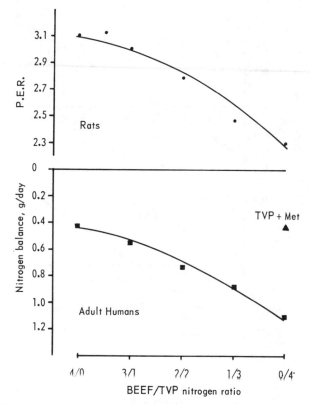

FIG. 5.10.   PROTEIN QUALITY OF MIXTURES OF TVP/BEEF DE-
TERMINED IN RATS AND ADULT HUMANS

to obtain the quality value. In the first place, extrapolating the regression line to an intake of 0 gives the total sum of endogenous nitrogen excreted. On the other hand, the regression line intercepts the nitrogen equilibrium line at different points of absorbed nitrogen, which is an indication of protein quality, the best proteins giving the lower values and the poorer ones, the higher intakes. Using absorbed nitrogen and assuming that it has the same amino acid pattern as ingested nitrogen, the amino acid composition of absorbed and retained nitrogen can be calculated. The latter is an indication of the amino acid needs for maintenance and would also indicate which amino acids are deficient.

As an example, data are shown in Table 5.21 from studies with children (Bressani 1972A) in which common corn, common corn supplemented with lysine and tryptophan, or Opaque-2 corn were fed. The data presented indicate that for nitrogen equilibrium a greater intake of nitrogen is needed from common corn than from common corn supplemented with lysine and

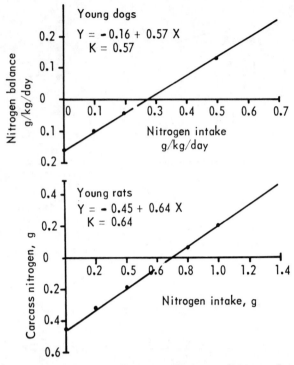

FIG. 5.11.   Relationship Between Nitrogen Balance Index
(NBI) in Dogs and Nitrogen Growth Index (NGI) in Rats
Fed on Casein

tryptophan and that less is needed from Opaque-2 corn. These intakes correspond to 272, 158, and 99 mg of absorbed nitrogen per kg body wt per day. Since biological value represents the amount of nitrogen retained from that which is absorbed, correction of the absorbed values by the biological value gives the amount of nitrogen utilized at nitrogen equilibrium. Assuming that absorption is high and equal for all amino acids, the pattern of amino acids absorbed and utilized can be calculated in a similar manner as that used for the nitrogen calculation. This is also shown in the table. These figures can be considered as amounts of amino acids needed for maintenance purposes, which are similar, with a few exceptions, to the values obtained by the same calculation on the figures for nitrogen equilibrium shown in Table 5.20. For most of the amino acids, values are approximately half the requirement levels as given in the FAO/WHO 1973 joint report for children 10–12 yr old.

TABLE 5.22

REGRESSION EQUATIONS OF PROTEIN INTAKE ON WEIGHT GAIN IN WEANLING
RATS AND NITROGEN ABSORBED ON NITROGEN BALANCE IN CHILDREN

Protein	Regression Equations	
	Rats	Children
INCAP 9[1]	$Y = -11.86 + 1.96\,X$	$-29.4 + 0.49\,X$
INCAP 14[1]	$Y = -15.18 + 2.26\,X$	$-37.2 + 0.62\,X$
INCAP 15[1]	$Y = -\ 9.80 + 2.13\,X$	$-36.7 + 0.47\,X$
Milk	$Y = -\ 9.86 + 3.49\,X$	$-40.8 + 0.73\,X$
Cassava/soya[1]	$Y = -\ 9.50 + 2.99\,X$	$-39.8 + 0.67\,X$
IRL[1]	$Y = -12.88 + 2.68\,X$	$-30.7 + 0.58\,X$

Source: Bressani (1975).
[1] Protein supplied by: cottonseed flour, 38%, corn flour, 58%, Torula yeast, 3%, Min. Vit. Suppl., 1% (INCAP 9); by: soybean flour, 38%, corn flour, 58%, Torula yeast, 3%, Vit. Min. Suppl., 1% (INCAP 14); by: cottonseed flour, 19%, soybean flour, 19%, corn flour, 58%, Torula yeast, 3%, Min. Vit. suppl., 1% (INCAP 15); by: skim milk, 10%, wheat flour, 28%, chick pea flour, 28%, split pea flour, 24% (IRL); and by: cassava flour, 70%, soybean flour, 30% in cassava/ soya mixture.

RELATIONSHIP BETWEEN HUMAN AND ANIMAL PROTEIN QUALITY ASSAYS

Several reviews on this subject have suggested quite strongly that protein quality assays in humans classify proteins in the same order as assays using experimental animals (such as the rat) classify them. A few examples showing that there is good agreement between human and animal protein assay results will be given. In Fig. 5.10, the results of human (Kies and Fox 1973) and rat tests (Bressani et al. 1975B) to evaluate the quality of mixtures of textured soybean and meat protein are shown. In the human study, the response was measured by the nitrogen balance method on diets where the protein was derived from mixtures of the textured vegetable protein (TVP) and meat in the proportions of 100:0, 75:25, 50:50, 25:75, and 0:100. The same approach was used with growing rats. The figures show in both cases that, as TVP replaced meat protein, a linear decrease in quality was obtained.

The agreement between human and rat assays can be even better if the assay technique used is the same. For example, the method used in humans could be the nitrogen balance index while for animals the assay technique could be the protein intake–growth index. An experimental example is shown in Fig. 5.11. In this case casein was assayed in growing dogs by the NBI method while the protein-growth index was used with young rats. In both cases, regressions of nitrogen intake were calculated, either on nitrogen balance or on weight gain converted into nitrogen (wt × 2.54). The two

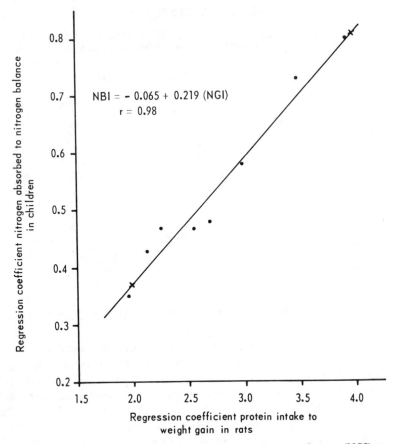

FIG. 5.12. RELATIONSHIP BETWEEN NITROGEN GROWTH INDEX (NGI) IN
RATS AND NITROGEN BALANCE INDEX (NBI) IN CHILDREN

regression coefficients are algebraically expressing the same relationship,
therefore, they should be the same. The values obtained were indeed very
similar (0.57 and 0.64).

Using a similar approach, various high protein-containing foods, tested
in children using the NBI method, were also tested in rats. Table 5.22 shows
the regression equations calculated from the measurements made (Bressani
1975A). In general, the coefficients of regression classified the proteins in
the same order. A regression of one coefficient on the other was then calculated. The results are shown in Fig. 5.12 from which one can predict the
NBI in children from the value obtained with rats. Therefore, the agreement
can be quite high, not only qualitatively but quantitatively as well, particularly when the assay techniques used are well standardized.

Because of the complexity of human assays for protein quality evaluation, these are not recommended for monitoring food development work, quality control or processing conditions. For these activities, traditional protein quality assay techniques, particulary PERs (protein efficiency ratios), are quite acceptable. Human assays should be used as confirmatory to animal results and in the evaluation of the protein quality of the final product, if such a test is required.

BIBLIOGRAPHY

ALLISON, J. B. 1955. Biological evaluation of proteins. Physiol. Rev. *35*, 664.

BRESSANI, R. 1971. Amino acid supplementation of cereal grain flours tested in children. *In* Amino Acid Fortification of Protein Foods (Rep. Intern. Conf., MIT, Sept. 16–18, 1969). N. S. Scrimshaw, and A. M. Altschul (Editors). The MIT Press, Cambridge, Mass.

BRESSANI, R. 1972. Prospects for other foods. *In* Nutritional Improvement of Maize (Proc. Intern. Conf. Instit. Nutr. of Central Am. and Panama, Guatemala City, March 6–8, 1972). R. Bressani, J. E. Braham, and M. Béhar (Editors). INCAP, Guatemala, C.A.

BRESSANI, R. 1973. Evaluación nutricional del maíz Opaco-2 en niños y adultos. *In* Simposio sobre Desarrollo y Utilización de Maíces de Alto Valor Nutritivo. (Memoria) Junio 29 y 30, 1972, Centro Médico Nacional del IMSS, México, D. F. Secretaría de Agricultura y Ganadería, Chapingo, México.

BRESSANI, R. 1974. Deficiencia proteinica en las dietas alimenticias en América Latina y su relación con la crisis mundial de alimentos. Presented at: IX Reunión Latinoamericana de Fitotecnia celebrada en Panamá del 10 al 16 de marzo de 1974.

BRESSANI, R. 1975A. Laboratory evaluation of protein-rich mixtures. *In* Nutrition, Vol. 4 (Proc. 9th Intern. Congr. Nutr., México, 1972). S. Karger, Basel, Switzerland.

BRESSANI, R. 1975B. Improving maize diets with amino acid and protein supplements (Proc. CIMMYT-Purdue Symp. Protein Quality in Maize, El Batán, Mexico, 1972). *In* High-Quality Protein Maize. Dowden, Hutchinson and Ross, Stroudsburg, Pa.

BRESSANI, R., ALVARADO, J., and VITERI, F. 1060. Evaluación en niños de la calidad de la proteína del maíz Opaco-2. Arch Latinoamer. Nutr. *19*, 129.

BRESSANI, R., and BRAHAM, J. E. 1964. Effect of water intake on nitrogen metabolism in dogs. J. Nutr. *82*, 469.

BRESSANI, R., GÓMEZ BRENES, R. A., and ELÍAS, L. G. 1972A. Nitrógeno urinario de perros adultos alimentados con una dieta sin nitrógeno y con diversas ingestas de calorías. Arch. Latinoamer. Nutr. *22*, 451.

BRESSANI, R., NAVARRETE, D. A., and ELÍAS, L. G. 1976. Valor proteínico de mezclas de proteína texturizada de soya y carne, y de harina de soya y leche. Arch. Latinoamer. Nutr. (in press).

BRESSANI, R., and VITERI, F. 1971. Metabolic studies in human subjects. *In* SOS/70 (Proc. 3rd Intern. Congr. Food Sci. Technol., Washington, D.C., Aug. 9–14, 1970). Institute of Food Technologists, Chicago.

BRESSANI, R., VITERI, F., WILSON, D., and ALVARADO, J. 1972B. The quality of various animal and vegetable proteins with a note on the endogenous and fecal nitrogen excretion of children. Arch. Latinoamer. Nutr. *22*, 227.

BRICKER, M., MITCHELL, H. H., and KINSMAN, G. M. 1945. The protein requirements of adult human subjects in terms of the protein contained in individual foods and food combinations. J. Nutr. *30*, 269.

CALLOWAY, D. H., and MARGEN, S. 1971. Variation in endogenous nitrogen excretion and dietary nitrogen utilization as determinants of human protein requirement. J. Nutr. *101*, 205.

CLARK, H. E., ALLEN, P. E., MEYERS, S. M., TUCKETT, S. E., and YAMAMURA, Y. 1967. Nitrogen balances of adults consuming Opaque-2 maize protein. Am. J. Clin. Nutr. *20*, 825.

CLARK, H. E., HOWE, J. M., and LEE, C. 1971. Nitrogen retention of adult subjects fed a high protein rice. Am. J. Clin. Nutr. *24*, 324.

CLARK, H. E., YANG, S. P., REITZ, L. L., and MERTZ, E. T. 1960. The effect of certain factors on nitrogen retention and lysine requirements of adult human subjects. I. Total calorie intake. J. Nutr. *72*, 87.

EDWARDS, C. H., BOOKER, L. K., RUMPH, C. H., WRIGHT, W. G., and GANAPATHY, S. N. 1971. Utilization of wheat by adult man: nitrogen metabolism, plasma amino acids and lipids. Am. J. Clin. Nutr. *24*, 181.

FAO/WHO. 1973. Energy and Protein Requirements (Rep. FAO/WHO Ad Hoc Expert Committee, Rome, Mar. 22–Apr. 2, 1971, WHO, Geneva, Switzerland (WHO Tech. Rept. Ser. *522*).

FORBES, R. M., VAUGHAN, L., and YOHE, M. 1958. Dependence of biological value on protein concentration in the diet of the growing rat. J. Nutr. *64*, 291.

HAWLEY, E. E., MURLIN, J. R., NASSET, E. S., and SZYMANSKI, T. A. 1948. Biological value of six partially purified proteins. J. Nutr. *36*, 153.

HENRY, K. M., and KON, S. K. 1957. Effect of level of protein intake and of age of rat on the biological value of proteins. Brit. J. Nutr. *11*, 305.

HOFFMAN, W. S., and McNEIL, G. C. 1949. The enhancement of the nutritive value of wheat gluten by supplementation with lysine as determined from nitrogen balance indices in human subjects. J. Nutr. *38*, 331.

HUANG, D. C., CHONG, N. E., and RAND, W. M. 1972. Obligatory urinary and fecal nitrogen losses in young Chinese men. J. Nutr. *102*, 1605.

INOUE, G., FUJITA, Y., KISKI, K., YAMAMOTO, S., and NIIYAMA, Y. 1974. Nutritive values of egg protein and wheat gluten in young men. Nutr. Rept. Intern. *10*, 201.

INOUE, G., FUJITA, Y., and NIIYAMA, Y. 1973. Studies on protein requirements of young men fed egg protein and rice protein with excess and maintenance energy intakes. J. Nutr. *103*, 1673.

KIES, C. V., and FOX, H. M. 1973. Effect of varying the ratio of beef and textured vegetable protein nitrogen on protein nutritive value for humans. J. Food Sci. *38*, 1211.

KIES, C., WILLIAMS, E., and FOX, H. M. 1965. Determination of first limiting nitrogenous factor in corn protein for nitrogen retention in human adults. J. Nutr. *86*, 350.

LEE, C., HOWE, J. M., CARLSON, K., and CLARK, H. E. 1971. Nitrogen retention of young men fed rice with or without supplementary chicken. Am. J. Clin. Nutr. *24*, 318.

MITCHELL, H. H. 1923–24. A method of determining the biological value of proteins. J. Biol. Chem. *58*, 873.

MITCHELL, H. H. 1924. The nutritive value of proteins. Physiol. Rev. *4*, 424.

MURLIN, J. R., EDWARDS, L. E., HAWLEY, E. E., and CLARK, L. C. 1946. Biological value of proteins in relation to the essential amino acids which they contain: I. The endogenous nutrition of man. J. Nutr. *31*, 533.

NAVARRETE, D. A., DAQUI, V. R. DE, LACHANCE, P. and BRESSANI, R. 1975. A rapid method for protein quality evaluation in humans. Presented at IFT Annual Meeting, Chicago, Ill., 8–12 June, 1975.

SCRIMSHAW, N. S., HUSSEIN, M. A., MURRAY, E., RAND, W. M., and YOUNG, V. R. 1972. Protein requirements of man. Variation in obligatory urinary and fecal nitrogen losses in young adults. J. Nutr. *102*, 1595.

SIRBU, E. R., MARGEN, S., and CALLOWAY, D. H. 1967. Effect of reduced protein intake on nitrogen loss from the human integument. Am. J. Clin. Nutr. *20*, 1158.

THOMAS, K. 1909. Ueber die Biologische Wertigkert die Stickstoffsubstanzen in Vershieden Nahrungsmitteln. Arch. Anat. Physiol. Abstr., 219.

TRUSWELL, A. S., and BROCK, J. G. 1962. The nutritive value of maize protein for man. Am. J. Clin. Nutr. *10*, 142.

VITERI, F. E., and BRESSANI, R. 1972. The quality of new sources of protein and their suitability for weanlings and young children. Bull. World Health Organ. *46*, 827.

YOUNG, V. R., OZALP, I., CHOLAKOS, B. V., and SCRIMSHAW, N. S. 1971. Protein value of Colombian Opaque-2 corn for young adult men. J. Nutr. *101*, 1475.

YOUNG, V. R., and SCRIMSHAW, N. S. 1968. Endogenous nitrogen metabolism and plasma free amino acids in young adults given a protein free diet. Brit. J. Nutr. *22*, 9.

YOUNG, V. R., TAYLOR, Y. S., RAND, W. M., and SCRIMSHAW, N. S. 1973. Protein requirements of man: Efficiency of egg protein utilization at maintenance and submaintenance levels in young men. J. Nutr. *103*, 1164.

CHAPTER 6

C. E. Bodwell | Biochemical Indices in Humans

Several biochemical parameters have been suggested to be potentially useful, in animal bioassays, as indirect indices of the nutritional value of dietary proteins. These have been the subject of several reviews (McLaughlan 1963; McLaughlan and Morrison 1968; Kiriyama 1970; Den Hertog and Pol 1972; Eggum 1970; Young and Scrimshaw 1972; Pion 1973; Bodwell 1975). The various parameters suggested are listed in Table 6.1, together with an assessment of their potential usefulness and the feasibility of their application in human studies. Some of the potentially more useful parameters cannot be readily studied in humans, e.g., free amino acids in muscle; liver xanthine oxidase activity, and kidney transamidinase activity. Those parameters which can be studied in humans are the subject of this review and include amino acid levels (plasma or serum, "blood cells," urine, feces), various metabolites (blood, serum or plasma urea or urea nitrogen, urinary urea or urea nitrogen, urinary creatinine as a percentage of total

TABLE 6.1

BIOCHEMICAL PARAMETERS SUGGESTED AS INDICES OF PROTEIN NUTRITIONAL VALUE IN ANIMAL STUDIES

Parameter	Assessment of Potential	Applicability in Humans
Amino Acid Levels		
Plasma (serum)	Promising[1]	Applicable
Blood "cells"	Uncertain	Applicable
Muscle	Promising	Not applicable
Urinary	Uncertain	Applicable
Fecal	Poor	Applicable
Ileal contents	Uncertain	Not readily applicable
Metabolites		
Plasma (serum, blood) urea levels	Excellent	Applicable
Urinary urea	Uncertain	Applicable
Urinary creatinine and total nitrogen	Promising	Applicable
Allantoin	Poor	Applicable
Enzyme Activities		
Liver arginase	Poor	Not applicable
Liver xanthine oxidase	Excellent[2]	Not applicable
Kidney transamidinase	Excellent[2]	Not applicable
Plasma amino transferases	Uncertain	Applicable
Protein Synthesis (Muscle Ribosomes)	Promising	Not applicable

[1]For estimating "limiting" amino acids; also, see text.
[2]Limited data available.

urinary nitrogen, urinary sulfate), and the levels of amino transferase activities (plasma, red blood cells).

AMINO ACID LEVELS

Plasma or Serum

Various dietary, physiological and pathological factors affect plasma amino acid levels in both animals and humans. Reports on these factors have been extensively reviewed (Almquist 1964; Longenecker 1961, 1963; McLaughlan 1963; Gitler 1964; Harper 1964, 1968; McLaughlan and Morrison 1968; Anon. 1969; Berry 1970; Den Hartog and Pol 1972; Young and Scrimshaw 1972). Likewise, the extensive number of animal studies concerned with evaluating the relationship of plasma amino acid levels and protein nutritional value have been recently reviewed elsewhere (Bodwell 1975) and, except for some selected references, will not be discussed. It should be noted, however, that results from studies with animals have been variable and often conflicting.

In human plasma, the ratio of essential to nonessential (or to total) amino acids or ratios between specific groups of amino acids have been studied relative to their possible use in assessing nutritional status (Berry 1970; Young and Scrimshaw 1972). Plasma levels have been used to estimate the requirement for specific amino acids in subjects maintained on crystalline amino acid diets containing different levels of the amino acid under study (Young *et al.* 1971, 1972; Tortisirin *et al.* 1973). In attempts to evaluate the nutritional value of proteins, postprandial changes (response curves) in plasma amino acid levels have been used to calculate indexes for predicting the limiting amino acids of various ingested proteins. Response curves *per se* have also been used to detect changes in availability.

To estimate the sequence in which amino acids in a protein become limiting, Longenecker and Hause (1959, 1961) developed the plasma amino acid (PAA) Ratio defined as

$$\text{PAA Ratio} = \frac{\text{average postprandial PAA concentration minus fasting PAA concentration}}{\text{amino acid requirement}} \times 100$$

where plasma amino acid levels are expressed as mg per 100 ml and requirement levels as gm amino acid per 16 gm of ingested nitrogen. Estimates of postprandial PAA concentrations were based on analyses of samples taken hourly for 5 hr. The ratio was based on the premise that the rate at which each amino acid supplied by an ingested protein were removed from the blood was proportional to the requirement for that amino acid. In experiments with dogs, the three most limiting amino acids in wheat gluten were indicated to be lysine, methionine, and arginine (in order); in gelatin, tryptophan, methionine, and histidine; in casein, arginine, methionine, and isoleucine. In studies with two human subjects who ingested test loads (67.4 gm) of gluten protein (Longenecker and Hause 1961), variations in the calculated PAA Ratios were very large. However, in five tests, lysine was always indicated to be the most limiting amino acid. Subsequent studies with human subjects (unspecified numbers) indicated that cystine and methionine (in order) were limiting in casein; lysine, tryptophan, and valine, in corn gluten; methionine and cystine, in soy protein concentrate (Longenecker 1963).

McLaughlan et al. (1968) used a modification of the approach of Longenecker and Hause (1961) in which PAA Ratios were determined for only four amino acids (lysine, threonine, methionine, and tryptophan). When nine subjects ingested 19 gm of protein from each of four sources (baked halibut, cereal, cereal + milk, boiled egg), plasma levels generally peaked at 1–2 hr postprandially. The calculated PAA Ratios indicated that methionine was clearly limiting in the baked halibut while either lysine or methionine was indicated as being limiting in the other three sources. The variability of their plasma response curves among the different subjects was very high. The "average" standard errors of the mean PAA Ratios (calculated from the response curves) expressed as a percentage of the means varied from about 11–68% for the lysine PAA Ratios, 8–32% for methionine, 11–175% for threonine and 17–87% for tryptophan. As pointed out by McLaughlan et al. (1963), such variability would cause the results to be regarded with uncertainty.

In studies with rats, Whitaker and Patrick (1971) used ½ hr postprandial (postintubation) plasma amino acid levels to calculate a "PAA Index" in a manner similar to that used by Oser (1951) to calculate Essential Amino Acid Indexes. The PAA Index was used to predict biological value and for the three protein sources studied (casein + lactalbumin, yeast protein, wheat gluten), the predicted values agreed well with published values. Although it has not been adequately tested in either animals or humans, the PAA Index approach has a major advantage in that it could be used in short-term studies.

McLaughlan (1963) suggested that although "it does not appear to be practical to use the magnitude of the plasma amino acid response as an indicator of protein quality," the approach could be useful for evaluating nutritionally related changes in specific amino acids, caused by heat or other processing treatments, in a single protein or food product. This application was used by Morrison and McLaughlan (McLaughlan 1963) to show differences in lysine or methionine availability in baked or canned salmon and two different fish flours (Table 6.2).

Using six adults as subjects, Vaughan et al. (1974) fed test meals con-

TABLE 6.2

PEAK PLASMA LYSINE AND METHIONINE LEVELS
FOLLOWING INGESTION OF TWO "PROCESSED" PROTEIN SOURCES

Protein Source	No. of Subjects	Lysine (μg/ml)	Methionine (μg/ml)
Salmon			
Baked	8	60[1]	7.7[1]
Canned	8	53	6.5
Fish flour			
A	6	47	8.7
B	6	40[2]	7.7[2]

Source: Data of Morrison and McLaughlan (McLaughlan 1963).
[1]Values for baked and canned salmon significantly different ($P < 0.01$).
[2]Significantly lower ($P < 0.05–0.07$) than values for flour A; fish flour B was known to contain unavailable methionine (rat bioassay) and less total lysine.

taining no protein, lactalbumin or lactalbumin which had been autoclaved at 120°C for 30 min. Most of the plasma amino acids increased markedly following ingestion of the unheated lactalbumin. Following ingestion of meals that were either protein-free or contained heated lactalbumin, with the exception of tryptophan levels, postprandial decreases were generally observed.

Using nitrogen balance techniques with infants, Graham and Placko (1973) could not detect known deficiencies of methionine in mixed protein diets. Postprandial levels of plasma methionine, particularly those at 4 hr, clearly reflected the deficiency (Fig. 6.1). Although observed variations were large from infant to infant, mean methionine values were markedly decreased from fasting levels when dietary methionine was limiting, but not when dietary lysine or threonine were limiting.

In studies with fasted dogs, Longenecker and Hause (1958) found that addition of lysine to a wheat gluten test meal greatly increased plasma lysine levels throughout 5 hr postprandially compared to test meals of only wheat gluten. Similar results were obtained when gelatin test loads, with or without tryptophan supplementation, were fed to dogs and when humans (unspecified number of subjects) were fed gelatin or gelatin supplemented with 0.5% tryptophan, wheat gluten or wheat gluten supplemented with 2% lysine monohydrochloride, and bread or bread supplemented with lysine (Longenecker 1963).

Results of a study in which a similar approach was used, with a single different subject in each of two experiments, have been reported by Longenecker and Lo (1974). Plasma lysine or methionine responses were measured following ingestion of meals containing test protein, heated test protein, and heated test protein supplemented with varying levels of lysine

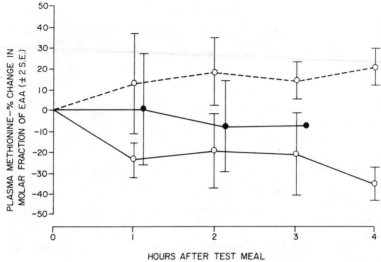

From Graham and Placko (1973)

FIG. 6.1. POSTPRANDIAL CHANGES IN PLASMA FREE METHIONINE IN IN-
FANTS FED MEALS SUPPLYING PROTEIN LIMITING IN METHIONINE (OPEN
CIRCLES, SOLID LINE), LIMITING IN LYSINE OR THREONINE (OPEN CIRCLES,
BROKEN LINE), OR NOT LIMITING IN ANY AMINO ACID (CLOSED CIRCLES,
SOLID LINE)

Reprinted with the permission of the authors and of the Journal of Nutrition.

or methionine (Table 6.3). The amount of supplemental lysine or methionine required to "restore" the postprandial levels, following ingestion of
heated protein to those observed following ingestion of unheated protein
was used to predict the availability of either lysine or methionine. As shown
in Table 6.3, the authors calculated that lysine availability was decreased
by 54% by baking a protein mixture (protein, corn oil, sucrose, and starch).
Likewise, they calculated that methionine availability was decreased 46%
by steam heating a soy protein concentrate. The validity of the approach
used cannot be evaluated on the basis of the limited data. However, the
approach may be useful in following and possibly in quantitating changes
in amino acid availability due to heat or other processing treatments.

Blood "Cells"

In studies with chicks, Stephens and Evans (1972) found that the levels
of aspartic and glutamic acids (including the amides, in both cases) differed
in the nonplasma or "cells" fraction of blood following ingestion of various
levels of egg, casein or gluten protein. They suggested that analyses of amino
acid constituents in cells could provide a rapid test for evaluating protein
quality. As discussed elsewhere (Bodwell 1975), when the cells glutamic

TABLE 6.3

USE OF POSTPRANDIAL PLASMA LYSINE OR METHIONINE LEVELS
TO ESTIMATE LYSINE OR METHIONINE AVAILABILITY IN A
HEATED PROTEIN MIXTURE OR HEATED SOYBEAN CONCENTRATE

Protein Source	Lysine Content (gm/16 gm N)	Postprandial Change in Plasma Lysine Levels[1] (mg/100 ml)
Mixture (wheat gluten, dried skim milk, and whole dried egg)[2]	4.60	0.52
Heated mixture[3]	3.71	0.11
Heated mixture, 1.25 gm L-lysine/16 gm N added after heating	4.96	0.25
Heated mixture, 2.50 gm L-lysine/16 gm N added after heating	6.21	0.60

$$\text{"lysine availability" in heated mixture} = \frac{4.6 - 2.5}{4.6} \times 100 = 46\%$$

	Methionine Content (gm/16 gm N)	Postprandial Change in Plasma Methionine Level[2] (mg/100 ml)
Soybean concentrate[4]	1.30	0.29
Heated soybean concentrate[5]	1.11	0.08
Heated soybean concentrate, 0.30 gm L-methionine/16 gm N added after heating	1.41	0.15
Heated soybean concentrate, 0.60 gm L-methionine/16 gm N added after heating	1.71	0.36

$$\text{"methionine availability" in heated concentrate} = \frac{1.3 - 0.6}{1.3} \times 100 = 54\%$$

Source: Longenecker and Lo (1974); data based on samples from a single subject.
[1] Average of 1, 3, and 5 hr postprandial levels minus the fasting level.
[2] 49 gm of protein ingested (24.5 gm from wheat gluten, 14.7 gm from dried skim milk, 9.8 gm from dried whole egg).
[3] Protein ingredients mixed with 20 gm corn oil, 10 gm sucrose, 10 gm starch, and 65 ml water to give a soft dough, spread in a thin layer in a flat pan, baked for 1 hr at 170°C.
[4] 55.8 gm protein (93 gm concentrate).
[5] Concentrate spread in a thin layer in flat pan and exposed to live steam (autoclave) at 105°C for 8 hr.

acid levels are evaluated in terms of dietary intake, the cells levels reported appear to reflect glutamic acid intake levels provided by the different proteins and not nutritional value. Aspartic acid levels of the cells fraction, however, appear to clearly reflect nutritive value and not intake levels. Further studies, including studies with humans, are needed to evaluate the usefulness of the approach.

TABLE 6.4

MEAN URINARY "FREE" ESSENTIAL AMINO ACID EXCRETION LEVELS
IN FIVE MALE SUBJECTS CONSUMING PROTEINS OF VARIED BIOLOGICAL VALUE

| Protein Source | Biological Value | Excretion of "Free" Essential Amino Acids[1] | |
		mg/Day	Ingested Amino Acid (%)
Nonprotein	—	48.56	—
		49.44	—
Wheat gluten	42	57.2	8.53
Casein	68	64.1	7.36
Dried beef	67	64.1	7.28
Fresh egg	95	71.6	6.61

Source: Nasset and Tully (1951).
[1]Recalculated from authors' data and including isoleucine, leucine, lysine, methionine, phenylalanine, threonine, tryptophan, and valine as essential amino acids.

Urine

Numerous studies have been conducted with rats to investigate possible relationships between urinary excretion of amino acids and the nutritional value of various sources of amino acids or proteins. These studies have been reviewed (Kiriyama 1970). Kiriyama's general conclusion would appear to be valid: "It may be said with reservation that, in spite of many investigations, we have not obtained conclusive data to suggest the definite correlation between the amino acid excretion pattern and the quality and quantity of dietary protein."

With respect to studies with humans, various authors (Bigwood et al. 1959; Soupart 1962; Albanese and Orto 1963; Efron 1965A, 1965B; Snyderman et al. 1968; Kiriyama 1970; Mackenzie 1971; Young and Scrimshaw 1972) have discussed the effects on amino acid excretion of level of protein intake, nutritional status, pathological conditions and nonnutritional diseases. The possible relationship between nutritional value of dietary protein and urinary amino acid levels, however, has not been extensively investigated.

Nasset and Tully (1951) determined the levels of "free" amino acids excreted by human subjects consuming 15.25–33.3 gm of protein per day (~0.25 to ~0.5 gm per kg body weight per day). In general the excretion of "free" essential amino acids, when expressed as a percentage of the essential amino acids ingested (Table 6.4), paralleled the biological value of the proteins ingested. However, both Nasset and Tully (1951) and Steele et al. (1947) concluded that when protein intake levels were held relatively constant the levels of essential amino acids excreted did not appear to be related to the nutritional value of dietary protein. In both studies, microbiological assays were used to estimate amino acid levels; in the one case, unhydrolyzed urines were analyzed (Nasset and Tully 1951), and in the other, complete hydrolysis was probably not achieved with the techniques used. Thus, levels of total (free and conjugated) essential amino acids excreted probably were not determined.

As reported by Kiriyama (1970), Isobe observed a higher ratio of amino acids excreted to those ingested from protein of poor nutritional value fed to three young adults than from protein of higher nutritional value. Metabolism of amino acids and proteins differs in many respects between humans and rats; in the human, urinary excretion of amino acids may be related to the quality of dietary protein. However, a definitive study, utilizing modern analytical techniques for amino acid analyses, is needed.

Feces

In studies with rats, Kuiken and Lyman (1948) and Kuiken (1952) estimated essential amino acid availability in various protein sources (including cottonseed meal steamed or autoclaved for various times) by measuring amino acid levels in the protein ingested and in the feces. Corrections were made for "metabolic" fecal amino acid levels. Inclusion of sulfasuxidine in one of the diets to inhibit microbial action in the gut did not significantly alter the estimated amino acid availability values.

Watts *et al.* (1958A, 1959B, 1960) used a similar technique in studies with humans. During the low nitrogen intake periods, the average fecal excretions of the essential amino acids plus cystine and tyrosine appreciably exceeded intake levels, which suggested that a large part of the fecal amino acid excretion was bacterial or endogenous in origin. Further, the amount of "metabolic" fecal amino acid excretion was affected by other components of the diets ingested. For total diets, quantitative estimates were reported for the availability of the various amino acids. The significance of such data is difficult to assess since, even optimally, such estimates would appear to be indicative of protein digestibility and would not reflect differences in utilization of absorbed amino acids. The analytical difficulties as well as the problems associated with correcting for fecal amino acids of microbial or endogenous origin would appear to preclude any general usefulness of the approach in studies of protein nutritional value in humans.

METABOLITES

Blood, Plasma or Serum Urea (or Urea Nitrogen) Levels

Using rats and pigs as test animals, Munchow and Bergner (1967) reported the first systematic investigations of the possible relationship between blood urea levels and the nutritional value of dietary proteins. To predict the biological value of each test protein, the blood urea level observed following feeding of a reference protein was expressed as a ratio to the level observed following feeding of each test protein. This reciprocal blood urea value was then multiplied by the biological value of the reference protein to give a predicted biological value. The rats were fed the reference protein or each test protein for at least 10 days; for the pigs, the length of feeding of each protein was not clearly indicated [in a subsequent study with pigs, a 14-day feeding period was used (Bergner *et al.* 1971)]. Whether the animals were fasted prior to obtaining blood samples was, likewise, not specified. Whole egg powder was used as the reference protein (assumed biological value of 100; experimentally determined biological value of 96.2) for the rat studies; fish meal (experimentally determined biological value of 81.4) for pig studies. The blood urea levels, experimentally determined biological values and the predicted biological values (the above reciprocal ratio times the biological value of the respective reference proteins) are listed in Table 6.5. Omitting the values for gelatin (the animals did not

TABLE 6.5

BLOOD UREA LEVELS, EXPERIMENTALLY DETERMINED BIOLOGICAL VALUES, AND BIOLOGICAL VALUES PREDICTED FROM BLOOD UREA LEVELS FOLLOWING FEEDING OF VARIOUS PROTEINS TO RATS OR PIGS

Protein Source	Blood Urea (mg %)	Predicted Biological Value Using Blood Urea Ratio[1]	Experimentally Determined Biological Value
Rats			
Whole egg powder	16.4	(100)	96.2
Dried skim milk	20.7	79.2	79.9
Fish meal	24.1	67.8	71.8
Moleirak	25.9	63.2	68.9
Whole egg powder	13.7	(100)	96.0
Rosenthaler yeast	25.9	53.1	49.8
Yeast "50"	26.6	51.6	49.2
Yeast "25"	44.4	30.9	33.4
Gelatin	29.2	47.0	8.2
Nitrogen-free diet	37.6		
Pigs			
Nitrogen-free diet	10.3	—	—
Fish meal	13.6	(81.4)	81.4
Peanut residue	22.5	49.0	53.6
Nitrogen-free diet	10.7	—	—
Gelatin	41.3	26.7	4.6
Barley	22.7	48.6	49.0
Moleirak	14.4	76.7	77.0
Nitrogen-free diet	8.7	—	—

Source: Data from Munchow and Bergner (1967); values represent averages of values for groups of 6–12 rats or 4 pigs (only 2 pigs per group fed gelatin or barley).
[1]Ratio defined as (blood urea level after feeding reference protein/blood urea level after feeding test protein) × biological value of reference protein; reference protein for studies with rats = whole egg powder and for studies with pigs = fish meal.

TABLE 6.6

DESCRIPTION OF STUDIES USED FOR EVALUATION OF THE
RELATIONSHIP BETWEEN ESTIMATED DIETARY PROTEIN VALUE
AND SERUM UREA CONCENTRATION

Protein Sources	Protein Intake Levels Studied (g/kg Body wt/Day)	Energy Levels Studied
Wheat gluten ± 2.25% L-lysine	0.27, 0.73	Adequate, Restricted[1]
Chick-pea ± 2.25% L-methionine	0.27	Adequate, Restricted
Chick-pea and rice (70:30)[2] ± 2.25% L-methionine	0.65	Adequate, Restricted
Dried skim milk	0.4, 0.5	Adequate, Restricted
Wheat gluten and chick-pea (85:15)[2]	0.2	Adequate
Wheat gluten, chick-pea and dried skim milk[2]	0.4	Adequate
Wheat gluten, chick-pea, dried skim milk and nonspecific nitrogen[2]	0.4	Adequate
Whole dried egg	0.2, 0.3, 0.4, 0.5	Adequate

Source: Data from Taylor *et al.* (1974).
[1] Adequate energy levels = sufficient calorie intake to maintain body weight; restricted energy levels = 20% less calories than provided for adequate energy level.
[2] Values given in parenthesis are ratios of protein supplied by each source; no ratios given for wheat gluten, chick-pea and dried skim milk diet or for wheat gluten, chick-pea, dried skim milk, and nonspecific nitrogen diets.

readily consume the gelatin diets), the correlation coefficient was 0.99 between the predicted and experimental biological values.

Eggum (1970) reported a regression coefficient of $r = -0.95$ between the experimentally determined biological values of 42 protein sources and the blood urea levels in the same rats following ingestion of the test protein for 9 days. In this study, food was removed 4–5 hr prior to obtaining blood samples. Although the overall relationship was very good, for predictive purposes, specific erroneous observations were extant. For instance, at blood urea levels of 16.0, 16.2, and 16.4 mg %, determined biological values were 65.7, 57.0, and 75 (shrimp meal, linseed meal, and oats, respectively). Such errors might have been caused by variations, between groups of rats, in the amount of diet eaten immediately prior to removal of the food.

In general, however, blood urea levels in pigs and rats, appear to be closely related to the nutritional value of dietary protein. The relationship also appears to be similar in pigs when the same protein is fed with or without supplementation with different levels of one or more limiting amino acids (Brown and Cline 1974).

Taylor *et al.* (1974) reported a relationship between the concentration of serum urea nitrogen and net protein utilization. Data from 13 different

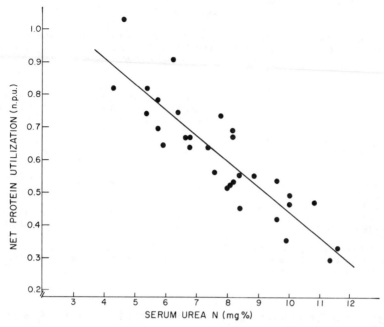

From Taylor et al. (1974)

FIG. 6.2. RELATIONSHIP BETWEEN SERUM UREA NITROGEN AND NET PROTEIN UTILIZATION IN HUMAN SUBJECTS CONSUMING VARIED SOURCES OF NITROGEN

Reprinted by permission of the authors and of the British Journal of Nutrition.

experiments were analyzed; in each experiment, from 6–11 subjects were studied. Protein intake was constant within a single experiment but varied from 0.2–0.65 gm per kg body weight per day in the various experiments and was consumed in two or three meals. Amino acid supplementation or sources of nonprotein nitrogen (diammonium citrate and glycine) were included in some of the experiments. The mean values for nitrogen balance were negative in 26 of the 31 dietary periods. Protein sources and protein and energy intake levels used in the different experiments are listed in Table 6.6.

Based on mean values of each diet group, the correlations between serum urea nitrogen levels and net protein utilization or biological value were −0.89 and −0.88, respectively. The regression of net protein utilization on serum urea nitrogen is shown in Fig. 6.2. Although a significant relationship is apparent, the predictive accuracy was not completely satisfactory. For instance, at 8–8½ mg % serum urea nitrogen levels, the net protein utilization varied from about 45–72; at 5½–6 mg % serum urea nitrogen levels,

TABLE 6.7

EFFECTS OF DIETARY ENERGY INTAKE LEVEL, NUMBER OF MEALS AND
AMINO ACID SUPPLEMENTATION ON MEAN SERUM UREA NITROGEN LEVELS
AND MEAN NET PROTEIN UTILIZATION VALUES

	Number of Dietary Periods	Mean Serum Urea Nitrogen (mg %)	Mean Net Protein Utilization
Dietary Energy Intake			
Adequate Calories	11	7.66	0.59
Restricted Calories	11	9.44	0.43
Number of Meals[1]			
Two meals	4	8.4	0.54
Three meals	4	8.3	0.57
Amino Acid Supplementation			
No supplementation	8	8.7	0.49
Supplementation	8	8.3	0.54

Source: Data from Taylor *et al.* (1974).
[1]Comparisons of effects of feeding protein in two or three meals for four different diets; all other diets were supplied in three meals.

net protein utilization values varied from about 64–83. As shown in Table 6.7, the effects on serum urea nitrogen values of dietary energy intake, number of meals, and amino acid supplementation were paralleled by corresponding effects on net protein utilization. Consuming the protein in either two or three meals, as well as amino acid supplementation, had little effect on either serum urea nitrogen levels or estimated nutritional value. Restriction of calories, as would be expected, resulted in a decrease in mean net protein utilization; this was paralleled by an increase in mean serum urea nitrogen levels.

The serum urea nitrogen levels, however, reflected protein intake more closely than net protein utilization (Table 6.8). For example, at protein intakes of 0.4, 0.5 and 0.65 gm per kg body weight per day (with restricted energy intake levels), serum urea nitrogen levels were 8.3, 9.9 and 10.5 mg %, respectively; the respective net protein utilization values were 45, 48, and 43. From the data given by the authors, correlations of 0.94 and 0.95 can be calculated for the relationships between level of protein intake and mean serum urea nitrogen levels for the "adequate" and "restricted" energy level groups, respectively. It is well known that net protein utilization values generally decrease with increasing protein intake levels. Conversely, blood urea levels increase with increased levels of protein intake. The reported correlations between serum urea nitrogen level and net protein utilization ($r = -0.89$) or biological value ($r = -0.88$) may thus, in part, reflect the varied levels of protein intake studied.

Bodwell and Schuster (1974) reported results of some preliminary ob-

TABLE 6.8

EFFECTS OF PROTEIN INTAKE LEVEL ON SERUM UREA NITROGEN LEVELS
AND NET PROTEIN UTILIZATION IN SUBJECTS MAINTAINED
ON ADEQUATE OR RESTRICTED ENERGY INTAKE LEVELS

Protein Intake (gm/kg Body wt/ Day)	Adequate Energy Intake Levels			Restricted Energy Intake Levels		
	No. of Dietary Periods	Serum Urea Nitrogen[1] (mg %)	Net Protein Utiliza- tion[1]	No. of Dietary Periods	Serum Urea Nitrogen[1] (mg %)	Net Protein Utiliza- tion[1]
0.2	2	4.5	92	—	—	—
0.27	4	5.8	75	4	7.8	53
0.3	1	6.4	89	—	—	—
0.4	6	6.8	65	2	8.3	45
0.5	2	8.3	65	2	9.9	48
0.65	2	8.8	52	2	10.5	43
0.73	2	9.9	35	2	11.6	27

Source: Taylor *et al.* (1974).
[1]Values are averages (expressed as whole numbers) calculated from the mean values given by the authors for each dietary period (6–11 subjects/period).

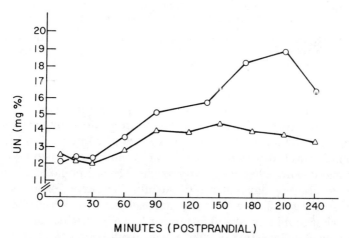

MINUTES (POSTPRANDIAL)

From Bodwell and Schuster (1974)

FIG. 6.3. POSTPRANDIAL CHANGES IN PLASMA UREA NITROGEN LEVELS IN A SINGLE SUBJECT (SUBJECT B) FOLLOWING INGESTION OF 42 AND 15 GM GELATING PROTEIN (UPPER AND LOWER CURVES, RESPECTIVELY).

servations on postprandial levels of plasma urea nitrogen in two or three human subjects following ingestion of test loads of various protein sources. Postprandial plasma urea nitrogen curves for a single subject, following ingestion of 15 or 42 gm of gelatin protein (0.19 and 0.54 gm protein per kg body weight, respectively), are shown in Fig. 6.3. The marked dependence

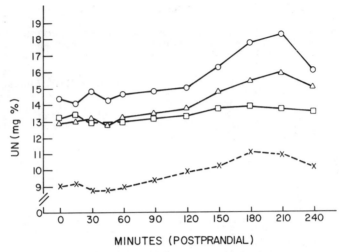

From Bodwell and Schuster (1974)

FIG. 6.4. POSTPRANDIAL RESPONSE IN PLASMA UREA NITROGEN
LEVELS IN THREE HUMAN SUBJECTS INGESTING VARIOUS
AMOUNTS OF SPRAY DRIED WHOLE EGG

Subject A, 28 gm of protein, ~0.5 gm per kg body wt (open circles);
Subject B, 42 gm of protein, ~0.5 gm per kg body wt (open diamonds)
and 15 gm protein, ~0.2 gm per kg body wt (open squares); and Subject
C, 25 gm of protein, ~0.3 gm per kg body wt (x's).

of the rise in urea nitrogen level on level of protein ingested is quite apparent. Similar curves, from data obtained from three subjects ingesting differing levels of spray dried whole egg, are presented in Fig. 6.4. The postprandial urea nitrogen response was proportional to the grams of protein ingested per kilogram of body weight. The postprandial plasma urea nitrogen levels were maximal at 150–240 min. The curves for subject B and the curves in Fig. 6.3 were from the same subject. For this subject, at the same level of protein intake (0.54 gm per kg body weight), the maximum change following ingestion of gelatin was about 6.8 mg %, that following ingestion of the egg protein, about 3.1 mg %.

A series of 8 protein sources were ingested by each of two subjects (0.54 gm protein per kg body weight for one subject; 0.75 gm protein per kg body weight for the other). The subjects were maintained on a relatively constant, but not strictly controlled, daily protein intake. Fasting values were subtracted from the subsequent postprandial values. The sum of the values at 120, 180, and 240 min, following ingestion of the egg protein, were expressed as a ratio to the sum of the corresponding values following ingestion of each test protein. The resulting ratios (× 100) generally paralleled the assumed nutritional value of the proteins ingested (Table 6.9). Exceptions

TABLE 6.9

RATIOS OF POSTPRANDIAL PLASMA UREA NITROGEN CHANGES IN
TWO SUBJECTS USING SPRAY DRIED WHOLE EGG AS THE REFERENCE PROTEIN

Protein Source	Ratios[1]
Spray dried whole egg	(100)
Tuna	112
Nonfat dried skim milk	91[2]
Fish protein concentrate	76
Soy protein concentrate[3]	51
Textured soy protein[3]	51
Peanut flour[3]	44
Gelatin	42

Source: Data from Bodwell and Schuster (1974).
[1]See text for definition.
[2]Based on values for one subject suspected to be lactose-intolerant.
[3]Cooked products.

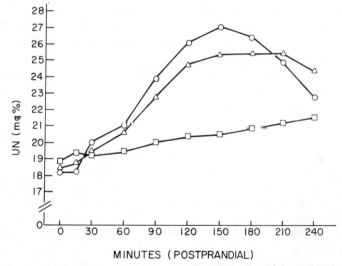

MINUTES (POSTPRANDIAL)

From Bodwell and Schuster (1974)

FIG. 6.5. EFFECTS OF TEMPERATURE OF PROTEIN WHEN INGEST-
ED AND OF HIGH LEVELS OF SUCROSE

(~25 gm) on postprandial plasma urea nitrogen levels in a single
subject (Subject A) ingesting 42 gm of gelatin protein at 40–45°C (open
circles), at 25°C (open diamonds) or at 25°C dissolved in lemonade
concentrate (open squares).

were the value for tuna (112) which was higher than that for spray dried
whole egg, the value for nonfat dried skim milk (91, based on values from
one subject) which appeared to be too high and the value for peanut flour
(44) which appeared to be too low.

In these preliminary studies, the postprandial plasma urea nitrogen response was affected by the temperature of the protein when ingested, by the presence of high levels of simple carbohydrates and by large variations in the fasting plasma urea nitrogen levels (prior to ingesting the test protein load). The effects of temperature and of high levels of sucrose (lemonade concentrate) on the postprandial rise in plasma urea nitrogen in a single subject following ingestion of gelatin protein are shown in Fig. 6.5.

Two further studies have been conducted (Bodwell and Schuster 1975; Bodwell *et al.* 1976), each with subjects maintained on defined diets providing a constant daily nitrogen intake. In the first study, four male subjects were maintained on a basal diet providing 0.55 gm protein per kg body weight per day. Following an overnight fast, test proteins were consumed at a level of 0.45 gm per kg body weight. Plasma urea nitrogen levels were determined in finger prick samples taken from each subject in the fasting state and 3½ hr after ingesting test protein. During a 3-day adaptation period, a mixed protein was consumed as the test load. On days 4–7 and 9–12, various proteins were consumed as the test load in a random order by each subject. The mixed protein was also ingested on the 8th and 13th day by each subject.

In the second study, four male subjects consumed a basal diet containing 0.20 gm protein per kg body weight per day. Test loads of 0.50 gm protein per kg body weight were consumed as in the previous study and postprandial changes in plasma urea nitrogen levels determined. In this study, canned tuna was ingested as the test protein during a 5-day adaptation period and on alternate days thereafter. Six test proteins were ingested in a randomized order by each subject on the other days.

The data were expressed both as mg % change from fasting levels and as a ratio [(change observed following ingestion of the reference protein per change observed following ingestion of the test protein) × 100]. Results are given in Table 6.10. In both studies, the mg % change increased, postprandially, with decreasing nutritional value. The calculated ratios generally decreased with decreasing nutritional value. In Study I, the responses observed following ingestion of spray dried egg white were anomalous (this may have been due to a lack of solubility of the preparation used). Likewise, the responses observed following ingestion of gelatin did not follow the general pattern (difficulty was experienced by some of the subjects in ingesting the specified quantity of gelatin protein). For the mixed protein (50% of the protein from spray dried egg white and 50% from wheat gluten), the mg % change was 3.6. This approximated an average between the changes observed following ingestion of spray dried egg white alone (1.4 mg %) and wheat gluten alone (4.9 mg %). In Study II (Table 6.10), the mg % changes, following ingestion of test loads of tuna protein, during the

TABLE 6.10

POSTPRANDIAL CHANGES IN PLASMA UREA NITROGEN LEVELS IN HUMAN SUBJECTS CONSUMING TWO LEVELS OF PROTEIN AND RATIOS OF CHANGES USING VALUES FOR TUNA OR SPRAY DRIED WHOLE EGG (SDWE) AS THE REFERENCE PROTEIN

| Protein Source | Δ mg % | | Ratios | | |
	Study I[1]	Study II[2]	Study I[1] $\frac{\Delta \text{(Tuna)}}{\Delta \text{(Other)}} \times 100$	Study II[2] $\frac{\Delta \text{(Tuna)}}{\Delta \text{(Other)}} \times 100$	Study II[2] $\frac{\Delta \text{(SDWE)}}{\Delta \text{(Other)}} \times 100$
Spray dried egg white	1.4	—	221	—	—
Spray dried whole egg	—	2.5	—	(118)	(100)
Tuna	3.1	3.0	(100)	(100)	84
Fish protein concentrate	3.2	3.4	97	91	77
Cottage cheese I	3.5	—	89	—	—
Cottage cheese II	—	4.4	—	68	57
Hamburger	3.6	—	86	—	—
Mixed protein[3]	3.6	—	86	—	—
Peanut flour[4]	3.9	4.1	80	72	60
Soy protein isolate[4]	—	4.2	—	70	60
Wheat gluten	4.9	5.5	63	54	46
Gelatin	4.5	—	69	—	—

Source: Data from Bodwell and Schuster (1975) and Bodwell et al. (1976); postprandial change, (Δ) = difference in plasma urea nitrogen level between fasting level and the level observed 3½ hr after ingestion of a test protein load.
[1] Subjects maintained on 1 gm/kg body weight/day protein intake with daily test protein loads contributing 0.45 gm/kg body weight/day.
[2] Subjects maintained on 0.7 gm/kg body weight/day protein intake with daily test protein loads contributing 0.5 gm/kg body weight/day.
[3] Wheat gluten + spray dried egg white protein (1:1).
[4] Cooked products.

adaptation period and on alternate days throughout the 15-day study were essentially identical.

When the ratio values from the two studies were compared (using tuna as the reference protein in both studies), values were similar for the three proteins ingested in both studies; i.e., 97 and 91 for fish protein concentrate, 80 and 72 for peanut flour, and 63 and 54 for wheat gluten. When spray dried whole egg was used as the reference protein in calculating the ratios from the data in Study II and the value for mg % change in plasma urea nitrogen following ingestion of spray dried whole egg was assigned a value of 100, the other ratios approximated the assumed biological values (84 for tuna, 77 for fish protein concentrate, 60 for peanut flour or soy protein isolate, 57 for cottage cheese, and 46 for wheat gluten).

A study of the relationship between protein nutritional value and serum or plasma urea nitrogen levels in human subjects under conditions comparable to those used by Taylor *et al.* (1974), but utilizing identical levels of protein intake for the protein sources studied would be of value. The results of the approach using postprandial changes must be verified by comparison with results from a standard method (i.e., determination of net protein utilization or of biological value by using nitrogen balance techniques). The use of changes in postprandial plasma urea nitrogen as possible indices of protein nutritional value has potential as a short-term procedure for the estimation of protein nutritional value directly in human subjects.

Urinary Urea (Urea Nitrogen)

Urinary urea or urea nitrogen excretion has been suggested to reflect nutritional value of the dietary protein fed to animals (Brown and Cline 1974; Prior *et al.* 1975; Kiriyama 1970). For the most part, in these studies with animals, the effects of adding one or more specific essential amino acids to diets inadequate in those amino acids have been investigated. Likewise, using young men as subjects, Nakagawa and Masana (1967) studied the effects of lysine, tryptophan or methionine deficiencies in otherwise adequate diets in which crystalline amino acids were used as the source of nitrogen and amino acids. Following consumption of diets deficient in any of the three amino acids for 8 days, urea nitrogen excretion markedly increased. Similar observations were reported by Rose *et al.* (1950, 1951) for diets deficient in valine, methionine or threonine.

The basal diets in the selected studies referred to above were usually identical and the changes observed in urea excretion levels, upon adding supplementary amino acids, may not be typical of differences induced by feeding diets which contain proteins varying widely in their general amino acid composition and/or nutritional value.

In the previously described studies on the relationship between serum

TABLE 6.11

CORRELATIONS BETWEEN ESTIMATED NET PROTEIN UTILIZATION
OR PROTEIN INTAKE IN YOUNG MEN AND
EXCRETION LEVELS OF URINARY NITROGEN

	Correlations			
	Net Protein Utilization[1]	Gm Protein Intake/kg Body Weight/ Day[1]	Net Protein Utilization[2]	Gm Protein Intake/kg Body Weight/ Day[2]
Gm protein intake/kg body weight/day	−0.74	—	−0.82	—
Gm urinary urea nitrogen/day	−0.87	0.90	−0.90	0.90
Total urinary nitrogen	−0.87	0.90	−0.88	0.91
Gm urinary urea nitrogen/day expressed as % of total urinary nitrogen/day	−0.90	0.88	−0.60	0.49
Gm urinary urea nitrogen/day per gm protein intake/kg body weight/day	−0.65	—	−0.33	—
Gm urinary urea nitrogen/day (expressed as % of total urinary urea nitrogen/day) per gm protein intake/kg body weight/day	− 0.59	—	−0.61	—

[1] Correlations calculated from mean data of Taylor *et al.* (1974).
[2] Correlations calculated from mean data (Table 6.12) given by Taylor *et al.* (1974) for groups of subjects consuming diets adequate in calories and not containing supplementary amino acids or nonprotein nitrogen and from mean data given by Young *et al.* (1975).

urea nitrogen levels and net protein utilization, Taylor *et al.* (1974) observed a close relationship between mean serum urea nitrogen levels and mean urinary urea nitrogen excretion ($r = 0.87$ or 0.93 between serum urea nitrogen and grams urea nitrogen excreted per day or grams urea nitrogen per day expressed as the percentage of total urinary nitrogen output, respectively). Using the mean data reported by the authors, correlations can be calculated of −0.87 between grams urea nitrogen excreted per day and net protein utilization and of −0.90 between grams urinary urea nitrogen expressed as a percentage of total urinary nitrogen and net protein utilization (Table 6.11). However, correlations of 0.90 and 0.88 can be calculated between protein intake level and mean urea nitrogen excretion expressed as grams per day or as a percentage of the total urinary nitrogen, respectively. Between grams urea nitrogen per day and grams urea nitrogen per day expressed as a percentage of total urinary nitrogen, $r = 0.92$.

When the same protein source is consumed at different intake levels (all below the maintenance nitrogen requirement level), net protein utilization is not a linear function of intake. Under the same conditions, urinary urea nitrogen excretion usually would appear to be directly proportional to intake levels. If the mean urinary nitrogen excretion data of Taylor *et al.* (1974) are expressed on a per grams of protein intake basis, the correlations are −0.65 between net protein utilization and grams urinary urea nitrogen excreted per day per gram of protein intake per kg body weight per day and −0.59 between net protein utilization and urinary urea nitrogen expressed as a percentage of total urinary nitrogen per gram protein intake per kilogram body weight per day (Table 6.11).

The data of Taylor *et al.* (1974) include replicates in which the same protein was fed but either calories were restricted or supplementary amino acids added (with adequate calories, supplementation had little effect on estimated protein nutritional value; see Table 6.7). Urinary urea nitrogen excretion data from those studies in which energy levels were not restricted and amino acid supplementation or nonprotein nitrogen sources were not used and similar data from Young *et al.* (1975) are given in Table 6.12, together with protein sources and intake levels, balance data, and estimates of nutritional value. As shown by these data, as the level of protein intake increased, nitrogen equilibrium was approached and estimates of nutritional value decreased. Urea excretion also increased but this increase was not always accompanied by a comparable increase in the percentage of total urinary nitrogen excreted as urea (see data for canned "strained" beef and whole wheat). In the data for canned "strained" beef, nitrogen excretion was not directly proportional to nitrogen intake.

Correlations, calculated from the data in Table 6.12, are also listed in Table 6.11. The correlations between grams urinary urea nitrogen per day or total urinary nitrogen excreted per day and net protein utilization or protein intake are similar to those discussed above. However, the correlations between grams urinary urea nitrogen per day, expressed as a percentage of total urinary nitrogen, and net protein utilization or protein intake are much lower. Likewise, for grams urea nitrogen per day and grams urea nitrogen per day expressed as a percentage of total urinary nitrogen, $r = 0.64$. The differences in correlation values between the two sets of data are partly due to the fact that in subjects consuming increasing levels of the beef protein, the increase in total nitrogen was much greater than the corresponding increase in urea nitrogen excretion levels.

Since urinary urea nitrogen excretion and net protein utilization are both related to nitrogen intake level, it is difficult to evaluate the significance of the apparent relationships noted above between urea excretion and protein nutritional value. An investigation of these relationships with

TABLE 6.12

MEAN URINARY UREA NITROGEN EXCRETION LEVELS AND NITROGEN BALANCES IN YOUNG MEN CONSUMING VARIOUS LEVELS OF PROTEINS OF DIFFERING ESTIMATED NUTRITIONAL VALUE

Protein Source	Protein Intake Level (gm/kg Body wt/Day)	Mean Urinary Urea Nitrogen Excretion (gm/Day)	% of Total Urinary Nitrogen	Nitrogen Balance (gm/Day)	Biological Value	Net Protein Utilization
Spray dried whole egg	0.2 (11)[1]	1.54	54	−0.71 ± 0.41[2]	107	103
	0.3 (11)	1.71	59	−0.05 ± 0.48	93	89
	0.4 (7)	2.93	69	−0.44 ± 0.34	65	64
	0.4 (8)	2.75	65	−0.32 ± 0.86	65	61
	0.5 (11)	2.37	71	0.85 ± 0.75	72	71
Canned "strained" beef[3]	0.2 (7)	2.07[4]	88	−1.84 ± 0.50[4]	79	79
	0.3 (6)	2.34[4]	73	−1.33 ± 0.51[4]	70	70
	0.4 (7)	2.93[4]	62	−0.60 ± 0.61[4]	67	65
Dried skim milk	0.5 (7)	3.51[4]	59	−0.06 ± 0.56[4]	62	61
	0.4 (7)	2.84	70	−0.31 ± 0.19	68	64
	0.5 (7)	2.95	70	−0.25 ± 0.35	69	66
Chick-pea + wheat gluten + dried skim milk	0.4 (6)	2.31	60	−0.31 ± 0.71	76	67
Wheat gluten + chick-pea (85:15)[5]	0.2 (6)	1.53	54	−1.45 ± 0.46	95	80
Chick-pea	0.27 (7)	1.61	57	−0.97 ± 0.29	90	72
Chick-pea + rice (70:30)[5]	0.65 (8)	4.04	76	−0.65 ± 0.41	62	52
Wheat gluten	0.27 (6)	2.22	65	−1.31 ± 0.40	73	72
Wheat gluten	0.73 (8)	7.01	83	−0.68 ± 0.62	31	31
Whole wheat[3]	0.3 (8)	2.57[4]	69	−1.39 ± 0.48[4]	69	65
	0.4 (8)	3.48[4]	72	−1.38 ± 0.71[4]	52	48
	0.5 (8)	4.11[4]	76	−0.82 ± 0.34[4]	48	45
	0.65 (7)	5.12[4]	79	−0.32 ± 0.56[4]	46	43

Source: Except where otherwise noted, data from Taylor et al. (1974); also see Scrimshaw et al. (1973), Taylor et al. (1973), Young et al. (1973), and Scrimshaw et al. (1966).
[1]Numbers of subjects given in parenthesis.
[2]Means ± standard deviations.
[3]Data from Young et al. (1975).
[4]Recalculated from Young et al. (1975).
[5]Ratios of protein supplied by each source; ratio not given by authors for ratio of protein supplied by each source in the chick-pea + wheat gluten + dried skim milk mixture.

subjects consuming various proteins at constant nitrogen intake levels would be of value.

In the preliminary studies previously described above, in which post-prandial changes in plasma urea nitrogen levels were studied in two or three subjects (Bodwell and Schuster 1974; also see Bodwell 1975), urinary urea nitrogen excretion levels were determined for a 4-hr (8–12 a.m.) postpranidal period. The excretion levels, following ingestion of the reference protein (spray dried whole egg), were expressed as a ratio to those observed following ingestion of the test proteins. There was general agreement between the urea nitrogen excretion and the plasma urea nitrogen ratios previously discussed. Given the difficulty of short-term standardization of urinary output in human subjects, the agreement was surprisingly good. The 8–12 a.m. time period is one of relatively low urinary nitrogen output (Powell *et al.* 1961) and urea nitrogen excretion during this time interval may be more reflective of the nutritional value of ingested protein than urea excretion during a 24-hr period.

Urinary Creatinine Nitrogen Percentage

Murlin *et al.* (1948) reported a linear relationship (r = >0.90; derived from the authors' data) between creatinine nitrogen percentage (creatinine nitrogen excretion expressed as a percentage of the total urinary nitrogen) and biological value in a study using 6–8 dogs. A consistent relationship between creatinine excretion (alone or expressed in terms of urinary nitrogen excretion) and protein nutritional value has not been observed with rats (Rippon 1959; Kiriyama and Ashida 1964; Yokota 1964A, 1964B; Kean 1967; Kiriyama 1970). However, creatinine excretion levels in rats have been reported to be affected by level of dietary protein (Yokota 1964A, 1964B), source of protein (Kiriyama and Ashida 1964), and amino acid supplementation (Yokota 1964A, 1964B). Also, Fisher (1965) found that rats fed purified amino acid diets excreted markedly higher creatinine levels than rats fed an equivalent amount of nitrogen from casein.

Although Calloway and Margen (1971) reported, in male subjects fed creatine-free diets, a continuous fall in creatinine excretion levels during an 88-day period, in most studies with humans, creatinine excretion levels have been constant. Ingestion of foods derived from muscle tissues results in elevated levels of estimated urinary creatinine (Murlin *et al.* 1953; Watts *et al.* 1959B; Young *et al.* 1975). In this case, although usually not done, analytical corrections can be made (Murlin *et al.* 1953).

Murlin *et al.* (1953) reported a correlation coefficient of 0.97 between creatinine nitrogen percentage and biological value in human subjects consuming ten different sources of protein (Fig. 6.6). The determination

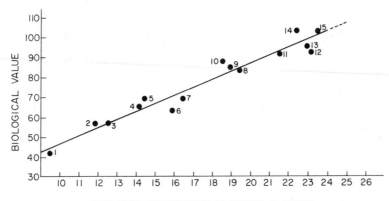

PERCENT CREATININE NITROGEN IN URINE

Adapted from Murlin et al. (1948)

FIG. 6.6. RELATIONSHIP BETWEEN BIOLOGICAL VALUE AND PERCENTAGE OF URINARY CREATININE NITROGEN IN HUMAN SUBJECTS CONSUMING VARIOUS PROTEIN SOURCES

1—Wheat gluten, 2—Peanut, 3—Raw casein, 4—Beef protein (corrected), 5 and 7—Casein (cooked), 6—Beef protein (uncorrected), 8—50% Wheat germ and 50% fresh whole egg, 9—Fresh whole egg, 10—Wheat germ, 11—Beefsteak, 12—Egg albumen, 13—Whole egg powder. 14 and 15—Whole fresh egg.

Reprinted with the permission of the Journal of Nutrition.

of total urinary nitrogen excretion levels is necessary in nitrogen balance studies and since creatinine excretion levels are often determined as a check on the completeness of collections, this relationship has presumably been examined and discarded. However, it is of interest to examine the data in those cases in which total urinary nitrogen, creatinine and estimates of nutritional value have been reported. As shown in Table 6.13, by using such data and an equation derived from the data of Murlin *et al.* [biological value = 11.53 + 3.50 (creatinine nitrogen percentage)], the resulting predicted biological values are comparable to the experimentally determined net protein utilization and biological values. However, the data used in the above calculations were from studies in which nitrogen excretion levels were well stabilized. It may not be possible to obtain meaningful creatinine nitrogen percentage data in experiments of shorter duration than nitrogen balance studies. Nevertheless, the approach appears to warrant further investigation.

Urinary Sulfate

Miller and Naismith (1958) suggested that most human diets were nutritionally limited by their levels of sulfur-containing amino acids. Subse-

TABLE 6.13

REPORTED NET PROTEIN UTILIZATION VALUES AND BIOLOGICAL VALUES
CALCULATED FROM CREATININE NITROGEN PERCENTAGE (Cr N %) VALUES

Protein Source	Protein Intake Level (gm/kg Day)	Net Protein Utilization	Biological Value	Biological Value Calculated from Cr N %
Wheat	0.3	65[1]	69[1]	70
	0.4	48[1]	52[1]	55
	0.5	45[1]	48[1]	48
	0.65	43[1]	43[1]	44
Wheat gluten	0.27	72[2,3]	73[2,3]	77
	0.73	31[2,3]	31[2,3]	38
Spray-dried whole egg	0.2	103[3,4]	107[3,4]	100
	0.3	89[3,4]	93[3,4]	87
	0.4	65[4,5], 61[3,4]	65[4,5], 65[3,4]	64, 65
	0.5	71[3,4]	72[3,4]	65
White flour[6]	0.9	—	—	36
	0.9	—	—	36
Peanut butter[7]	1.0	—	—	39
Pork[7]	1.0	—	—	46
Canned "strained" beef	0.2	79[1]	79[1]	83
	0.3	70[1]	70[1]	77
	0.4	65[1]	67[1]	71
	0.5	61[1]	62[1]	65

Source: "Equation" from Murlin et al. (1948) used to calculate biological values
from Cr N %; Cr N % calculated from data reported in references cited.
[1] Young et al. (1975); biological values calculated from authors' data.
[2] Scrimshaw et al. (1973).
[3] Taylor et al. (1974).
[4] Young et al. (1973).
[5] Scrimshaw et al. (1966).
[6] Bolourchi et al. (1968).
[7] Watts et al. (1959B).

quently, Miller and Donoso (1963) proposed that the ratio of sulfur to nitrogen was a useful indicator of protein nutritive value.

Pellett (1963) fed three diets containing varied ratios of sulfur to total nitrogen to five human subjects for 4 days. Urines were collected on the third and fourth days. As shown in Table 6.14, the ratios of dietary sulfur to nitrogen, and of urinary levels of inorganic sulfate to urinary levels of nitrogen, paralleled estimates of nutritional value obtained from rat feeding studies. However, with respect to the other essential amino acids, the sulfur-amino acids were probably limiting in all three diets studied.

Sabry et al. (1965) fed diets in which the sulfur amino acids, at levels ranging from 0.8–4 gm per day, were supplied by bread plus egg, uncooked rice plus baked beans with pork or peanut butter plus bread. Three adult and three adolescent males were used as subjects. The excretion of sulfate

TABLE 6.14

RELATIONSHIP BETWEEN DIETARY SULFUR AND NITROGEN INTAKE
AND URINARY SULFUR AND NITROGEN EXCRETION IN FIVE HUMAN SUBJECTS

Protein Sources	Protein Intake (gm/Day)	Urinary Sulfate / Urinary nitrogen (×1000)	Dietary Sulfur / Dietary Nitrogen (×1000)	Net Protein Utilization$_{(op)}$
Oatmeal (10%) + skim milk powder (28%) + cooked beans (52%)[1]	67	42.8 (56)[2]	60	61
Oatmeal (10%) + skim milk powder (42%) + soy protein (45%)	70	51.5 (67)	65	71
Oatmeal (10%) + skim milk powder (34%) + eggs (45%)	71	76.4 (100)	100	90

Source: Data of Pellett (1963); net protein utilization$_{(op)}$ estimated by rat assays.
[1] % of total dietary protein.
[2] Relative ratios.

per gram creatinine per 16 gm of nitrogen ingested was similar for both groups and appeared to be affected by the nutritional value of the dietary protein fed; a relationship which appeared to be dependent on methionine plus cystine being the limiting amino acids. When the peanut butter plus bread diet was supplemented with methionine, however, sulfate excretion exceeded the excretion levels expected relative to sulfur-amino acid intake. The authors suggested that the increased sulfur excretion reflected a deficiency in dietary lysine.

The limited data available suggest that urinary sulfate excretion increases with increasing adequacy of sulfur amino acids when these are limiting, and also, when the sulfur amino acids are present in excess or when other amino acids are limiting. With controlled dietary conditions, relative to sulfur amino acid levels, it is conceivable that urinary sulfate excretion levels (together with urinary nitrogen or creatinine excretion levels) may be a useful approach for predicting protein nutritive value.

ENZYME ACTIVITIES

Amino Transferases

In a study with pigs, Bergner *et al.* (1966) suggested that a useful relationship existed between the biological value of ingested protein and serum alanine aminotransferase activity. Das and Waterlow (1974) noted that liver aspartate and alanine aminotransferase activities were markedly higher in rats fed casein than in rats fed gelatin. Differences occurred within 24 hr after the source of dietary protein was changed from casein to gelatin. However, in a study in which 3–5 subjects were maintained for 4-day periods on diets providing a protein intake level of 1 gm per kg body wt per day, no relationship was observed between nutritive value and levels of plasma or red blood cell aspartate or alanine aminotransferase activity levels (Schuster and Bodwell 1975). The protein sources used included spray dried whole egg, tuna, fish protein concentrate, soy protein concentrate with 0.75% L-methionine added, peanut flour, soy protein concentrate and wheat gluten. At the high levels of protein intake used, differences were not expected. However, the large day-to-day variations in enzyme activities of these enzymes in humans may have little value regardless of the level of protein intake.

SUMMARY

The standard method for estimating protein nutritional value in humans involves the use of nitrogen balance experiments. An "ideal" evaluation using nitrogen balance techniques would involve trials at several different levels of protein intake. The technical difficulties and costs associated with such studies preclude determinations on large numbers of proteins or protein foods. More rapid and less costly evaluation procedures are needed. With the continuously increasing diversity of food products supplying dietary protein, the advent of nutritional labeling, and the increased awareness of consumers, attempts to utilize biochemical indices for this purpose are particularly appropriate. Accordingly, this discussion has focused on an evaluation of the various biochemical parameters which may be utilized in human studies as potential indices of protein nutritional value.

BIBLIOGRAPHY

ALBANESE, A. A., and ORTO, L. A. 1963. Proteins and amino acids. *In* Newer Methods of Nutritional Biochemistry, Vol. I, A. A. Albanese (Editor). Academic Press, New York.

ALMQUIST, H. J. 1954. Utilization of amino acids by chicks. Arch. Biochem. *52*, 197.

ANON. 1969. Factors causing changes in plasma amino acid patterns. Nutr. Rev. *27*, 241.

BERGNER, H., MUNCHOW, H., and REISCHUCK, M. 1971. Proteinbewertung unter Proxisbedingugen mit Hilfe von Blutaharnstoffkonzentration-suntersuchungen an wachsenden Schweinen. Arch. Tierernahrung. *21*, 133.

BERGNER, H., WIRTHGEN, B., and MUNCHOW, H. 1966. Unterschungen zur Proteinbewertung von Futtermitteln. I. Mittellung. Arch. Tierernahrung. *16*, 507.

BERRY, H. K. 1970. Plasma amino acids. *In* Newer Methods of Nutritional Biochemistry, Vol. IV, A. A. Albanese (Editor). Academic Press, New York.

BIGWOOD, E. J., CROKAERT, R., SCHRAM, E., SOUPART, P., and VIS, H. 1959. Amino aciduria. Advan. Clin. Chem. *2*, 201.

BODWELL, C. E. 1975. Biochemical parameters as indices of protein nutritional value. *In* Protein Nutritional Quality of Foods and Feeds, Part 1. Assay Methods-Biological, Biochemical, and Chemical, M. Friedman (Editor). Marcel Dekker, New York.

BODWELL, C. E., and SCHUSTER, E. M. 1974. Plasma and urinary urea levels in humans after ingestion of proteins of different biological value. Federation Proc. *33*, 711.

BODWELL, C. E., and SCHUSTER, E. M. 1975. Changes in postprandial plasma urea N levels in human subjects as potential indices of protein nutritional value in short-term studies. Federation Proc. *34*, 929.

BODWELL, C. E., SCHUSTER, E. M., BROOKS, B., WOMACK, M., and DADE, R. 1976. Postprandial plasma urea nitrogen levels in adult men ingesting proteins of varied nutritional value. (Unpublished data.)

BOLOURCHI, S., FEURIG, J. S., and MICKELSON, O. 1968. Wheat flour, blood urea concentrations, and urea metabolism in adult human subjects. Am. J. Clin. Nutr. *21*, 836.

BROWN, J. A., and CLINE, T. R. 1974. Urea excretion in the pig: an indicator of protein quality and amino acid requirements. J. Nutr. *104*, 542.

CALLOWAY, D. H., and MARGEN, S. 1971. Variation in endogenous nitrogen excretion and dietary nitrogen utilization as determinants of human protein requirement. J. Nutr. *101*, 205.

DAS, T. K., and WATERLOW, J. C. 1974. The rate of adaptation of urea cycle enzymes, aminotransferases and glutamic dehydrogenase to changes in dietary protein intake. Brit. J. Nutr. *32*, 353.

DEN HARTOG, C., and POL, G. 1972. Assays based on measurements of plasma-free amino acids. *In* Protein and Amino Acid Functions, E. J. Bigwood (Editor). Pergamon Press, New York.

EFRON, M. L. 1965A. Aminoaciduria. New Engl. J. Med. *272*, 1058.

EFRON, M. L. 1965B. Aminoaciduria. New Engl. J. Med. *272*, 1107.

EGGUM, B. O. 1970. Blood urea measurement as a technique for assessing protein quality. Brit. J. Nutr. *24*, 983.

FISHER, H. 1965. Variations in the urinary creatinine excretion of rats fed diets with different protein and amino acid content. J. Nutr. *85*, 181.

GITLER, C. 1964. Protein digestion and absorption in nonruminants. *In* Mammalian Protein Metabolism, Vol. I, H. N. Munro, and J. B. Allison (Editors). Academic Press, New York.

GRAHAM, G. G., and PLACKO, R. P. 1973. Postprandial plasma free methionine as an indicator of dietary methionine adequacy in the human infant. J. Nutr. *103*, 1347.

HARPER, A. E. 1964. Amino acid toxicities and imbalances. *In* Mammalian Protein Metabolism, Vol. II, H. N. Munro, and J. B. Allison (Editors). Academic Press, New York.

HARPER, A. E. 1968. Diet and plasma amino acids. Am. J. Clin. Nutr. *21*, 358.

KEAN, E. A. 1967. The relationships between nutritive value of dietary protein and activity of liver arginase and kidney transamidinase enzymes. Brit. J. Nutr. *21*, 29.

KIRIYAMA, S. 1970. Biological quality of dietary protein and urinary nitrogen metabolites. *In* Newer Methods of Nutritional Biochemistry, Vol. IV, A. A. Albanese (Editor). Academic Press, New York.

KIRIYAMA, S., and ASHIDA, K. 1964. Effect of the quality of dietary protein on nitrogen compounds in the urine of rats. J. Nutr. *82*, 127.

KUIKEN, K. A. 1952. Availability of the essential amino acids in cottonseed meal. J. Nutr. *46*, 13.

KUIKEN, K. A., and LYMAN, C. M. 1948. Availability of amino acids in some foods. J. Nutr. *36*, 359.

LONGENECKER, J. B. 1961. Relationship between plasma amino acids and composition of ingested protein. III. Effect of dietary protein on plasma amino acids and clinical chemistry of dogs. *In* Progress in Meeting Protein Needs of Infants and Preschool Children. Publ. *843*, National Research Council-National Academy of Sciences, Washington, D.C.

LONGENECKER, J. B.   1963.   Utilization of dietary proteins.   *In* Newer Methods of Nutritional Biochemistry, Vol. I, A. A. Albanese (Editor).   Academic Press, New York.

LONGENECKER, J. B., and HAUSE, N. L.   1958.   Rate of absorption of supplementary free amino-acids during digestion.   Nature *182*, 1739.

LONGENECKER, J. B., and HAUSE, N. L.   1959.   Relationship between plasma amino acids and composition of the ingested protein.   Arch. Biochem. Biophys. *84*, 46.

LONGENECKER, J. B., and HAUSE, N. L.   1961.   Relationship between plasma amino acids and composition of the ingested protein.   II.   A shortened procedure to determine plasma amino acid (PAA) ratios.   Am. J. Clin. Nutr. *4*, 356.

LONGENECKER, J. B., and LO, G. S.   1974.   Protein digestibility and amino acid availability assessed by concentration changes of plasma amino acids.   *In* Nutrients in Processed Foods, Proteins, P. L. White, and D. C. Fletcher (Editors).   Publishing Sciences Group, Acton, Mass.

MACKENZIE, J. C.   1971.   Nutrition and dialysis.   *In* World Review of Nutrition and Dietetics, Vol. 13, G. H. Bourne (Editor).   S. Karger, Basel, Switzerland.

MCLAUGHLAN, J. M.   1963.   Relationship between protein quality and plasma amino acid levels.   Federation Proc. *22*, 1122.

MCLAUGHLAN, J. M., and MORRISON, A. B.   1968.   Dietary factors affecting plasma amino acid concentrations.   *In* Protein Nutrition and Free Amino Acid Patterns, J. H. Leathem (Editor).   Rutgers Univ. Press, New Brunswick, N.J.

MCLAUGHLAN, J. M., NOEL, F. J., MORRISON, A. B., and CAMPBELL, J. A.   1963.   Blood amino acid studies.   IV.   Some factors affecting plasma amino acid levels in human subjects.   Can. J. Biochem. Physiol. *41*, 191.

MILLER, D. S., and DONOSO, G.   1963.   Relationship between the sulphur/nitrogen ratio and the protein value of diets.   J. Sci. Food Agr. *14*, 345.

MILLER, D. S., and NAISMITH, D. J.   1958.   A correlation between sulphur content and net dietary-protein value.   Nature *182*, 1786.

MUNCHOW, H., and BERGNER, H.   1967.   Untersuchungen zur Protein-bewertung von Futtermitteln. 2.   Mitteilung. Arch. Tierernahrung. *17*, 141.

MURLIN, J. R., HAYES, A. D., and JOHNSON, K.   1953.   Correlation between the biological value of protein and the percentage of creatinine in the urine.   J. Nutr. *41*, 149.

MURLIN, J. R., SZYMANSKI, T. A., and NASSET, E. C.   1948.   Creatinine nitrogen percentage as a check on the biological values of proteins.   J. Nutr. *36*, 171.

NAKAGAWA, I., and MASANA, Y.   1967.   Assessment of nutritional status of men: protein.   J. Nutr. *93*, 135.

NASSET, E. S., and TULLY, III, R. H.   1951.   Urinary excretion of essential amino acids by human subjects fed diets containing proteins of different biological value.   J. Nutr. *44*, 477.

NATL. ACAD. SCI.–NATL. RES. COUNCIL.   1963.   Evaluation of Protein Quality.   Natl. Res. Council-Natl. Acad. Sci. Publ. *1100*.

OSER, B. L.   1951.   Method for integrating essential amino acid content in the nutritional evaluation of protein.   J. Am. Dietet. Assoc. *27*, 396.

PELLETT, P. L.   1963.   *Cited by* Natl. Acad. Sci.–Natl. Res. Council Publ. *1100*.

PION, R.   1973.   The relationship between the levels of free amino acids in blood and muscle and the nutritive value of proteins.   *In* Proteins in Human Nutrition, J. W. G. Porter, and B. A. Rolls (Editors).   Academic Press, New York.

POWELL, R. C., PLOUGH, I. C., and BAKER, III, E. M.   1961.   The use of nitrogen to creatinine ratios in random urine specimens to estimate dietary protein.   J. Nutr. *73*, 47.

PRIOR, R. L., MILNER, J. A., and VISEK, W. J.   1975.   Urea, citrate and orotate excretions in growing rats fed amino acid-deficient diets.   J. Nutr. *105*, 141.

RIPPON, W. P.   1959.   A comparison of several methods for estimating the nutritive value of proteins.   Brit. J. Nutr. *13*, 243.

ROSE, W. C., HAINES, W. J., WARNER, D. T., and JOHNSON, J. E.   1951.   The amino acid requirements of man.   II.   The role of threonine and histidine.   J. Biol. Chem. *188*, 49.

ROSE, W. C., JOHNSON, J. E., and HAINES, W. J.   1950.   The amino acid requirements of man.   I.   The role of valine and methionine.   J. Biol. Chem. *182*, 541.

SABRY, Z. I., SHADAREVIAN, S. B., COWAN, J. W., and CAMPBELL, J. A. 1965. Relationship of dietary intake of sulphur amino acids to urinary excretion of inorganic sulphate in man. Nature *206*, 931.

SCHUSTER, E. M., and BODWELL, C. E. 1975. Fasting human aminotransferase activity after short-term consumption of proteins of different biological value. Federation Proc. *34*, 928.

SCRIMSHAW, N. S., YOUNG, V. R., SCHWARTZ, R., PICHE, M. L., and DAS, J. B. 1966. Minimum dietary essential amino acid-to-total nitrogen ratio for whole egg protein fed to young men. J. Nutr. *89*, 9.

SCRIMSHAW, N. S., TAYLOR, Y., and YOUNG, V. R. 1973. Lysine supplementation of wheat gluten at adequate and restricted energy intakes in young men. Am. J. Clin. Nutr. *26*, 965.

SNYDERMAN, S. E., HOLT, L. E., NORTON, P. M., and ROITMAN, E. 1968. Effect of high and low intakes of individual amino acids on the plasma aminogram. *In* Protein Nutrition and Free Amino Acid Patterns, J. H. Leathem (Editor). Rutgers Univ. Press, New Brunswick, N.J.

SOUPART, P. 1962. Free amino acids of blood and urine in the human. *In* Amino Acid Pools, J. T. Holden (Editor). Elsevier Publishing Co., Amsterdam.

STEELE, B. F., SAUBERLICH, H. E., REYNOLDS, M. S., and BAUMANN, C. A. 1947. Amino acids in the urine of human subjects fed eggs or soybeans. J. Nutr. *33*, 209.

STEPHENS, A. G., and EVANS, R. A. 1972. The distribution of free amino acids netween plasma and blood cells of chicks fed on different proteins. Proc. Nutr. Soc. *31*, 50A.

TAYLOR, Y. S. M., SCRIMSHAW, N. S., and YOUNG, V. R. 1974. The relationship between serum urea levels and dietary nitrogen utilization in young men. Brit. J. Nutr. *32*, 407.

TAYLOR, Y. S. M., YOUNG, V. R., MURRAY, E., PENCHARZ, P. B., and SCRIMSHAW, N. S. 1973. Daily protein and meal patterns affecting young men fed adequate and restricted energy intake. Am. J. Clin. Nutr. *26*, 216.

TONTISIRIN, K., YOUNG, V. R., MILLER, M., and SCRIMSHAW, N. S. 1973. Plasma tryptophan response curve and tryptophan requirements of elderly people. J. Nutr. *103*, 1220.

VAUGHAN, D. A., WOMACK, M., and MCCLAIN, P. E. 1974. Plasma free amino acid levels in human subjects after consuming meals containing lactalbumin, heated lactalbumin or no protein. Federation Proc. *33*, 712.

WATTS, J. H., ALLEN, C. H., and BOOKER, L. K. 1960. Biologic availability of essential amino acids to human subjects. III. Whole egg and beef muscle. J. Am. Dietet. Assoc. *36*, 42.

WATTS, J. H., BOOKER, L. K., MCAFEE, J. W., GRAHAM, D. C. W., and JONES, JR., F. 1959A. Biologic availability of essential amino acids to human subjects. II. Whole egg, milk and cottage cheese. J. Nutr. *67*, 497.

WATTS, J. H., BOOKER, L. K., MCAFEE, J. W., WILLIAMS, E. G., WRIGHT, W. G., and JONES, JR., F. 1959B. Biologic availability of essential amino acids to human subjects. I. Whole egg, pork muscle and peanut butter. J. Nutr. *67*, 483.

WHITAKER, T. R., and PATRICK, H. 1971. A plasma amino acid method for determining protein quality. W. Va. Univ. Agr. Exp. Sta., Bull. *605T*.

YOKOTA, F. 1964A. Effect of excess glycine on rats (report 1). Effect of glycine on the growth of rats. Jap. J. Nutr. *22*, 190. (Japanese)

YOKOTA, F. 1964B. Effect of excess glycine on rats (report 2). Amino acids and creatinine in urine of rats fed an excess glycine diet. Jap. J. Nutr. *22*, 193. (Japanese)

YOUNG, V. R., FAJARDO, L., MURRAY, E., RAND, W. M., and SCRIMSHAW, N. W. 1975. Protein requirements of man: comparative nitrogen balance response within the sub-maintenance-to-maintenance range of intakes of wheat and beef proteins. J. Nutr. *105*, 534.

YOUNG, V. R., HUSSEIN, M. A., MURRAY, E., and SCRIMSHAW, N. S. 1971. Plasma tryptophan response curve and its relation to tryptophan requirements in young adult men. J. Nutr. *101*, 45.

YOUNG, V. R., and SCRIMSHAW, N. S. 1972. The nutritional significance of plasma and urinary amino acids. *In* Protein and Amino Acid Functions, E. J. Bigwood (Editor). Pergamon Press, New York.

YOUNG, V. R., TAYLOR, Y. S. M., RAND, W. M., and SCRIMSHAW, N. S.   1973.   Protein requirements of man: efficiency of egg protein utilization at maintenance and submaintenance levels in young men.   J. Nutr. *103*, 1164.

YOUNG, V. R., TONTISIRIN, K., OZALP, I., LAKSHMANAN, F., and SCRIMSHAW, N. S.   1972. Plasma amino acid response curve and amino acid requirements in young men: valine and lysine.   J. Nutr. *102*, 1159.

CHAPTER 7

G. A. Miller
and P. A. Lachance

Techniques in Rat Bioassays

Protein quality assessment, with the rat as the experimental model, quite often suffers from poorly designed methodology. This situation creates problems of reproducibility and validity (Greenfield and Briggs 1971). The purpose of this chapter is to stress the need for specific attention to the experimental methodology in the assessment of protein quality. Investigators either choose to adopt specific methods for assessing protein nutritive value or are required by specific federal food labeling regulations to utilize the Association of Official Agricultural Chemists' (AOAC) rat bioassay method for determining the protein efficiency ratio of a food. Irrespective of the method chosen, the general guidelines provided are insufficient to ensure accurate and reproducible results. This chapter describes the basis for the various measures of protein nutritive value and discusses, in particular, the methodological parameters which can be sources of error. All the methods to be discussed refer to bioassays in which the rat is used as the experimental animal. Fisher (1973) has discussed the use of the chick and rabbit. Samonds and Hegsted (1973) have worked with the cebus monkey, and Allison (1949) has worked with dogs.

GENERAL CONSIDERATIONS

There have been many techniques developed to measure the biological and nutritive quality of proteins. Each method must attempt to evaluate the ability of a protein to furnish a mixture of amino acids that will promote synthesis of body tissue and maintenance of body tissue and function. To date, the primary focus of attention has been on methods which measure, or correlate with, the effect of a protein on nitrogen stores. None of the procedures developed have gained universal acceptance, and none is without significant problems (see Chapter 4). Many of the problems associated with protein quality assays can be minimized if care is taken in the protocol used to perform these procedures.

Environment of the Animal Room

Environmental conditions are important in the control of proper experimental conditions for the assessment of protein quality. The temperature of the animal room should be maintained at about the optimum for small rodents, 22–24°C, with adequate ventilation. The relative humidity should be held in the range of 50–60%. These conditions are necessary for the comfort and health of the animals. Lighting should be controlled to a 12 hr light–12 hr dark schedule and windows should be avoided (Lane-Petter and Pearson 1971).

Transient environmental disturbances (TED's) have been shown by Halberg (1959) to be a stressor. TED's are mild stressors such as noise, irregular entrances into the animal environment and inconsistent handling procedures. To decrease the variability induced by TED's, access to the animal facilities should be restricted. Time of entry and exit into and out of the animal room in relation to the light-dark schedule should be standardized, and the time span of human activity in the room should be kept to a minimum. The people who handle the animals should do so as similarly as possible and extraneous noises should be held to a minimum. This will not only decrease induced variability, but also make handling of laboratory animals much easier.

The maintenance of constant environmental conditions removes one source of variation that can be found in protein quality assessment tests. The animal laboratory should have a recording temperature and humidity device, and these records should be included in the data record book. Some institutions alter heat and air conditioning on weekends and holidays for economic reasons and, further, breakdowns do occur. Without records, the investigator cannot correlate and interpret data accordingly.

The type and size of caging can be of significance. Nolen and Black (1973) have shown that the size of the cage can affect the estimation of protein quality, and the standard size rat cage (7 in. × 9½ in. × 7 in.) should be used. Since rats defecate indiscriminately and cohrophagy can occur, wire screen bottom cages are suggested. Many materials have been utilized for the manufacture of caging. The type of caging material used is important. Galvanized steel has been used because of its relative inexpensiveness. The galvanized cage provides zinc to the rats through their gnawing on the cage. Since stainless steel has begun to replace galvanized steel, because of its strength and durability, there is a need for zinc to be added to mineral mixes of rat diets.

Feed dishes should be large enough to allow true *ad libitum* feeding, however, containers sufficient to hold 2–3 days' diet rather than several days' diet should be used. Food should be changed every other day, and residual food should be discarded. Further, a feeding system that reduces spillage, and decreases the potential of fecal and/or urinary contamination of food should be used. For this purpose there seems to be no perfect system at this time. Caging with special feeding tunnels are available but unless concomitant urine and fecal collection is desired, this type of metabolism caging is rarely used because of its expense.

The water bottle should be filled periodically with fresh clean water. The bottles, corks and tubes should be washed once a week and stopper guards should be employed to prevent the consumption of the bottle stoppers.

Handling of Laboratory Rats

The manner of handling of laboratory animals is very important. Gloves, forceps, or any other means, except the use of the hand, to pick up laboratory rats should be avoided. The rat should be picked up by placing the palm of the hand on the rat's back with the thumb and index finger being used to fold the forelegs under the chin. This method will prevent the rat from biting the handler. The body should not be squeezed because excess pressure on the rat can cause respiratory problems. The rat should not be picked up by the tail (Griffith 1949). Further, Antelman (1975) has shown that mild tail pinching rapidly and reliably induced eating, gnawing, or licking behavior. Therefore, rats being handled by the tail may be induced to eat, while those handled normally are not. Proper handling of rats (especially weanling animals) will lead to a "taming" of the rats and effects of handling, as a variable in the method, will be decreased.

Adaptation of Laboratory Rats

The duration of adaptation periods and diets used during protein quality work are rarely reported. Adaptation periods allow rats to adapt to all the environmental conditions present and the type of diets to be used. Further, considerable taming can occur during the adaptation period.

A four day adaptation period allows for the experimenter to determine whether any animal is diseased, and for adaptation of the rats to the protocol to be used. A semisynthetic diet identical in design to the diets used during the experimental period should be used. The protein should be of sufficient quality as to allow normal growth to occur. The choice of protein for the adaptation period diet should be chosen so that the same protein may be used in most of the studies conducted.

Diet

All dietary components should be carefully chosen, and all pertinent data concerning the ingredients should be known. Diets should not be mixed until needed, and proximate analysis of the mixed diets should be performed to assure no mixing error has occurred. Amino acid analysis of protein sources is quite useful and should be done whenever possible. This allows the researcher to troubleshoot problems before they occur. The vitamin mix, the protein, and the fat sources, as well as the mixed diet, should be stored in a refrigerator (4°C). This will increase the shelf stability of the components and the diets, and will decrease deterioration and loss of specific nutrients.

Control Groups

As in any analytical procedure, control groups or standards must be included to correct for routine experimental variations. In protein quality

TABLE 7.1

A COMPARISON OF INDISPENSABLE AMINO ACID COMPOSITIONS AND CHEMICAL
SCORES OF TWO LOTS OF LACTALBUMIN PURCHASED AT TWO SEPARATE TIMES
FROM A SINGLE SUPPLY SOURCE

Indispensable Amino Acid	Lactalbumin Lot 1 (mg/gm Protein)	Lactalbumin Lot 2 (mg/gm Protein)	FAO[1] Provisional Pattern
Isoleucine	45.1	33.2	40
Leucine	96.1	89.6	70
Lysine	78.0	65.6	55
Methionine and cystine	43.2	32.7	35
Phenylalanine and tyrosine	64.2	54.8	60
Threonine	43.0	41.9	40
Tryptophan	—	—	10
Valine	47.5[2]	34.9[2]	50
Chemical Score[3]	95%	70%	

[1] FAO (1973).
[2] Most limiting indispensable amino acid.
[3] Chemical score is the percentage of the standard (FAO) that the most limiting amino acid yields.

assessment this means the inclusion of an extra diet group. Usually casein is the protein source used in control group diets, but lactalbumin is also used. Lactalbumin as purchased from a supply house is not a consistent product, but is composed of various proteins, and the relative concentrations of these proteins varies from batch to batch. Table 7.1 demonstrates the variability found in the indispensible amino acid compositions of two lots of lactalalbumin purchased from the same supplier on two different occasions.

Animal Nutrition Research Council (ANRC) casein is a blended casein with a decreased variability in amino acid composition due to season, breed, processing, etc. (ANRC casein can be purchased from Sheffield Chemical, Lyndhurst, N.J. 07071.) We have found ANRC casein to be the most consistent source of casein. Investigators often use casein sources other than ANRC in spite of the specific AOAC guidelines. This practice should be avoided unless stringent quality control measurements are available to assure consistency from lot to lot.

Other problems exist in defining control groups for protein quality assessment. Morrison and Campbell (1960) have shown that different strains of rats give different protein efficiency ratios. Schemmel et al. (1970) have shown that rats of different strains have different growth rates. However, rat strain may only have a nominal effect on a 10% casein control group for protein efficiency ratios (Hegarty 1975; Hurt et al. 1975). The sex of the rats used can also affect growth rates, with males showing a more rapid growth rate than females (Osborne and Mendel 1912). Further, the age of the rats used will have an effect on protein quality assessment. Chapman *et al.* (1959) reported that 29-day-old rats gave lower protein efficiency ratios than 21- to 23-day-old rats.

Is is not sufficient to define a controlled experiment by age, sex, strain, environmental conditions and diet fed of the control group. The use of a genetic potential (GP) curve of the control group will help the investigator determine whether or not the experiment was truly controlled. The regression of weight of rat and age of rat should be developed for the defined control groups used in all experiments. Any significant deviation from the GP curve in any one study would indicate that a stressor has become involved in the experimental procedure. In that case reproducibility and validity will suffer greatly. GP curves take time to develop; however, institutions providing rats to a laboratory can provide a base of data for initial comparisons.

Reporting of Data

The reporting of protein quality data is often insufficiently detailed. All the general environmental conditions discussed above should be included in the material and methods section of the publication, as well as an unambiguous and concise description of all experimental diets. A description of a biochemical technique would include every step and condition used, and this should be followed in nutrition methodology. This is necessary if protein quality work is to be reproducible within one and/or between several laboratories.

METHODS

Protein Efficiency Ratio (PER)

The PER developed by Osborne *et al.* (1919) is presently the most widely utilized procedure for the evaluation of protein quality, and it is the official method for the measurement of protein quality for nutritional labeling (FDA 1973). Several collaborative assays have been performed (Derse 1960, 1962), and a great deal of work has been done to standardize this procedure. However, the PER is often improperly performed.

The officially recognized procedure for the evaluation of protein quality is the PER method described by AOAC (1975). The diet suggested is described in Table 7.2, and the composition of the vitamin mix in Table 7.3.

The experimental animals required are male weanling rats, of the same strain, and in the age range of 21–28 days. The weight range should be less than 10 gm, and an acclimation period of 3–7 days is suggested for shipped rats.

TABLE 7.2

DIET COMPOSITION SUGGESTED FOR PER ASSAY

Ingredient	Quantity (%)
Protein	$X = 1.60 \times 100/\%$ N sample (10% protein)
Cottonseed oil	$8—X \times \%$ ether extract/100
Salt mixture (USD XIX)	$5—X \times \%$ ash/100
Vitamin mix (AOAC)	1
Cellulose	$1—X \times \%$ crude fiber/100
Water	$5—X \times \%$ moisture/100
Sucrose or cornstarch	To make 100

TABLE 7.3

AOAC VITAMIN MIX COMPOSITION

Ingredient	mg/gm Ration[1]
Vitamin A (dry stabilized)	2000 IU
Vitamin D (dry stabilized)	200 IU
Vitamin E (dry stabilized)	10 IU
Menadione	0.5
Choline	200
p-Aminobenzoic acid	10
Inositol	10
Niacin	4
Ca-pantothenate	4
Riboflavin	0.8
Thiamin, H Cl	0.5
Pyridoxine, H Cl	0.5
Folic acid	0.2
Biotin	0.04
Vitamin B-12	0.003
Glucose to make	1000

[1]Except for vitamins A, D, and E.

The PER is a 28-day assay with ANRC casein used as the reference protein. Groups should consist of 10 or more rats with a mean difference in weight between groups of 5 gm or less on the first day of the assay period. Body weight and food consumption should be measured regularly, and not less than every seventh day. Rats are caged individually, and provided food and water *ad libitum.*

The calculation of PER is given in the following equation:

$$PER = \frac{\text{weight gain}}{\text{protein consumed}}$$

This is done for each animal, and a mean is then calculated for each protein group. The test groups are corrected by multiplying the PER values of the test proteins by the following fraction.

$$\frac{2.5}{\text{PER of reference}}$$
$$\text{ANRC casein}$$

Another means for correcting PER data is to express the data as a percentage of the PER of casein. Because PER is not a linear function, a percentage casein PER value should not be interpreted as percentage of casein nutritive value.

This AOAC procedure has several problems associated with it. The diet composition is only suggested and many researchers change the diet as suits their need. For example, many food products have a fat level that is too high to obtain an 8% fat level in the final diet.

The main concern is that all diets in a PER assay be as similar as is possible. Hurt *et al.* (1975) has shown that the most significant dietary factor in the PER assay is the protein level. When other dietary factors were changed (i.e., level or type of fat, moisture level) the corrected PER was not significantly affected. However, until a specific diet is established that can be used more universally than the present AOAC (1975) *suggested* diet, problems of reproducibility and precision will continue to occur.

The weight range of 5 gm between test groups may be too large. Attempts should be made to reduce the mean weight difference of the test groups on the first day of assay. A goal of 1 gm or less difference between each group is a more acceptable goal.

Net Protein Ratio (NPR)

The NPR was developed by Bender and Doell (1957) in an attempt to resolve some of the theoretical problems associated with the PER. The diet suggested for the NPR, the characteristics of the test animals and characteristics of the dietary groups should be the same as described above for the PER. The NPR is only a 10-day assay, and a no-protein group is included to estimate the maintenance requirement. The use of a casein control group is suggested. The NPR can be calculated by the following formula.

$$\text{NPR} = \frac{\begin{array}{cc}\text{weight gain} & \text{weight loss} \\ \text{(test protein)} & \text{(no protein)}\end{array}}{\text{test protein consumed}}$$

The weight loss factor is calculated by determining the mean of weight lost in the no-protein group. The NPR is then calculated for each animal and the mean value is then expressed as a percentage of the corresponding value for the casein control group. NPR can be routinely included in PER tests by the inclusion of the no-protein test group.

Relative Protein Value (RPV)

Relative nutritive value (RNV) was developed by Hegsted and Chang (1965), and Hegsted *et al.* (1968) by using a slope-ratio technique. Samonds and Hegsted (see Chapter 4) modified this procedure with the deletion of the no-protein test group. This procedure is called the relative protein value (RPV), and the most detailed description is presented in the Protein Advisory Group (PAG) Bulletin (PAG 1975).

The diet is composed of vegetable oil, 10%, salt mix, 3% (Bernhardt and Tomeralli 1966), vitamin mix, 1% (Hegsted and Chang 1965), and variable protein levels (e.g., 2, 5, and 8% protein or 0.3, 0.8, and 1.3% N). The rest of the diet is made up to 100% with corn starch. The fat and fiber levels should be adjusted to include the amounts present in the test material.

Weanling rats (21- to 23-days-old) of a single strain are placed in individual cages and adapted with a control diet of 1.3% N. ANRC casein is suggested as the reference control by PAG (1975), and lactalbumin is suggested by Samonds and Hegsted (in press). The adaptation period is of 2-days duration. The rats are then divided into groups of four rats of equal weight and sex distribution. Weight variation between groups should be kept at a minimum, and should not exceed 1 gm difference between group means at the beginning of the assay period.

For each protein tested, at least three groups of four rats are needed with each group being fed a different dietary level of nitrogen. Food consumption and weight gain must be recorded regularly and at least weekly. The test period suggested by PAG (1975) is 14 days while Samonds and Hegsted (see Chapter 4) suggest 21 days.

The regression of weight gain on nitrogen intake is calculated for each protein, and the slope of the regression line is used to calculate the RPV as follows.

$$\text{RPV} = \frac{\text{slope of test material}}{\text{slope of reference protein}}$$

When calculating the slopes one must be sure that the data used is located in the linear portion of the weight gain to nitrogen intake response. Either too high or too low a dietary intake level of protein can displace the response to a curvilinear portion of the relationship. This will create errors in the interpretation of the data. The RPV method is relatively new, and more complete and specific protocols seem necessary to improve its reproducibility.

Nitrogen Balance Techniques (Biological Value; Nitrogen Balance)

Thomas (1909) described the first quantitative method for biologically evaluating dietary proteins. This method, biological value (BV), was developed using adult human subjects, is tedious because it requires precise collection and measurement of food and excreta. BV was expressed by Thomas (1909) by the following formula.

$$BV = \frac{\text{nitrogen retained}}{\text{nitrogen absorbed}}$$

Mitchell (1923–1924) adapted the method to growing and adult rats and further defined the formula as follows.

BV =

$$\frac{\text{N intake} - (\text{fecal N} - \text{metabolic N}) - (\text{urinary N} - \text{endogeneous N})}{\text{N intake} - (\text{fecal N} - \text{metabolic N})}$$

Metabolic N and endogenous N are measured when test animals are fed a nitrogen-free diet, but endogeneous N can be estimated from body weight (Mitchell 1923–1924; Tagle and Donoso 1965). The length of balance periods can be as short as 4 days (Henry 1965), and as long as 7 days (Mitchell 1923–1924). At least ten rats should be included for each protein. Weanling rats of the same strain are used as are individual metabolism cages.

Biological value is affected by the level of protein fed (Mitchell 1123–1924). Henry and Kon (1957) have shown that a dietary level of 8–10% protein is best when growing rats are used. Therefore, diets similar to the PER diets as suggested by AOAC (1975) or the RPV diets as suggested by PAG (1975) could be used. A control reference protein should be evaluated with each test as in other protein quality tests. At least 3 days of test diet feeding should elapse before the balance period is begun with the collection of urine and feces. Food and water are provided *ad libitum*. Collection of urine and feces should be done no less than every other day. Feces and urine can be frozen prior to Kjedahl analysis for N. Markers can be used as indicators of when a dietary sample has begun to be excreted in the feces, and when the dietary sample has cleared the gastrointestinal tract. Markers should be chemicals that are not affected or do not affect the gastrointestinal tract. Davignon *et. al.* (1968) has used Cr_2O_3 in humans as a marker as has Snook (1973) in rats. Carmine dye (Oser 1965) has also been used as a marker. Many other substances are used with no perfect system of marking yet designed, and quite often feces are collected on a time basis.

This method is tedious and has a problem of cumulative errors that decrease precision. Problems occur in completely separating urine, feces, and food, which further affects the precision of the method.

A simpler though less quantitative procedure is nitrogen balance (NB) where:

$$NB = N \text{ intake} - (\text{urinary, fecal, and skin N losses})$$

In contrast to BV this method does include digestion. However, the assumption is made that endogenous and metabolic nitrogen will not differ significantly from animal to animal, and thus the method is less rigorous than BV. Very carefully controlled conditions must be maintained for reproducibility and precision. Normally, a 4-day balance period is preceded by a 3-day adaptation period. Generally, this procedure is not used in estimating protein nutritive value because more precise rat bioassay methods are available, such as PER, NPR, and net protein utilization (NPU) (McLaughlan 1972).

Net Protein Utilization (NPU)

Previously NPU was derived from balance sheet techniques by the following formula.

$$NPU = BV \times \text{true digestibility}$$

Bender and Miller (1953) developed a direct carcass analysis technique. In this approach male weanling rats of the same strain are used. They are fed diets similar to that described for the PER (AOAC 1975). A group of 10 rats, individually caged, are necessary as well as a no-protein group of 10 rats. A casein control reference group is advised. The food and water are provided *ad libitum.*

The duration of the test is 10 days, at which time the rats are sacrificed and the carcass is analyzed for nitrogen content. NPU is calculated by the following formula.

NPU =

$$\frac{(\text{body N of test protein group} - \text{body N of protein free group})}{\text{N intake of test group}} \times 100$$

It should be noted that whole carcass analysis is tedious and precision can be a problem. Attempts to utilize body water as an indicator for body nitrogen, as suggested by Miller and Bender (1955), has been supported by the work of Middleton *et al.* (1960), Donoso and Yanez (1962), Hegsted *et al.* (1968), and the PAG collaborative studies (PAG 1964). However, Henry (1965) and Stucki and Harper (1962) found that there are significant differences in the nitrogen to water ratios in rats on different diets. Also, Forbes and Yohe (1955) found high body-water content in rats which previously had been moderately deficient in protein. Henry (1965) observed that these differences, though statistically significant, did not affect the accuracy of the procedure. Further, Lachance and Miller (1973) have shown that hind limb nitrogen concentration correlates with whole carcass nitrogen concentration when weanling rats are fed a diet surfeit in protein (11%) for 28 days. Bressani (1975) has shown the same correlation with a

10-day experiment period. While attempts to make the estimation of nitrogen retention easier may be useful, total carcass N is still the method of preference in most laboratories. Carcasses are prepared for analysis by making openings in the abdominal, thoracic, and cranial areas. The gastrointestinal tract does not need to be flushed of residual materials (Rasmussen and McCully 1972). The carcasses are then dried at 105°C for 2 days. The whole carcass is then ground to a homogenous mass, and samples taken for Kjeldahl analysis. This method provides more reproducible results, with lower variation in the determination of whole carcass nitrogen, than do methods utilizing whole fresh, or defatted, carcass procedures (Braham *et al.* 1967). The NPU method is tedious and little or no precision is gained over other methods (Henry 1965; Miller *et al.* 1973).

CONCLUSIONS

Various rat bioassay methods for the estimation of protein quality have been discussed. All methods discussed measure the efficiency of nitrogen retention, but from different perspectives. Precision is a problem with these methods and more specific protocols are necessary if reproducibility is to be gained.

BIBLIOGRAPHY

ALLISON, J. B. 1949. Biological evaluation of proteins. *In* Advances in Protein Chemistry, Vol. 5, M. L. Anson, and J. T. Edsall (Editors). Academic Press, New York.

ANTLEMAN, S. 1975. Tail pinch induces eating in sated rats which appears to be dependent upon nigrostrinal dopamine. Science *189*, 731.

AOAC. 1975. Official Methods of Analysis, 12th Edition. Assoc. of Official Agricultural Chemists, Washington D.C.

BENDER, A. E., and DOELL, B. H. 1957. Biological evaluation of proteins: A new aspect. Brit. J. Nutr. *11*, 140.

BENDER, A. E., and MILLER, D. S. 1953. New brief method of estimating net protein value. Biochem. J. *53*, vii.

BERNHARDT, F. W., and TOMARELLI, R. M. 1966. A salt mixture supplying the National Research Council estimates of the mineral requirements of rats. J. Nutr. *89*, 495.

BRAHAM, J. E., ELIAS, L. G., DEZAGHI, S., and BRESSANI, R. 1967. Effect of protein level and duration of test on carcass composition, net protein utilization and protein efficiency ratio. Nutr. Dieta. *9*, 99.

BRESSANI, R. 1975. Personal communication.

CHAPMAN, D. G., CASTILLO, R., and CAMPBELL, J. A. 1959. Evaluation of protein in foods. I. A method for the determination of protein efficiency ratios. Can. J. Biochem. Physiol. *37*, 679.

DAVIGNON, J., SIMMONDS, W. J., and AHRENS, E. H. Jr. 1968. Usefulness of chromic oxide as an internal standard for balance studies in formula fed patients and for assessment of colonic function. J. Clin. Invest. *47*, 127.

DERSE, P. 1960. Evaluation of protein quality (Biological method). J. Assoc. Offic. Agr. Chem. *43*, 38.

DERSE, P. 1962. Evaluation of protein quality (Biological method). J. Assoc. Offic. Agr. Chem. *45*, 418.

DONOSO, G., and YANEZ, E. 1962. Estudio sobre el méthodo de Miller y Bender para la determinación de la utilización proteica neta. Nutr. Bromatol. Toxicol. *1*, 37.

FAO. 1973. Energy and Protein Requirement. Report of a Joint Ad Hoc Expert FAO/WHO

Committee, Rome, Mar. 22–Apr. 2, 1971. Food and Agriculture Organization, Rome, Italy.

FISHER, H. 1973. Methods of protein evaluation: Assays with chicks and rabbits. *In* Proteins in Human Nutrition, J. W. G. Porter, and B. A. Rolls (Editors). Academic Press, New York.

FD. 1973. Federal Register *38,* 13, Part III, 2131.

FORBES, R. M., and YOHE, M. 1955. Net protein value of blood fibrin for the albino rat: Evaluation of nitrogen balance and carcass method. J. Nutr. *55,* 493.

GREENFIELD, H., and BRIGGS, G. M. 1971. Nutrition methodology in metabolic research with rats. Ann. Rev. Biochem. *40,* 549.

GRIFFITH, J. Q. 1949. General methods. *In* The Rat in Laboratory Investigations, J. Q. Griffith (Editor). Lippincott Co., Philadelphia, Pa.

HALBERG, F. 1959. Physiologic 24 hour periodicity; general and procedural considerations with reference to the adrenal cycle. Z. Vitamin-Hormon-Fermentforsch. *10,* 225.

HEGARTY, P. V. T. 1975. Some biological considerations in the nutritional evaluation of foods. Food Technol. *29,* 52.

HEGSTED, D. M., and CHANG, Y. 1965. Protein utilization in growing rats. J. Nutr. *85,* 159.

HEGSTED, D. M., NEFF, R., and WORCHESTER, J. 1968. Determination of relative nutritive value of protein. Factors affecting precision and validity. J. Agr. Food Chem. *16,* 190.

HENRY, K. 1965. A comparison of biological methods with rats for determining the nutritive value of proteins. Brit. J. Nutr. *19,* 125.

HENRY, K., and KON, S. D. 1957. Effect of level of intake and age of rat on biological value of proteins. Brit. J. Nutr. *11,* 305.

HURT, H. D., FORSYTHE, R. H., and KRIEGER, C. H. 1975. Factors which influence the biological evaluation of protein quality by the protein efficiency ratio method. *In* Protein Nutritional Quality of Foods and Feeds. Part I. Assay Methods-Biological, Biochemical, and Chemical, M. Friedman, (Editor). Marcel Dekker, New York.

LACHANCE, P. A., and MILLER, G. A. 1973. Protein quality assessment in the rat: Correlation between whole carcass and hind limb nitrogen concentration. Nutr. Rept. Int. *7,* 25.

LANE-PETTER, W., and PEARSON, A. E. G. 1971. The Laboratory Animal Principles and Practice. Academic Press, New York.

MCLAUGHLAN, J. M. 1972. Effects of protein quality and quantity on protein utilization. *In* Newer Methods of Nutritional Biochemistry, Vol. V, A. A. Albanese, (Editor). Academic Press, New York.

MIDDLETON, E. J., MORRISON, A. B., and CAMPBELL, J. A. 1960. Evaluation of proteins in foods. VI: Further factors effecting the PER of foods. Can. J. Biochem. Physiol. *38,* 865.

MILLER, D. S., and BENDER, A. E. 1955. The determination of net protein utilization by a shortened method. Brit. J. Nutr. *9,* 383.

MILLER, G. A., MOLINA, M. R., MARTINEZ, M. L., and LACHANCE, P. A. 1973. Questionable importance of rat carcass nitrogen concentration in net protein utilization. Nutr. Rept. Intern. *8,* 153.

MITCHELL, H. H. 1923–1924. A method for determining the biological value of protein. J. Biol. Chem. *58,* 873.

MORRISON, A. B., and CAMPBELL, J. A. 1960. Evaluation of proteins in food. V. Factors influencing the protein efficiency ratio of foods. J. Nutr. *70,* 112.

NOLEN, G. A., and BLACK, D. L. 1973. The effect of cage size on the determination of protein quality by protein efficiency ratio or slope ratio assay. Federation Proc. *32,* 911.

OSBORNE, T. B., and MENDEL, L. B. 1912. Maintenance experiments with isolated proteins. J. Biol. Chem. *13,* 233.

OSBORNE, T. B., MENDEL, L. B., and FERRY, E. L. 1919. A method for expressing numerically the growth promoting value of a protein. J. Biol. Chem. *37,* 223.

OSER, B. L. 1965. Hawk's Physiological Chemistry, 14th Edition. McGraw-Hill Book Co., New York.

PAG. 1964. Collaborative study on protein evaluation. Nutr. Doc. R. 6/Ad. 3. Unipub Inc., New York.

PAG. 1975. PAG Guideline (No. 16) on protein methods for cereal breeders as related to human nutritional requirements. Protein Advisory Group Bull. 5.

RASMUSSEN, A. E., and MCCULLY, M. T. 1972. Evaluation of techniques used to assess the utilization of amino acids from protein by the weanling rat. Univ. Delaware Agr. Expt. Sta. Bull. 388.

SAMONDS, K. W., and HEGSTED, D. M. 1973. Protein requirements of young cebus monkeys. Am. J. Clin. Nutr. 26, 30.

SAMONDS, K. W., and HEGSTED, D. M. A collaborative study to evaluate four methods of estimating protein quality: protein efficiency ratio, net protein ratio, protein value and relative protein value. In Evaluation of Protein Foods (Revision of Publ. 1100), Natl. Acad. Sci., Washington, D.C. (in press).

SCHEMMEL, R., MICKELSON, O., and GILL, J. L. 1970. Dietary obesity in rats: Body weight and body weight accretion in seven strains of rats. J. Nutr. 100, 1041.

SNOOK, J. T. 1973. Protein digestion. In World Review of Nutrition and Dietetics, Vol. 18. G. H. Bourne (Editor). S. Karger, Basel, Switzerland.

STUCKI, W. P., and HARPER, A. E. 1962. Effect of altering the ratio of indispensable to dispensable amino acids in diets for rats. J. Nutr. 78, 278.

TAGLE, M. A., and DONOSO, G. 1965. Net protein utilization in short and long-term experiments with rats. J. Nutr. 87, 173.

THOMAS, K. 1909. Ueber die biologische wertigkert der stickstoff-substanzen in vershieden nahrungsmitteln. Arch. Anat. Physiol. Abstr. 219.

CHAPTER 8

C. V. Kies

Techniques in Human Nitrogen Balance Studies

The nitrogen balance method has long been favored as the research approach to studying amino acid/protein requirements of human adults, children, and infants. Bioassay of protein quality of food products also most commonly uses this method when human beings are employed directly as test organisms. Unlike animal studies, methods based on growth rate (growing subjects) or repletion rate (adult subjects) have not proved popular in human studies because of the placement of substantial physiological stress on the individuals involved—an obvious ethical and practical concern in working with humans.

Nitrogen balance type studies are done with animals as well as with humans. Basically the same formula [i.e., nitrogen balance = nitrogen intake − nitrogen excretion (urine nitrogen + stool nitrogen)] is used for both. In some laboratories, sweat, hair, and skin nitrogen losses are also determined or estimated as part of the nitrogen balance formula. These procedures are difficult, time-consuming and so unwieldy as to be unpractical for routine use. Other refinements in the nitrogen balance formula have been suggested but the aforementioned formula is most frequently used. Techniques used for obtainment of data in the formula are quite different when applied to humans or when applied to animals. Because animal experimentation is far more widespread than is human experimentation, animal study nitrogen balance techniques are more universally understood than are those related to human studies. This has led to some misunderstandings in interpretations of results of human nitrogen balance studies.

In this chapter techniques used in human nitrogen balance studies done in the Department of Food and Nutrition, University of Nebraska—Lincoln, will be described in some detail. Techniques of the nitrogen balance method certainly did not originate at the University of Nebraska, nor is the University of Nebraska the only institution where the procedures are currently in use. Such studies have been done almost continuously at the laboratory for over 30 yr under the direction of several research scientists. In describing the techniques currently in use which evolved over this period of time, the objective is not to define some sort of a standard by which others could grade their own approaches. Furthermore, it certainly is not meant as a guide to novices attempting to initiate human subject research programs of their own. Such individuals are urged to spend some time at one or more of the several institutions which also have laboratories competent in this research area; e.g., The University of Wisconsin—Madison, University of California—Berkeley, Massachusetts Institute of Technology—Cambridge. The true objective of this chapter is to inform the user of human nutrition research information in how nitrogen balance data are obtained in one laboratory so as to better appreciate the inherent strengths and weaknesses of such information. Several manuals on how human nitrogen balance studies are conducted have been published (DeHaas and Morse 1968; Leichsenring et al. 1958; Foman 1967). Discussion here will be primarily limited to laboratory-controlled, open-subject studies. Techniques involved in out-patient clinical studies and to locked-ward hospital studies are somewhat different.

RESEARCH PLAN

Obviously, the research plan of any study is designed as an expression of its objective. Unlike the PER method for judging protein quality using inbred strains of white rats, agreement on application of the nitrogen balance in judging protein quality in humans has not been reached. Some similarities in design of human nitrogen balance studies do exist regardless of objective.

Dietary nitrogen intake of subjects while receiving their pre-experimental, self-selected diets is usually unknown but is assumed to be different than that level chosen for the experimental diet regime. For this reason, studies usually start with an introductory period to allow subjects to adjust to the new dietary nitrogen level. Depending upon the subject and the change in dietary nitrogen involved, it may require 8–12 or more days for an individual to reach a relatively steady-state of urinary nitrogen excretion. We have found that initial feeding of a very low nitrogen diet (0.5–0.8 gm nitrogen per subject per day) can hasten this adjustment and shorten the length of this introductory period. During this period, education of subjects and determination of energy intake for the weight maintenance of each individual also takes place.

Following this introductory period, a series of experimental periods follow. Nitrogen balance studies involving humans nearly always include some kind of cross-over design so that each individual subject receives all experimental treatments and can act as his/her own control. Difference in genetic background of humans influencing quantitative nitrogen balance are great. Numbers of individuals per group would have to be very large in order for statistically meaningful data to be collected in a group comparison-type study as is usually done with inbred animals. The simplest approach involves comparison of the protein in question against a known standard protein. Standard proteins frequently used include albumin and casein. Mixtures of purified L-amino acids patterned after the amino acid composition of egg or milk or according to recommendations of Food and Agriculture Organization (FAO 1973), National Research Council–National Academy of Sciences (Natl. Res. Council–Natl. Acad. Sci. 1974), Rose (1957), Leverton (1959), or others are also sometimes used for this purpose. If a food source of protein rather than a protein per se is desired, whole dried egg and dried skim milk have frequently been employed.

A study involving one experimental product in comparison with a control product would probably involve two experimental periods. Regardless of the number of experimental periods used, to minimize the effects of order of presentation and of time, the order of experimental periods is randomized for each subject. Pattern of response, rather than actual quantity response then becomes of importance in interpretation of results.

Length of experimental periods is an area of controversy among researchers doing human nitrogen balance studies. Under even the most controlled, favorable conditions, nitrogen balance figures for an individual show shifting tendencies. This suggests use of long experimental periods. The cost in time, effort, and money encourages use of the shortest possible experimental periods for obtainment of valid data. In our laboratory, a minimum length of 4 days for each experimental period is set when nitrogen intakes are kept constant from one experimental period to the next. If dietary nitrogen intake varies from one experimental period to the next, then the minimum is set at 7 days. When possible, longer periods are used.

Number of experimental subjects needed per study is also a matter of some disagreement. Large numbers of subjects are advantageous in establishment of statistically significant results. The great expense of human studies of this type is directly proportional to the number of subjects used suggesting use of small groups. Although many important studies have been reported using four to six subjects, we prefer to use groups of 10 subjects. It would be nice to say that experimental objectives usually determine the number of subjects used. In reality, such practicalities as room in the metabolism unit and current finances become the deciding factors.

SUBJECTS

In any human metabolism study, the success of the project is largely in the hands of the subjects. Hence, the selection, training and motivation of subjects is of utmost importance. In order to meet minimum standards of morality, all subjects must be true volunteers. They must understand that they are subjects for research and the true meaning of their participation. No direct or indirect pressure should be applied. While such procedures are necessary from legal and ethical standpoints, they are also of practical importance. True volunteers are most cooperative and more understanding which leads to greater probability of success in a research project.

In our laboratory, several techniques are used to obtain subjects regardless of source. Basically the groups we use can be classified as (1) inmates of the Nebraska Penal Correctional Complex for Men, (2) University of Nebraska students and employees, other college-level students, and townspeople from Lincoln, Nebraska, and (3) adolescent boys from Lincoln, Nebraska. Word-of-mouth advertising from ex-subjects is possibly the most important form of gaining volunteers when any of these three groups are used. This is advantageous in that prospective subjects come to us with a fairly clear idea of what will be expected of them and how their life styles may be disrupted. Disadvantages are cliquishness and sometimes the passing along of misinformation, particularly if experimental plans pertaining to subject responsibilities are altered.

About two weeks before the start of a study, posters are placed on bulletin boards in areas frequented by prospective subjects. Sometimes announcements are made in classes and/or advertisements are placed in newspapers. Information is given on study objectives, subject responsibilities, pertinent dates and financial rewards. Interested individuals are asked to telephone our laboratory. When the initial contact is made, prospective subjects' names are placed on a list in strict order of time of making this first contact. Usually more individuals volunteer than can be employed. All other factors being equal, subjects are selected in order of first indicating an interest in participating. At this point, details pertaining to the study are given to the prospective subject. The individual is "invited" (in fact, this is a requirement) to a "trial day."

The trial day is a pre-day in which prospective subjects eat the experimental diet so as to give each individual a better idea of exactly what he or she is volunteering to do. It also gives a chance for any questions to be answered. Since these are done with groups of individuals, questions are sometimes asked and answered for one individual which are of benefit to the group. A prospective subject, as an individual, sometimes doesn't know what to ask or is sometimes shy about this. Since the group is usually a mixture of individuals with past experience and no experience as subjects, this event affords an occasion for exchange of information and clearing-up of doubts or worries. At the end of this day, subjects are asked to make a decision in writing on whether or not they wish to participate. At this time, they usually are asked to fill out medical history forms and general background forms.

Medical approval for each prospective subject must be obtained for participation from a neutral physician or from a physician biased in favor of the individuals considering this activity. For prisoners, the medical officer of the Penal Complex performs this assignment. In the case of students, physicians of the Student Health Division are involved. When adolescent boys are subjects, their own personal physicians are contacted for the physical examinations. Subjects are told to contact these physicians if they

TABLE 8.1

SUBJECT CONSENT FORM

I agree to become a volunteer subject for a research project dealing with (brief statement of objective), under the direction of Dr. Constance Kies and Dr. Hazel Fox. I understand my responsibilities for the study to include the following:

(a) Eating all assigned foods and nothing else.
(b) Making complete collections of urine and stools according to direction.
(c) Giving (number) small blood samples (50cc each).
(d) Filling out various forms.

I understand that I may withdraw from the study at any time. I agree that information dealing with this study about me may be published but that I will not be identified or identifiable. Risks of volunteering for a project of this kind have been explained to me. I understand that the diet food is boring and rather unpalatable. I also understand that participation on projects of this kind also may temporarily result in some alteration in my life style.

Date	Signature

feel ill during the course of the study. Prior consent from the project directors is not needed and all costs are borne by the laboratory.

Subjects are required to sign consent forms as a condition of participating in the study. While these do not relieve the investigator of legal responsibility if damage is done to a subject, it does place the investigator in a better ethical position. This is also a requirement as part of meeting standards of ethics set by such granting agencies as the National Institute of Health. An example of the form used for a specific study from our laboratory is given in Table 8.1.

Subject/subject and subject/research personal relationships are extremely important in maintenance of morale. Development of a feeling of rapport, companionship, and loyalty among members of a subject group is important in giving individuals the inner strength necessary to carrying through to successful completion of studies of this type. This is particularly true during depression periods, not necessarily caused by participation in the project.

In our laboratory, an attempt is made to make subjects feel that they are a part of the research team. This is more easily accomplished with our college students, townspeople and adolescent boy subjects than with the prisoner subjects. Most laboratory personnel have had experience of being subjects themselves—a great help in their developing an empathy with subjects in on-going studies. Selection of personnel on the basis of their ability to relate and sympathize with subjects is important. Both Dr. Fox (my co-reseacher) and I spend a good deal of time directly working with subjects. We feel that the real secret in successful open-laboratory studies

TABLE 8.2

SUBJECT ACTIVITY SHEET

Date_____   Subject No._____

1. What time did you get up this morning?_____ How many hours of
    sleep did you have last night and yesterday?_____

2. How did you feel physically yesterday? (Please check).

| Much better than usual | Better than usual | As usual | Poor | Very poor |

If worse than usual, please explain._____

Did you experience any nausea, cramping, diarrhea, distention, gas, vomiting,
regurgitation?_____ If yes, please explain._____

3. Please describe your physical activities for yesterday. (Please check).

| Much more active than usual | More active than usual | As usual | Less active than usual | Much less active than usual |

4. How would you rate your mental spirits yesterday? (Please check).

| Much better than usual | Better than usual | As usual | Worse than usual | Much worse than usual |

Are you becoming discouraged with the study?   If yes, is there
anything we can do to help? (Please describe)_____.

5. Are all of your urine collections for yesterday complete?_____
    Did you have a stool collection yesterday?_____

is in the day-to-day, meal-to-meal contact between the study directors and
the subjects. This time spent in encouraging, praising and *listening* to the
concerns of subjects is essential. The investigator must develop an instinct
for knowing who needs encouragement, when and how it should be given.
Subjects differ in their support needs. Researchers also vary in their abilities
to relate to subjects. The personality of the investigator must honestly mesh
with these subjects' support needs if a study is to be successful.

Although not as important as direct subject–investigator contacts in establishment of day-to-day emotional/physiological well being, subjects are requested to fill out "activity" sheets each morning pertaining to various aspects of their feelings, health and life style of the day before. An example of the activity sheet used in our laboratory is given in Table 8.2. In some laboratories and our own in the past, subjects were asked to keep diaries. Diaries offer the advantage of an open-ended expression from subjects which are useful in evaluations of projects. However, the check list approach from the activity sheet gives faster feed-back to the researchers, is easier to quantify relative to the answers given, gives information on specific points in which the researchers may have an answer and gives subjects better protection of personal privacy.

Subject protection should be always foremost in the mind of an investigator. To be absolutely honest and fair with subjects and to be obviously concerned with their well-being "pays off" in terms of subject response. To get honesty, one must be honest in dealing with subjects. Individuals dealing with federal government grants and contracts are aware of the necessity of proving safety and fairness of research projects involving human subjects before neutral protection committees. While this approach is valuable both to subjects and to researchers, legal and moral protection of subjects is the responsibility of the researcher.

DIETS

Diets in human nitrogen balance studies are formulated and fed differently than those of animal nitrogen balance studies. Although formula diets are sometimes employed, mixed food diets are more commonly used in human studies.

The basal food diet used in our laboratory is shown in Table 8.3. Depending upon the experimental plan, the protein resource might be a mixture of purified L-amino acids, casein, dried skim milk, or test product. In our laboratory, dried skim milk is usually used in one period for reference purposes as a positive control. In a human study, the decision on how much protein and how much total diet each individual subject will consume per day is made prior to the start of the feeding phase as part of the experimental planning. It is desirable for subjects to be in slight negative balance if comparisons are to be made on relative protein quality values of different food products. In our laboratory, we have found that feeding at approximately 4.0 gm nitrogen per subject per day places nitrogen balance in good testing range. In some laboratories, the controlled level of nitrogen intake is tied to weight of each individual subject; i.e., the test product is fed to provide a pre-set number of milligrams of nitrogen from the test product per kilogram of body weight of the subject per day. While protein/amino acid needs are roughly correlated to body weight, this is by no means a perfect correlation, particularly among groups of approximately the same

TABLE 8.3

MENU CHECK SHEET

SUBJECT NO. _____

DATE _____

	Breakfast			Lunch			Supper	
Subject Check		Amount Assigned	Subject Check		Amount Assigned	Subject Check		Amount Assigned
____	Test product	1	____	Starch bread	1 slice	____	Starch bread	1 slice
____	Starch bread	1 slice	____	Test product	1	____	Test product	1
____	Applesauce	1	____	Peaches	1	____	Pears	1
____	Orange Juice	1	____	Vitamin capsule	1	____	Jelly	1
____	Butter oil	1	____	Mineral capsule	1	____	Butter oil	1
____	Jelly	1	____	Butter oil	1	____	Soft drink	1
			____	Jelly	1			
			____	Soft drink	1			

type (for example, adult young men, normal weight for height) which are usually used in controlled laboratory studies. From the standpoint of laboratory management, this latter approach is less efficient usage of time since test products can be prepared only after subject selection is made. Otherwise, products can be prepared before the start of the study, evening out work in the diet laboratory at a considerable cost reduction.

In a nitrogen balance study, caloric intake for each individual is geared to the individual's assumed needs for weight maintenance (adults) or weight gain (infants and children). In our laboratory, subjects weigh in each morning before breakfast. Different philosophies and approaches are used in various laboratories to achieve this general objective. Over short term periods, a range of energy intakes allows for general weight maintenance in the adult.   In several laboratories the phraseology "energy intake to allow for weight maintenance" means gearing caloric intake at the high end of the maintenance scale so that weight gain over the long-term basis is actually occurring. This allows for maximum energy sparing of protein. This approach is useful in situations such as establishment of minimum amino acid requirements, particularly if purified amino acids are being employed as the protein source. In our laboratory, energy to meet maintenance needs is pegged at the lower end of the scale. Probably over a long period of time, weight loss would occur in the adult subjects. Since much of our work currently deals with evaluation of various aspects of cereal and plant products as suppliers of protein, practical application of the results are more likely to be of concern among marginally fed populations in which neither protein nor calories are at optimal levels. Of less importance is that the normal-health people we use in our studies frequently become very disturbed at any hint of weight gain. They know that weight loss is not permitted, but weight gain for many Americans is not a desirable situation.

Sometimes caloric intake is determined by weight of the subjects, e.g.: 35 kcal per kg body wt. This level is maintained unless subjects show great weight loss or gain. More typically in our laboratory, male subjects initially are placed on diets containing about 2600 kcal per day and female subjects are placed on diets containing about 1800 kcal. These are adjusted up or down as needed for weight maintenance.

Usually a starch bread, based on the method of Steele et al. (1965) is used in our laboratory as the principal source of energy. Starch cookies or wafers are frequently employed in other laboratories. Intake of soft drinks, butter oil, jelly and hard candy are used to make necessary adjustments in energy intake.

All food items are purchased from the same lots prior to the beginning of the study. Daily portions of each diet item for each individual are weighed. Subjects' trays are carefully checked to make sure that all items are completely eaten. Reminders to "eat everything" are made in a friendly manner but stressing the importance and necessity of such action.

It is fairly simple to check whether or not subjects eat the diet completely. To determine whether or not subjects eat other items is somewhat more difficult to ascertain. Part of the answer is in establishing good investigator/subject rapport. The other is in analysis of excreta. For example, a gross change in nitrogen excreta in comparison to other days within a period for an individual makes it advisable to closely question the subject. In general, individuals who sign up for research of this type do so with the best of intentions. If proper encouragement is given, the incidences of cheating are rare. In our laboratory, individuals are encouraged to report incidences of failure. These rare reports are greeted with disappointment but understanding. The individual is given the choice of continuing with days added for readjustment or terminating participating in the project; usually their reaction is to take the former course.

COLLECTION, SAMPLING, PRESERVATION AND ANALYSES OF EXCRETA AND FOOD

Subjects are told in our laboratory that from the first day of the study all urine and stools must be saved. This is one of the hardest items in human nitrogen balance studies to really convince subjects of the necessity of doing ("Save everything!"). Subjects are directed to make urine collections in glass jars to which a small amount (about 1 ml per quart jar) of toluene has been added (see Table 8.4). Stool collections are made in plastic-lined freezer boxes (see Table 8.4). Jars and boxes are carried by subjects wherever they go in carrying bags (currently airline flight bags are used).

Urine for nitrogen balance studies in our laboratory is collected, processed and analyzed on the basis of total excretion for 24 hr. The division is made when a urine collection is made before breakfast (called "rising collection"). This marks the end of collections made for a specific 24 hr. In our laboratory, all urine collections for the past 24 hr are removed from the collection refrigerators where they are left by the subjects and are taken to the urine volume room. Here, all collections for each individual are lined up on the laboratory bench. The time that the "rising collection" was made is recorded in a data book in order to determine whether or not the collections made by the individual truly represent a 24-hr period. The daily collections for each individual are then poured into separate 2000 ml polyvinyl cylinders and the nondiluted volume is recorded. Each collection jar and lid is rinsed with approximately 10 ml of distilled water and the rinse water is added to the collections in the cylinders. If the amount of fluid in the cylinder is 1880 or less, 20 ml of concentrated hydrochloric acid is added and the total volume is made up to 2000 ml with distilled water. If more than 1880,

TABLE 8.4

DIRECTIONS FOR SUBJECTS

I. SUBJECT RESPONSIBILITIES

Basically responsibilities include consuming the test diets and eating *nothing* else, giving blood (small samples), making complete collections of urine and stools, and filling out various questionnaires.

II. MEDICAL EXAMS

Clearance for participation will be needed for each subject from the NU Student Health Center. Medical history forms will be given to them— whether or not additional medical exams are needed will be determined by physicians of that department. (We'll let you know). Naturally, the Dept. of Food and Nutrition will pay for this. If you feel ill at any time during the study, report to Student Health, ask for Cindy, identify yourself as a FN subject and follow her directions. Again, the FN department will pay all costs within reason.

III. FORMS

Signed subject consent forms, medical history and diet history forms will be needed at the beginning of the project. Activity record forms will be needed on a daily basis.

IV. PAYMENTS

Money payments will be made only to subjects who complete the project unless excused from participation for illness as determined by a physician of the NU Student Health Center.

Payments:
1. $4.00 per day on controlled part of study. Diet consumption and excreta collections must be correctly done for payments to be made.
2. $2.00 for each blood sample.

V. MEALS

All meals will be served in Room 21 in the basement of Filley Hall.
1. Be sure to eat everything provided by the diet and nothing else except for the following: gum and water.
2. You will be assigned particular quantities of jelly, butter oil, carbonated beverages, Lifesavers to eat each day to balance energy intake to your particular energy needs.
3. In order to keep track of the items assigned and consumed at each meal, fill out the diet sheet at each meal.
4. We really want you to eat meals in the laboratory. If you need a bag meal other than the usual time, please sign up for these AS SOON AS YOU CAN on the forms posted in the laboratory. Bagged meals will be placed in the refrigerator.
5. Usual times for meals are as follows:
   Breakfast 7:30
   Lunch   12:00
   Supper   5:00
   Please sign up for other times.
6. WARNING—DO NOT attempt to swallow the large white calcium pill whole. Chew them up.

VI. URINE COLLECTIONS

1. Collect all urine in the glass quart jars which are provided. Be sure the jars are marked with your subject number.
2. Date all jars by writing on the tape on the jars. Dating of urine jars is somewhat confusing. After breakfast on the 1st day of the study, mark all jars of urine collected that day, Sept. 10. Also, date all bottles collected that night, Sept. 10. The last collection dated Sept. 10 should be the one you make when you get up on Thursday morning,

TABLE 8.4 (*Continued*)

Sept. 11, just before breakfast. This collection should also be marked
R.C. (for rising collection) and the time should be indicated. Following
breakfast on Thursday, Sept. 11, mark all collections Sept. 11 through
the R.C. collection made on Friday morning. Continue this system
throughout the study. The rising collection should be made at the same
time each morning.

3. Bring all collections to meals to turn in. Pick up clean bottles at this
   time.
4. Take bottles with you wherever you go. Remember: all urine must be
   saved.
5. Bags for carrying bottles will be provided.
6. Continue to make urine collection through the morning collection
   made on Sept. 30.

VII. STOOL COLLECTIONS
1. Collect all stools in freezer boxes. Place freezer box in plastic baggie.
   Use room spray for odor control. Be sure freezer box is marked with
   your subject number.
2. Stool boxes are dated somewhat differently than are urine collections.
   Simply write the date and time (indicate morning or afternoon), the
   collection is made.
3. Remember, save all stools. *Do not use laxatives.*
4. Continue to make stool collections at end of study until dye marker
   shows.

VIII. BLOOD SAMPLES
Blood samples will be drawn several times during the study. Do not eat
breakfast before blood samples are taken. Report to the laboratory at
6:00 on the mornings blood samples are to be drawn.
See attached calendar for dates blood samples will be drawn.

IX. OTHER DIRECTIONS
1. Each morning please fill out the activity sheet pertaining to activities,
   health feelings of the day before. Ask about medications.
2. Please weigh yourself each morning before eating and record your
   weight on the chart beside the scales. Weigh with shoes on or off but
   be consistent on which you do.
3. Place all excreta collections (urine and stools) in assigned refrigerators
   in basement of Filley Hall, southwest end. Clean bottles and boxes will
   be located on racks in the same area. Be sure they are correctly marked
   with your subject numbers.
4. Remember that you are a research subject. While we think that the
   risks for you in participating are very small, they do exist. FOR
   FEMALES ONLY—please be sure not to be or become pregnant during the course of the study.
5. In case of emergency need for meal preparation or for anything else,
   please do not hesitate to contact the project directors:

Dr. Constance Kies   Diet laboratory
Home phone 466-1162   Food and Nutrition Building
Office phone 472-2444   472-2444

Dr. Hazel Fox   Chemistry laboratory
Home phone 466-3862   Food and
Office phone 472-3716   Nutrition Building
                              472-2444

acidification at the 1% level and dilution with distilled water to the nearest 1000 ml level is maintained. The cylinders are then emptied into plastic buckets and are well mixed by stirring. The amount of urine saved for analysis depends upon the dictates of the experimental plan. Usually, two 80-ml samples are taken from each subject's 24-hr collection—one for use in immediate analysis and the other to be frozen for analysis to be done later and for rechecking of analysis. (In our laboratory, it is customary for 10% of all analyses to be redone by different technicians as a check on the accuracy of the originally reported values.)

Stool collections are pooled in lots of 4–10 days depending upon lengths of the experimental periods. For separation into lots, divisions are made on the basis of use of fecal dye markers, although sometimes glass beads are used—either concurrently or independently.

Carmine and brilliant blue are two dyes frequently reported as being used for this purpose. In our laboratory, a No. 1 gelatin capsule of carmine was used. Recently, on advice from Clark (1974), our laboratory has changed from use of carmine to brilliant blue. According to the directions of Clark (1974), which have also been successful for us, 50 mg of brilliant blue is mixed with 200 mg of mucilose flakes and is fed in a No. 1 gelatin capsule. The brilliant blue marker seems to give a more definite division than does the carmine marker. Choice of desirability of marker is probably somewhat determined by the composition of the experimental diet and the natural color of the resulting stool. A word of warning—carmine may become *Salmonella* contaminated so each batch must be checked.

When glass beads are used as markers, we have found it useful to alternate colors used in different periods. Bead markers tend to "spread" throughout several collections and period lots may overlap. In general, fecal dye markers "show" before beads indicating a difference between transit spread of the water and solid phases. A decision must be made as to which marker to use. Because more precise division is possible with dye markers, this is the one usually used in our laboratory. However, the inherent general lack of precision possible in division of stools into period lots is a major source of error in human (or animal) nitrogen balance studies.

Subjects make stool collections in plastic-lined cardboard freezer boxes. They are requested to mark their subject numbers, the date and the times the collection was made on the box. The box is then placed in a plastic bag with a few "spurts" of room deodorant for favorable environment control to be carried by the subject to the laboratory refrigerators. All fecal collections for each subject for each period are placed in tared 2-qt glass jars, the division between periods being made on the basis of the fecal marker. If fecal markers are given at breakfast of the day of a start of a new period, then at the first sign of the marker, a new period lot is started. Weight of stools is determined by difference weighing. If only nitrogen analyses are to be done on the stools, acid hydrolysis is used. Concentrated hydrochloric acid is combined with the stools (on the basis of volume: 1 to 3). These are allowed to slowly digest at room temperature under a hood or the jars are placed in a water bath set at about 90°C for 24 hr. Weight of the acidified stool mass is determined by difference. The acidified stools are then placed in a heavy-duty blender. After thorough blending, two 80-ml samples are taken for immediate analysis and for back-up analysis. If such additional analyses are to be done, then a water, rather than an acid hydrolysis, may be necessary. Acid hydrolysate samples may be stored at room temperature; however, water hydrolysates require freezer temperature storage if analyses are not to be done within a day or so.

Food composites are prepared by combining all dietary constituents for one day by weight, blending in a heavy-duty blender, sampling and preserving an adequate amount, for later laboratory analyses, by freezing. Food composites are made at least two times per study and whenever case lots of food are changed.

Analyses of excreta and food is less confusing than other aspects of human nitrogen balance studies in that well-known laboratory procedures are employed. Creatinine content of each 24-hr urine collection for each subject is done by the method of Folin (1914), as a test of completeness of urine collections and of their accuracy of division into 24-hr lots. While creatinine excretion is not unaffected by diet, its consistency of excretion by a particular individual on the same diet makes it a valuable tool in nitrogen balance studies. Nitrogen content of urine, feces and stools is most frequently reported as being analyses by one of the modifications of the Kjeldahl method. In our laboratory, the Scales and Harrison (1920) modification is employed.

In the past, nitrogen balance studies were frequently reported in the form of case histories. This is no longer the case. Statistical analyses of data is needed. Analyses of variance and Duncan's Multiple Range Test are frequently used in our laboratory. However, this judgment is usually made by a statistician.

CONCLUSION

The nitrogen balance method has been known for many years. It is cumbersome, expensive, time-consuming and has many well-known limitations affecting accuracy. Nevertheless, it has been the mainstay for the establishment of information on human protein needs in the past and continues to be important in this area of research.

BIBLIOGRAPHY

CLARK, H.   1974.   Personal communication. Purdue University, West Lafayette, Ind.
DeHAAS, H., and MORSE, E. H.   1968.   Utilization of amino acids from protein, manual of procedures. Northeast Regional Res. Publ., Univ. Maine Agr. Exp. Sta., Tech. Bull. 33.

FAO. 1973. Energy and protein requirements, Report of a Joint FAO/WHO ad hoc expert Committee, Rome, Mar. 22–Apr. 2, 1971. Food and Agriculture Organization, Rome, Italy.

FOLIN, O. 1914. On the determination of creatinine and creatine in urine. J. Biol. Chem. *17*, 469.

FOMAN, S. J. 1967. Infant Nutrition. W. B. Saunders Co., Philadelphia, Pa.

LEICHSENRING, J. M., BIESTER, A., ROBERTS, H., SWANSON, P. P., GRAM, M. R., LEVERTON, R. M., BREWER, W., and BURRELL, L. M. 1958. Methods used for metabolic studies in the North Central region. North Central Regional Publ. *80,* Univ. Minn. Agr. Exp. Sta., Tech. Bull. *225.*

LEVERTON, R. M. 1959. Amino acid requirements of young adults. *In* Protein and Amino Acid Nutrition, A. A. Albanese (Editor). Academic Press, New York.

NATL. ACAD. SCI.–NATL. RES. COUNCIL. 1974. Improvement of Protein Nutriture. Committee on Amino Acids, Food and Nutrition Board, National Academy of Sciences, Washington, D.C.

ROSE, W. C. 1957. The amino acid requirements of adult man. Nutr. Abstr. Rev. *27,* 631.

SCALES, F. M., and HARRISON, A. P. 1920. Boric acid modification of the Kjeldahl method for crops and feeds. J. Ind. Eng. Chem. *12,* 350.

STEELE, B. F., HJORTLAND, M. C., and BLOCK, W. D. 1965. A yeast-leavened low-protein bread for research diets. J. Am. Dietet. Assoc. *47,* 445.

Factors Affecting Nutritional Value

CHAPTER 9

G. R. Jansen | ## Amino Acid Fortification

Amino acid fortification is a procedure by which the protein quality of plant proteins can be improved by the addition of the limiting amino acid(s). This subject has been reviewed many times in the past (Howe 1961; Jansen 1962; Jansen 1974; Vaghefi *et al.* 1974; Scrimshaw and Altschul 1972) and will not be reviewed in detail again. A general summary of the present situation specifically in respect to the amino acid fortification of cereals is as follows. Studies with experimental animals have demonstrated unequivocally that the protein quality of wheat, corn, and rice can all be improved substantially by the addition of lysine, lysine and tryptophan, or lysine and threonine. Studies carried out under controlled conditions have demonstrated that growth and/or nitrogen balance in human infants fed wheat or corn is significantly improved by the addition of lysine or lysine and tryptophan, respectively. Whether or not amino acid fortification of cereals will be of any practical value in human nutrition has not yet been demonstrated but is under active investigation (Jansen 1974). Major issues to be resolved include whether or not lysine is the limiting amino acid in any significant number of practical human diets and whether or not calorie deficiencies completely preclude beneficial responses from being obtained when the limiting amino acid is added.

As has been discussed in detail elsewhere (Jansen 1974) protein quality and quantity together define the net protein value of a diet. Amino acid fortification is just one method out of many by which the net protein value of a diet can be improved. Other approaches are (*1*) plant breeding programs, such as the one that led to the development of Opaque-2 corn, (*2*) protein fortification, for example the addition to cereals of protein concentrates such as soy or fish flour, and (*3*) educational programs that encourage the consumption of legumes with cereals. Recently the concept that the protein value of cereal diets needs to be improved has been challenged. Harper *et al.* (1973) suggest that primary protein deficiency in young children fed cereal diets is most unlikely to be the cause of malnutrition if the supply of calories is adequate. They therefore seriously question the development of protein-rich food, amino acid fortification, the genetic improvement of cereal protein, and efforts to increase legume production and use. McLaren (1974) has referred to these efforts in protein improvement that have been carried out over the last 20 yr as "The Great Protein Fiasco." Payne (1975) concluded that 2–3 yr old children need only 5% of calories in the form of utilizable protein, and cereals can by themselves supply this protein need.

The above discussion suggests that the issues surrounding amino acid fortification can be divided into three general categories. The first includes the most fundamental question as to whether or not protein improvement programs have any merit in the light of current knowledge about the nature of practical human diets. The second is whether or not protein quality improvement has merit, even if a need for additional usable protein in a diet can be demonstrated. The third is the most relevant to amino acid fortification and is whether adding a specific amino acid to a specific food staple has any practical value.

In this report the literature dealing with amino acid fortification of cereals and of legumes will be reviewed briefly, with the emphasis placed on cereals and on human studies. Next, the results obtained in several recent experiments dealing with maternal nutrition and protein quality-energy relationships will be presented. Finally, and based on the above, the present status of amino acid fortification will be discussed.

FORTIFICATION OF LEGUMES

Animal Studies

As is well known, the first limiting amino acid in legumes is methionine. Because cereals are first limiting in lysine, mixtures of legumes and cereals are better balanced in amino acid composition and biological value than either of the two components (Bressani and Elias 1974). In Table 9.1 data on the amino acid composition, chemical score and biological value of a number of legumes are summarized. The improvement in biological value of heat-processed soy protein is well documented (Borchers 1962; Barnes *et al.* 1962; Mattil 1974) and methionine fortification of soy-based products has been of considerable commercial utility for many years (Rosenberg 1959). Shurpalekar *et al.* (1961) reported that the protein efficiency ratio (PER) of a spray-dried soybean milk could be made equivalent to that obtained with modified cows milk by the addition of DL-methionine. Similar results were obtained by Parthasarathy *et al.* (1964C) for soybean

TABLE 9.1

AMINO ACID COMPOSITION (PARTIAL) AND NUTRITIVE VALUE OF HEAT PROCESSED LEGUMES

| Legume | mg/gm N | | | | Chemical Score[2] | Biological Value | Digestibility | NPU |
	Lysine	Sulfur Amino Acids[1]	Threonine	Tryptophan				
Arachis hypogaea	221	150	163	65	41	55	87	43
Cajanus cajan	481	93	182	35	26	57	78	52
Cicer arietinum	428	139	235	54	38	68	86	—
Glycine max	399	162	241	80	45	73	90	61
Lens esculenta	449	107	248	60	30	45	85	30
Phaseolus aureus	504	77	209	50	21	70	81	—
Phaseolus lunatus	465	141	231	50	39	67	78	52
Phaseolus vulgaris	450	119	218	63	33	58	73	38
Pisum sativum	470	127	254	56	35	64	88	47
Vigna sinensis	427	141	225	66	39	57	79	45
Reference Standard								
Whole Egg	436	362	320	93	100	94	97	94

Source: Data obtained from FAO (1970).

[1]Methionine + cystine.

[2]$CS = \dfrac{\text{limiting amino acid (mg/gm N) in sample}}{\text{Concentration of same amino acid (mg/gm N) in egg}} \times 100.$

meal. These workers also showed that methionine hydroxy analog (MHA) was equally as effective as methionine. This equivalency has been confirmed for the rat (Longenecker *et al.* 1964; Dreyer and Du Bruyn 1965; and Jenkins *et al.* 1975) and for the dog (Bressani and De Zaghi 1970). Schneider and Sarett (1969) reported that an isolated soy protein supplemented with methionine had 85% of the protein quality of milk protein when fed to baby pigs. Heat-processed peanut meal has been reported to be about equally limiting in lysine, threonine, and methionine (McOsker 1962; Howe *et al.* 1965).

As has been mentioned, legume seeds in general are deficient in methionine. Rat feeding studies have demonstrated that addition of methionine to many species of beans (*Phaseolus* vulgaris, *P. lunatus, P. angularis*), peas (*Pisum sativum*), lentils (*Lens esculenta*), cowpeas (*Vigna sinensis*) and chickpeas (*Cicer arietinum*) increased growth and protein efficiency, when the samples are properly heat processed (Jansen 1975). Pigeon peas (*Cajanus indicus*) require the addition of tryptophan with methionine for rat growth to be improved (Jansen 1975). The necessity for heat-processing legume seeds and products in order to destroy toxic and antigrowth factors has been stressed elsewhere (Liener 1969; also, see Chapters 12 and 14).

Human Studies

Parthasarathy *et al.* (1964A) studied the effect on protein utilization of adding DL-methionine or DL-methionine hydroxy analog to soy flour fed to 8–9 yr old children. The protein intake was 1.2 gm per kg and the supplementation level was 1.2 gm per 16 gm nitrogen. Methionine addition increased the biological value (BV) and net protein utilization (NPU) from 63.5 and 53.3 to 74.9 and 64.7, respectively, compared to corresponding values of 82.6 and 72.0 for skim milk. The hydroxy analog was nearly as effective as methionine itself. Korslund *et al.* (1973) compared the effects on nitrogen balance of 12–16 yr old boys of a textured soy protein (TVP) and a similar product supplemented with 1% DL-methionine. At a nitrogen intake of 5.0 gm per day methionine addition increased nitrogen balance from −0.08 to 0.48 gm per day. Kies and Fox (1971) carried out a similar study with TVP at two levels of nitrogen intake in adult men. At a nitrogen intake of 4.8 gm per day, methionine increased nitrogen balance from −0.70 to −0.45 gm per day. At a nitrogen intake of 8.8 gm per day, methionine addition had no effect on nitrogen balance.

From the standpoint of reducing the extent of protein-calorie malnutrition by improving the utilization of legumes, studies carried out in infants are more relevant than studies with older subjects. Graham (1971) has evaluated the effects on nitrogen retention of supplementing soy protein with methionine. In his experiments methionine addition to the commercial formula Sobee, a soy isolate or full fat soy flour was studied. In addition,

TABLE 9.2

METHIONINE SUPPLEMENTATION OF SOY PROTEIN STUDIES IN INFANTS

Age (Months)	Protein	DL-Methionine mg/kg/Day	Days	N Intake mg/kg/Day	N Retained mg/kg/Day
21	Sobee	—	6	240	42
	Sobee	11	12	232	70
23	Sobee	—	12	194	23
	Sobee	14	19	198	54
13	ProSobee[1]	—	9	320	95
	Sobee	—	15	320	79
13	ProSobee[1]	—	16	317	105
	Sobee	22	18	320	106
6	Soy isolate	—	10	238	12
	Soy isolate	20	9	240	44
8	Soy isolate	—	6	240	63
	Soy isolate	20	6	240	88
15	Soy isolate	—	9	239	27
	Soy isolate	20	9	242	57
21	Casein	—	11	320	107
	Soy isolate	—	15	320	77
21	Casein	—	9	320	137
	Soy isolate	16	6	320	107
19	Full fat soy Flour	—	32	280	69
	Full fat soy Flour	20	20	282	109

Source: Data of Graham (1971).
[1]ProSobee fortified with DL-methionine.

retention on Sobee with or without added methionine was compared to retention on ProSobee, a commercial formula enriched with methionine. As shown in Table 9.2, in all cases reported, methionine addition had a consistent and beneficial effect on nitrogen retention in infants ranging in age from 6–23 months.

A beneficial effect of methionine addition to soy protein fed to infants would be expected on the basis of the animal experiments (FAO 1970). In the United States at the present time it is common practice to add methionine to soy formulae fed to infants. It is interesting to note that this practice antedated the studies of Graham and was apparently based primarily on the prior animal experimentation. At the present time one would have to conclude that the desirability of adding methionine to soy formulae has not been conclusively demonstrated. Fomon *et al.* (1973) have convincingly shown that a methionine supplemented formula based on soy isolate with protein supplying 6.5% of calories when fed to 13 infants resulted in growth comparable to milk formulae supplying greater intakes of protein. However in previous work, Fomon (1959) reported that a soy formula without added methionine that supplied protein at 6.8% of calories when fed to four infants resulted in growth and nitrogen retention equivalent to that on human milk. The work of Graham is apparently the only published research in which the effects of soy with and without added methionine have been directly compared. Such direct comparisons are desirable because of many complications that result when different formulations are compared. For example, Theuer and Sarett (1970) have demonstrated marked differences in the level of trypsin inhibitors present in a series of commercial soy formulae. The Committee on Nutrition of the American Academy of Pediatrics (1963) stressed the differences in the adequacy of vitamin and mineral levels in commercial soy formulae that have been demonstrated. In considering the need and level of methionine addition to soy formulae several additional considerations should be kept in mind. Any beneficial effect from methionine addition would likely be very difficult to demonstrate at higher protein intakes. Also D-methionine is apparently not utilized to any significant extent by the human infant (Stegink et al. 1971).

FORTIFICATION OF CEREALS

Cereals are especially good potential candidates for amino acid fortification because they, generally speaking, would supply adequate amounts of dietary protein to meet the needs of even young children if the protein were higher in quality (Jansen 1974). In Table 9.3 amino acid composition data (FAO 1970) for 10 cereal grains are compared with the amino acid composition of whole egg protein and the most recent Food and Agriculture Organization pattern (FAO/WHO 1973) for the four amino acids of most concern, lysine, sulfur amino acids, threonine, and tryptophan. All of the cereals are first limiting in lysine with corn nearly as limiting in tryptophan. Although the beneficial effects on rat growth of adding lysine to wheat protein was demonstrated over 60 yr ago (Osborne and Mendel 1914), the practical value of lysine fortification in human nutrition has not yet been conclusively demonstrated. The following is a brief review of the literature dealing with amino acid fortification of cereals. A more detailed review has recently been published (Jansen 1974).

Animal Studies

Wheat.—The addition of lysine to whole wheat, wheat gluten, white flour, or white bread fed to rats greatly increases growth and doubles the protein efficiency ratio (PER). Rosenberg and Rohdenberg (1952) showed over 20 yr ago that the PER of white bread fed to weanling rats would be increased from 1.0 to 1.9 by the addition of 0.25% L-lysine monohydrochloride, based on flour weight. Bender (1958), Hutchison et al. (1959), and later Rosenberg et al. (1960B) showed that for maximum response in the rat both lysine and threonine are necessary. Jansen (1969) estimated that lysine fortified white bread was equal in protein value to bread fortified

TABLE 9.3

AMINO ACID PATTERNS OF CEREALS COMPARED WITH WHOLE EGG AND FAO PATTERNS

mg Amino Acid/gm N

Cereal	Lysine	Methionine and Cystine	Threonine	Tryptophan	Limiting Amino Acid	Chemical Score (Egg)	Chemical Score[1]
Barley	216	246	207	96	Lysine	50	64
Cornmeal	167	217	225	38	Lysine	38	49
Millet	214	302	241	106	Lysine	49	63
Oats	232	272	207	79	Lysine	53	68
Polished rice	226	229	207	84	Lysine	52	66
Ragi	181	357	263	105	Lysine	42	53
Rye	212	210	209	46	Lysine	49	62
Sorghum	126	181	189	63	Lysine	29	37
Teff	174	301	213	93	Lysine	40	51
Wheat bulgur	161	219	177	66	Lysine	37	47
Wheat flour (white)	130	250	168	67	Lysine	30	38
Standard							
Hen's Egg	436	362	320	93	—	—	—
FAO/WHO 1973	340	220	250	60	—	—	—

Source: Data obtained from FAO (1970).
[1]FAO/WHO (1973).

with 3% fish protein concentrate (FPC) or 8% toasted soy flour, and that lysine and threonine fortified white bread was equal in protein value to bread fortified with 6% FPC. Using a slightly different method, Stillings *et al.* (1971) estimated that lysine fortified white bread was equivalent in protein value to bread fortified with 5% FPC.

Corn.—Rosenberg *et al.* (1960A) reported the results of an extensive experiment in which white corn meal was fortified with graded levels of lysine and tryptophan. The diet was 90% corn meal and contained only 6.9% protein, dry weight. Addition of 0.05% L-lysine monohydrochloride significantly increased weight gain from 9 gm to 22 gm. A maximum weight gain of 44 gm was achieved with simultaneous addition of 0.20% L-lysine monohydrochloride and 0.02% L-tryptophan, based on weight of diet. These levels furnished dietary lysine and tryptophan levels of 0.35% and 0.063%, respectively, for a Lys:Try ratio of 5.5:1. Bressani *et al.* (1968) studied the supplementation of lime-treated corn as well as raw corn meal with lysine and tryptophan. They found small but insignificant responses to lysine addition alone; however, the levels chosen were higher than Rosenberg *et al.* (1960A) had shown to be desirable. Simultaneous supplementation with lysine and tryptophan greatly increased the PER's of both lime-treated and raw corn. For lime-treated corn 0.41% L-lysine monohydrochloride and 0.10% L-tryptophan increased the PER from 1.21 to 2.68. In the case of the raw corn meal similar addition levels increased the PER from 1.13 to 2.58. Hegsted (1969) using the slope-ratio assay, reported that the percentage of utilizable protein in yellow corn meal was increased from 3.0 to 3.7 and 5.1 by fortification with lysine, or lysine and tryptophan, respectively. Howe *et al.* (1967) carried out protein quality investigations with six varieties of corn. Protein content ranged from 8–12% with the highest protein sample having the lowest PER. Fortification with 0.1% L-lysine monohydrochloride raised the PER's to corrected values (casein = 2.5) ranging from 1.7–2.3.

Rice.—Pecora and Hundley (1951) reported that growth of rats fed rice was improved for fortification with lysine and threonine. The amino acid composition of rice protein does not suggest the need for supplemental threonine and it appears that the threonine in rice is less available biologically than is the case for wheat. Rosenberg *et al.* (1959) later reported that optimum growth performance in rats fed a 90% rice diet resulted when 0.42% L-lysine monohydrochloride and 0.36% DL-threonine were added to the diet. In this case, total weight gain for 5 weeks was 190 gm compared to approximately 70 gm on the unfortified rice diet.

Howe *et al.* (1967) emphasized the improvement in the protein quality of rice made possible by the addition of lysine alone. PER values of 2.2–2.7 for six varieties of lysine fortified rice were obtained compared with a value of 2.5 for casein.

Other Cereals.—Numerous rat feeding studies have been carried out demonstrating that, in agreement with chemical analysis, lysine is the first limiting amino acid in a wide variety of cereal grains and that the protein quality of such cereals can be improved by lysine fortification. These cereals include barley, millet, oats, ragi, rye, sorghum, and teff (Jansen 1974).

Cereal-concentrate Mixtures.—Two major research groups have been involved in the study of the amino acid fortification of cereal-concentrate mixtures developed primarily for use in infant feeding. These are the Institute of Nutrition of Central America and Panama (INCAP) in Guatemala, and the Central Food Technological Research Institute at Mysore in India. Their studies have been reviewed in detail by Bressani and Elias (1968, 1974) and Swaminathan (1967), respectively. As a general rule, it would appear that cereal legume mixtures in which 50% or more of the protein is of cereal origin are first limiting in lysine whereas mixtures in which legumes supply more than 50% of the protein are first limiting in methionine (Bressani and Elias 1974).

Human Studies

Wheat.—Bressani et al. (1960) studied the effect of lysine supplementation of wheat flour as measured by nitrogen retention in six young children ranging in age from 1 yr 5 months to 5 yr 9 months. Protein and calories were fed at 2 gm and 80–100 kcal per kg body wt per day, respectively. The data obtained showed that wheat protein can be improved markedly by the addition of lysine alone, and in some cases the retention approximated that of milk protein. These workers later demonstrated that maximal retention of nitrogen was obtained with the addition of 162–194 mg lysine per gram N to the basal wheat diet fed at 2–3 gm protein per kg body wt per day (Bressani et al. (1963A).

Barness and colleagues (1961) also evaluated lysine and potassium supplementation of wheat protein fed in the form of commercial cream of wheat to 22 underweight infants recently recovered from severe acute diarrhea. Protein and calories were fed at 1.2–4.0 gm and 75–120 kcal per kg body wt per day, respectively. L-Lysine monohydrochloride was added as 0.35% of the wheat to give a lysine to tryptophan ratio of 4. The results showed that the protein value of wheat protein supplemented with potassium and lysine was close to that of milk and was an adequate source of protein for the infants studied. The authors emphasized the need for adequate potassium. It may be that the recent severe diarrhea in these children, even though recovery occurred at least ten days prior to the start of the balance experiments, increased the need for potassium in these infants.

Graham et al. (1969) reported the results of experiments in which lysine enrichment of wheat flour was evaluated in six infants with ages ranging from 11–24 months. The white flour used was air classified and contained 21% protein. Protein and calories were fed at 1.5–2.0 gm and 90–125 kcal per kg body wt per day. The fortification levels employed were equivalent to 0.12%, 0.20%, and 0.40% additions of L-lysine monohydrochloride to ordinary white flour. Each child received all four wheat diets in random sequence for 15–36 days each, with intervening 9-day periods on casein. Nitrogen balances on each diet were determined in 9 to 15-day periods. Mean rates of weight gain as percentages of the casein value, were 67 ± 11.6, 83 ± 14.2, 97 ± 22.7, and 91 ± 15.0 for unfortified and incrementally forti-fied wheat diets, respectively. Corresponding values for nitrogen retention, again as percentages of the casein value, were 63 ± 11.9, 87 ± 9.6, 98 ± 11.0, and 106 ± 9.6, respectively, in good agreement with the weight gain data. It was estimated that the casein control diet had a biological value 76% of breast milk. In a later experiment these investigators fed these three ly-sine-fortified wheat diets as the sole source of dietary protein to six infants for up to 6 months (Graham *et al.* 1971). At 8% of protein calories, all three diets were equally effective in supporting normal linear growth, weight gain, nitrogen retention, serum proteins, plasma amino acids, and liver mor-phology. Between 6.4 and 7.3% protein calories it appeared that at least the 0.2% and possibly the 0.4% fortification level was required for normal growth. These workers recommended that wheat be enriched with at least 0.12% L-lysine monohydrochloride. In areas where wheat is the main source of protein for infants and small children and where dilution with nonprotein calories is the rule, a 0.2% enrichment with L-lysine monohydrochloride was recommended. Knapp *et al.* (1973) also have reported that lysine for-tified wheat was equivalent to milk in promoting growth when fed to infants as the sole source of protein for 2–3 months.

In contrast to the results obtained by the above workers, Reddy (1971) was unable to demonstrate any consistent effect of lysine fortification of wheat on nitrogen retention in six malnourished children ranging in age from 2–5 yr. The diet was based on whole wheat made into chappatis and supplied protein and energy at levels of 2 gm and 100 kcal per kg body wt, respectively. The basal and supplemented diet furnished 56 and 72 mg lysine per kg body wt, respectively. No significant effects on nitrogen re-tention were observed.

The above studies were all carried out under controlled conditions in a hospital or metabolic word. In addition a number of field studies on lysine fortification of wheat have been carried out and are reviewed next. Krut *et al.* (1961) carried out a field trial of a bread diet supplemented with lysine and fed to 45 institutionalized children, ages 2–8 yr old. Bread supplied 89% of the protein and 52% of the energy in the diet. The L-lysine monohydro-chloride was administered as a separate drink at a level equivalent to 0.27–0.30% of the bread. The gain in weight of the group supplemented with lysine was reported to be greater than that of the group supplemented with glycine.

Lysine fortification of bread fed to Haitian school children was evaluated by King et al. (1963). Breads made from lysine fortified flour or unfortified flour were fed to the children in a school lunch. It was estimated that the bread supplied 25% of the calories and 34% of the protein on the days in which it was fed. This was an estimate based on previous work and it wasn't known what other foods these children were eating during the experimental period. The supplemental bread was only fed 150 days out of a 261-day period. The response to lysine was very small in this study, and of doubtful significance. This is not surprising in view of the ages of the children and the relatively small percentage of the daily protein intake supplied by the bread.

A field trial on lysine fortification of bread has been carried out in Iran (Hedayat et al. 1971). The fortified or unfortified bread was fed to school children as part of a school lunch program to provide approximately half of the protein and calorie recommendations. No attempt was made to control the intake of the children at home, although based on household food consumption data, it was calculated that the diets were likely to be limiting in lysine. The supplemental school lunch feeding caused a significant increase in weight, compared to the control children. However, no advantage was found for the lysine supplemented group.

The above experiments carried out in Haiti and Iran were carried out in populations of school-age children. The protein needs of these children are less severe than those of preschool children, particularly in regards to the amino acid pattern. Pereira et al. (1969) have reported the results of an experiment in which lysine fortification of wheat was evaluated in 52 preschool children in an orphanage in India. The diet provided 2 gm protein and 100 kcal per kg body wt per day. The wheat in both control and experimental groups provided 54% of the calories and 85% of the protein. The results indicated that there was a statistically significant increase in height in the children fed lysine-supplemented wheat as compared with those fed wheat without added lysine. Significant differences in body weight or nitrogen retention were not observed. However, children in both groups lost weight during the last month of the trial and it was pointed out that this was the hottest month of the year. The experiment illustrated some of the difficulties of carrying out practical feeding studies, even under the relatively controlled conditions of an orphanage.

Corn.—Gomez et al. (1957) evaluated in four preschool children the effect of amino acid supplementation of a maize and bean diet on absorption and retention of nitrogen. In all cases both nitrogen absorption and retention were increased when the diet was supplemented with lysine and tryptophan. Lysine alone was not tried.

Scrimshaw et al. (1958) and Bressani et al. (1958) studied the influence of amino acid supplementation of corn masa on nitrogen retention of young children with ages from 1½–4½ yr old. Protein was fed at high (3 gm per kg body wt) and intermediate (1.5–2.0 gm per kg body wt) levels of intake. At either level lysine and tryptophan added individually were of no benefit. When they were added together, a marked increase in nitrogen retention occurred which could be further improved by addition of isoleucine. Methionine, added to the level of the 1957 FAO provisional pattern, had an adverse effect.

Additional studies with corn masa were carried out with four children 1½–5 yr of age (Bressani et al. 1963B). Nitrogen retention was doubled by addition of lysine and tryptophan, but was still lower than values obtained with milk. In two children lysine alone improved nitrogen balance. Hansen (1960) also has reported that nitrogen balance in children 1–4 yr of age can be increased by supplementing corn with lysine and tryptophan.

Rice.—Fewer studies have been carried out on the effects in young children of fortifying rice with amino acids than is the case for either wheat or corn. Bressani et al. (1971) studied the effects of fortification of rice with lysine, threonine and methionine in young children ranging in age from 2–4 yr who had recently recovered from protein-calorie malnutrition. The basal diet, consisting of rice flour 96%, cornstarch 1% and glycine 3%, was fed to supply 2 gm protein and 90–100 kcal per kg body wt. No consistent effects on nitrogen retention were observed as a result of amino acid fortification. Fecal nitrogen on the rice diet amounted to 18–24% of intake suggesting a relatively poor digestability of rice protein in the infants. In this study the rice protein was diluted with nonessential nitrogen in the form of glycine to the extent that only ⅔ of dietary nitrogen was in the form of rice protein. Since the proportion of amino acid nitrogen in the form of essential amino acids is already marginal in rice and other cereals, this dilution with glycine may also be another factor to consider in interpreting the results.

A study has been reported in which rice diets were evaluated with and without amino acid supplements in 8–9 yr old girls (Parthasarathy et al. 1964B). Daily intake was 250 gm of milled rice and 12 gm Tur dhal along with nonprotein foodstuffs. Nitrogen balance experiments indicated the net available protein (g per kg body wt) from the various diets were as follows: rice diet 0.71, rice diet + lysine 0.76, rice diet + lysine + threonine 0.85, rice diet + lysine + threonine + methionine 0.91, skim milk control diet 0.96–0.98. Recently, a field study was carried out in which the effects of fortification of rice with lysine and threonine on the growth of preschool children was evaluated in feeding trials at a residential orphanage and a village day-care center (Pereira et al. 1973). A total of 135 children ranging in age from 2–5 years were studied in the several experiments run. The basal diet supplied 2 gm protein per 100 kcal with rice furnishing 82% of the total energy and 78% of the protein. The diets were offered ad libitum with plate waste recorded. No effects of amino acid fortification were observed on body height, body weight or any of the blood parameters measured. Both control and experimental groups of children in the orphanage grew at rates comparable to those reported for North American children, suggesting that the basal rice diet used met their nutritional needs. In contrast a number of children in the village center were unable to consume enough food to meet their energy requirements.

Other Cereals.—Workers at Mysore have reported results of several experiments in which ragi diets were evaluated for protein value with and without amino acid supplements. Daniel and coworkers (1965) carried out balance experiments in groups of girls 11–12 yr of age with eight girls per group. Net available protein (g per kg body wt) were: ragi diet 0.60, ragi diet + lysine 0.70, ragi diet + lysine + threonine 0.80, skim milk diet 0.94. In an experiment carried out with boys 6–12 yr of age lysine added to a ragi diet improved nitrogen balance from 0.76 to 1.50 gm per child per day (Doraiswamy *et al.* 1969).

Similar studies have been conducted by this same group in which amino acid supplementation of kaffir corn (sorghum) was evaluated in young girls age 7–12. Daniel *et al.* (1966) reported the following values for net available protein (gm per kg body wt) for the various diets: kaffir corn diet 0.64, kaffir corn diet + lysine 0.69, kaffir corn diet + lysine + threonine 0.81, skim milk diet 0.93. In an extension of these studies Doraiswamy and coworkers (1968) evaluated the effect of supplementation of the kaffir corn diet with lysine alone when fed to school children for a 6-month period. The diet supplied 2.0 gm protein per kg body wt per day. The lysine content of the basal diet was 4 gm per 16 gm N and this was increased to 6.5 gm per 16 gm N by addition of L-lysine monohydrochloride. The experimental group and the control group each consisted of 24 girls 7–12 yr of age. The study was carried out in a boarding school in Mysore. The mean increases in height and weight were as follows: height—controls 1.82 cm, lysine supplemented 2.93 cm; weight—controls 0.80 kg, lysine supplemented 1.74 kg. Nitrogen retention data paralleled the weight change data. The authors concluded that lysine supplementation of this kaffir corn diet resulted in statistically significant increases in the growth and nitrogen retention of the children.

Bressani *et al.* (1963C) reported that nitrogen retention in young children fed oat protein at 2 gm per kg body weight per day could be increased to a level only slightly below that of milk by addition of lysine and threonine. Results were more variable, however than observed by these workers in the studies with wheat and corn.

RECENT EXPERIMENTAL STUDIES

Fortification During Pregnancy and Lactation

Almost all of the literature dealing with the amino acid fortification of cereals has been concerned with growth of the postweaning animal or infant (Jansen 1974). The implications of protein quality improvement of cereals

TABLE 9.4

EFFECT OF AMINO ACID FORTIFICATION OF BREAD
ON BIRTH AND WEANING WEIGHTS

Diet	Birth Wt (gm)	Total Litter Wt (gm)	Weaning Wt (gm)
Litter 1			
White bread	5.50 ± 0.14[1]	74.2 ± 3.9	17.0 ± 0.4
Bread + lysine	6.39 ± 0.09	74.5 ± 4.8	26.8 ± 0.2
Bread + lysine + threonine	6.54 ± 0.24	62.1 ± 6.0	39.8 ± 0.6
Casein	7.13 ± 0.16	68.9 ± 2.6	42.8 ± 0.8
Litter 2			
White bread	5.80 ± 0.19	46.5 ± 3.5	16.8 ± 0.9
Bread + lysine	5.84 ± 0.11	70.5 ± 2.2	25.4 ± 0.8
Bread + lysine + threonine	6.20 ± 0.14	80.6 ± 6.2	45.4 ± 0.9
Casein	6.34 ± 0.13	52.3 ± 5.7	43.6 ± 1.2

Source: Data from Jansen and Chase (1976).
[1]Mean ± standard error.

for maternal nutrition have been considered and the literature reviewed in a recent publication (Jansen 1973). Based on this review it was concluded that the value of adding lysine to cereals consumed during pregnancy or lactation has not yet been clearly established. Because the lysine need for maintenance in adults appears to be fairly low and the lysine content of muscle protein is quite high, it may be that the lysine need of the developing fetus or the lactating mammary gland can be met from maternal tissues with the resulting deficit made up subsequent to delivery or lactation. Recently we have studied the effects of fortifying white bread fed to rats during pregnancy and lactation with amino acids. The results to be described strongly suggest that protein quality improvement of cereals is of considerable value during pregnancy and lactation, as well as during postweaning growth.

The experimental procedures and the results have been described in detail elsewhere (Jansen and Chase 1976; Chase and Jansen 1976). Air-dried standard white bread fortified with 0.35% L-lysine monohydrochloride or 0.6% L-lysine monohydrochloride and 0.35% DL-threonine was fed to pregnant rats from conception until weaning. An isonitrogenous casein diet was also fed (2.1% N, 13% protein). All diets contained adequate levels of vitamins and minerals, and 4% corn oil. At weaning the pups were weighed, their brains removed, weighed, divided into major regions, and analyzed for DNA and protein. The mothers were kept on the same diets, rebred and the second litter of offspring analyzed at weaning for somatic and brain growth as above. Birth weights, total litter weights, and weaning weights of the offspring are listed in Table 9.4. Birth weights of first litter pups whose mothers were fed unfortified bread were significantly smaller than all other treatments (P < 0.001) but this was not true for second litters. The number of pups per litter and total litter weights did not vary significantly in first litters. However, in the second litters, litter size was significantly affected by protein quality and as a result total litter weight in mothers fed unfortified bread was only 46.5 ± 1.2 gm compared to 80.6 ± 1.6 gm in the lysine- and threonine-fortified bread group (P < 0.01). As shown in Table 9.4, weaning weights were significantly greater in the offspring of mothers fed amino acid fortified bread than in the offspring of mothers fed unfortified bread (P < 0.001). Weaning weights in the lysine and threonine group were substantially the same as found for the casein group in both first and second litters.

Brain growth on any diet was not significantly different in second than in first litter offspring. Therefore in Table 9.5 only first litter results are given with brain weight, protein, and DNA listed separately for whole brain, cerebellum, and cerebrum. Lysine addition significantly increased weight, protein, and DNA in whole brain, cerebellum, and cerebrum (P < 0.05) over values obtained in offspring fed unfortified bread. The addition of threonine with the lysine gave additional significant increases over values obtained with lysine alone in all cases except for total protein in the cerebrum which was unchanged. Brain weight, protein, and cellularity (i.e., DNA content) observed in the offspring of mothers fed lysine- and threonine-fortified bread in all cases were as high as values obtained in offspring of mothers fed casein.

Fortification During Energy Deficiency

The current debate concerning the value of protein improvement programs under conditions where the energy requirement may not be fully met has been mentioned. Several experiments have been carried out to investigate these relationships in young growing or pregnant rats. In the first two experiments weanling rats were fed diets of air-dried white bread, bread + 0.3% L-lysine monohydrochloride or bread + 0.5% L-lysine monohydrochloride, and 0.3% DL-threonine for 21 days at energy levels ranging from 55–100% of *ad libitum* intake. The protein:calorie ratio of the diet was held constant and the complete diet included vitamins, minerals, and 5% corn oil. The experimental procedures and results have been described in detail elsewhere (Jansen and Verburg 1976). The results for the first experiment are summarized in Table 9.6. In experiment 1 rats fed lysine fortified bread at 80% of *ad libitum* consumption gained twice as much weight and showed 220% and 50% increases in PER and NPR respectively over those fed unfortified bread *ad libitum* in spite of the fact that they consumed 10% less food (groups 15 versus group 17). The addition of threonine with lysine gave additional increases in these parameters also at a reduced food intake

TABLE 9.5

EFFECT OF AMINO ACID FORTIFICATION DURING PREGNANCY AND LACTATION ON BRAIN GROWTH

Part of Brain	Diet			
	Bread	Bread + Lysine	Bread + Lysine + Threonine	Casein
	Brain Weights (gm)			
Whole brain	1.212 ± 0.012[1]	1.359 ± 0.010	1.466 ± 0.013	1.466 ± 0.011
Cerebellum	0.133 ± 0.002	0.158 ± 0.003	0.178 ± 0.002	0.178 ± 0.003
Cerebrum	0.848 ± 0.010	0.931 ± 0.006	1.009 ± 0.009	1.007 ± 0.006
	Brain Protein (mg)			
Whole brain	93.52 ± 3.16	107.98 ± 3.40	115.79 ± 1.21	112.64 ± 1.89
Cerebellum	10.71 ± 0.32	13.96 ± 0.28	15.37 ± 0.25	15.74 ± 0.36
Cerebrum	69.77 ± 1.04	78.32 ± 1.29	80.94 ± 1.10	78.84 ± 1.04
	Brain DNA (mg)			
Whole brain	2.145 ± 0.030	2.286 ± 0.058	2.519 ± 0.058	2.442 ± 0.053
Cerebellum	1.006 ± 0.018	1.128 ± 0.015	1.201 ± 0.020	1.208 ± 0.022
Cerebrum	0.919 ± 0.018	0.975 ± 0.011	1.091 ± 0.0147	1.010 ± 0.012

Source: Data from Chase and Jansen (1976).
[1]Mean ± standard error.

TABLE 9.6

WEIGHT GAIN AND NITROGEN UTILIZATION AS A FUNCTION OF PROTEIN QUALITY AND ENERGY LEVEL (EXP.1)

Group	Diet	Energy Level % of ad libitum Consumption	Wt Gain[2] (gm)	Food intake (gm)	PER[3,4]	NPR[5,6]
1	Powdered Egg	100	86.0 ± 2.7[7]	250	3.44 ± 0.11	4.06 ± 0.11
2	White	90	65.3 ± 5.8	222	2.94 ± 0.26	3.64 ± 0.26
3		80	57.8 ± 1.9	198	2.92 ± 0.09	3.70 ± 0.09
4	ANRC Reference	70	46.5 ± 1.4	174	2.67 ± 0.08	3.56 ± 0.08
5	Casein	100	72.5 ± 5.7	230	3.15 ± 0.25	3.82 ± 0.25
6		90	48.3 ± 1.3	192	2.52 ± 0.11	3.32 ± 0.11
7		80	34 ± 1.7	171	2.54 ± 0.10	3.44 ± 0.10
8		70	35.3 ± 1.8	151	2.34 ± 0.12	3.36 ± 0.12
9	Bread + 0.5%	100	53.3 ± 4.2	205	2.60 ± 0.20	3.36 ± 0.20
10	L-lysine HCL +	90	37.5 ± 4.1	184	2.04 ± 0.22	2.88 ± 0.22
11	0.3% DL-	80	32.7 ± 2.3	163	2.00 ± 0.14	2.95 ± 0.14
12	threonine[1]	70	26.3 ± 1.3	143	1.84 ± 0.09	2.92 ± 0.09
13	Bread + 0.3%	100	25.8 ± 4.0	171	1.51 ± 0.23	2.41 ± 0.23
14	L-lysine HCL[1]	90	17.5 ± 1.4	154	1.14 ± 0.09	2.14 ± 0.09
15		80	15.8 ± 2.3	137	1.15 ± 0.17	2.28 ± 0.17
16		70	11.7 ± 1.1	123	0.95 ± 0.09	2.20 ± 0.09
17	Bread	100	8.0 ± 1.5	153	0.52 ± 0.09	1.53 ± 0.10
18		90	2.3 ± 1.1	131	0.18 ± 0.12	1.36 ± 0.08
19		80	0.3 ± 1.0	116	0.03 ± 0.23	1.36 ± 0.09
20		70	0.5 ± 1.3	107	0.05 ± 0.48	1.41 ± 0.12
21	Protein-free	100	−15.0 ± 1.8			

Source: Jansen and Verburg (1976).

[1] Amino acid levels expressed as percentages of the dry weight of the bread.
[2] Statistical comparisons for weight gain; groups 1–14 all greater than 17–20 at P < 0.001, 15 greater than 17–20 at P < 0.025. 12 greater than 14 or 15 at P < 0.001.
[3] Protein Efficiency Ratio (PER).
[4] Statistical comparisons for PER; groups 1–14 all greater than 17–20 at P < 0.001, 15 or 16 greater than 17–20 at P < 0.01, 12 greater than 14 or 15 at P < 0.001.
[5] Net Protein Ratio (NPR).
[6] Statistical comparisons for NPR; groups 1–16 all greater than 17–20 at P < 0.001, 12 greater than 14 or 15 at P < 0.001.
[7] Mean ± standard error, N = 6.

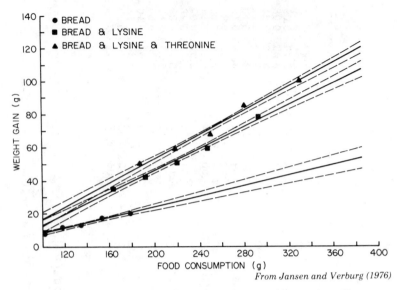

From Jansen and Verburg (1976)

FIG. 9.1.   WEIGHT GAIN VERSUS FOOD CONSUMED AS AFFECTED BY PROTEIN QUALITY (EXPERIMENT 2)
The regression lines with 95% confidence intervals for each diet are shown (n = 40 rats per group).

(group 12 versus group 17). Because rat growth in this experiment was less than that observed in previous work, the experiment was repeated with a fresh supply of bread, a different rat strain, more energy levels, and more animals per group. In this study growth on the bread diets was considerably improved, but the relative improvement in growth and nitrogen utilization with lysine-fortified bread fed at reduced energy level was substantially the same as had been observed in the first experiment. The regression relationship for weight gain and NPR for bread, bread plus lysine and bread plus lysine plus threonine are shown in Fig. 9.1 and 9.2, respectively. The improvements in these parameters with protein quality improvement even when dietary energy and protein were severely restricted is clearly apparent. These results strongly suggest that protein quality improvements is of potential value even if the dietary energy supply is not completely adequate.

Because of these results it was of considerable interest to study the effect of amino acid fortification of bread fed at varying levels of energy intake to rats during pregnancy and lactation. The experimental procedures and results obtained are described in detail elsewhere (Jansen and Monte 1976). Briefly, air dried white bread, bread + 0.3% L-lysine monohydrochloride, bread + 0.5% L-lysine monohydrochloride, and 0.3% DL-threonine were fed to pregnant rats during gestation and lactation at energy levels of 100%,

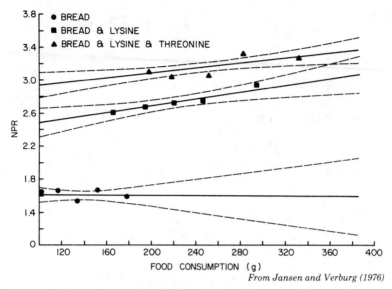

From Jansen and Verburg (1976)

FIG. 9.2.   NPR VERSUS FOOD CONSUMED AS AFFECTED BY PROTEIN QUALITY
(EXPERIMENT 2)
The regression lines with 95% confidence intervals are shown   (n = 40 rats per
group).

85%, and 70% of *ad libitum* intake. The results for the most pertinent
groups have been summarized in Table 9.7. Confirming earlier experiments,
the offspring of mothers fed lysine and threonine fortified bread showed
at weaning substantial and highly significant increases in body weight, brain
weight, and in the levels of DNA and protein in all major regions of the brain
(group 4 versus 1). Mother rats fed lysine and threonine fortified bread at
70% of *ad libitum* intake consumed 13% less food in pregnancy and lactation
than did mothers fed unfortified bread *ad libitum* (group 5 versus 1). In
spite of this reduced level of food intake, weaning weight, brain weight,
cerebellum weight, cerebrum weight, and brainstem weight of the offspring
were all significantly increased in the bread group fortified with amino acid
($P < 0.001$). This was also true for cerebellum, cerebrum and brainstem
protein as well as DNA ($P < 0.01$). The addition of lysine alone when
mothers were fed *ad libitum* increased these parameters significantly ($P
< 0.02$) over values obtained with unfortified bread (group 2 versus 1).
Weaning weights of the offspring of mothers fed lysine fortified bread at
70% of *ad libitum* consumption were significantly greater ($P < 0.001$) than
was the case for the offspring of mothers fed bread *ad libitum* in spite of
consuming 13% less food (group 3 versus 1). Brainstem and cerebellum
weight, protein and DNA levels also were significantly increased ($P < 0.05$)
in the lysine group under these conditions (group 3 versus 1). These results

TABLE 9.7

AMINO ACID FORTIFICATION OF BREAD FED TO PREGNANT OR LACTATING RATS AT DIFFERENT ENERGY LEVELS

Group Diet Level of Feeding[1]	1 Bread 100%	2 Bread + Lysine 100%	3 Bread + Lysine 70%	4 Bread + Lysine + Threonine 100%	5 Bread + Lysine + Threonine 70%
Food consumption-pregnancy (gm/day)	16.8 ± 1.3[2]	20.4 ± 0.5	14.5 ± 0.5	19.9 ± 0.5	14.6 ± 0.8
Food consumption-lactation (gm/day)	31.4 ± 1.4	36.5 ± 1.7	26.3 ± 0.9	38.5 ± 0.9	27.2 ± 0.1
Weaning weight (gm)	16.8 ± 0.4	26.4 ± 0.2	21.4 ± 0.2	38.8 ± 0.4	28.8 ± 0.3
Brain weight (gm)	1.235 ± 0.010	1.322 ± 0.008	1.256 ± 0.007	1.491 ± 0.008	1.344 ± 0.012
Cerebellum weight (gm)	0.148 ± 0.003	0.155 ± 0.001	0.154 ± 0.001	0.177 ± 0.001	0.159 ± 0.001
Cerebrum weight (gm)	0.847 ± 0.012	0.894 ± 0.008	0.843 ± 0.007	0.966 ± 0.010	0.882 ± 0.008
Brainstem weight (gm)	0.202 ± 0.004	0.208 ± 0.004	0.218 ± 0.005	0.235 ± 0.002	0.213 ± 0.002
Cerebellum protein (mg)	11.90 ± 0.20	14.38 ± 0.13	12.70 ± 0.10	16.34 ± 0.10	14.26 ± 0.08
Cerebrum protein (mg)	71.16 ± 0.99	78.13 ± 0.72	70.31 ± 0.56	81.12 ± 0.86	77.14 ± 0.70
Brainstem protein (mg)	16.23 ± 0.33	19.20 ± 0.36	17.28 ± 0.39	19.49 ± 0.13	18.22 ± 0.14
Cerebellum DNA (mg)	1.023 ± 0.019	1.136 ± 0.012	1.080 ± 0.009	1.467 ± 0.010	1.144 ± 0.007
Cerebrum DNA (mg)	0.922 ± 0.016	0.975 ± 0.010	0.927 ± 0.012	1.088 ± 0.014	0.973 ± 0.013
Brainstem DNA (mg)	0.231 ± 0.005	0.264 ± 0.005	0.247 ± 0.006	0.281 ± 0.002	0.258 ± 0.002

Source: Data from Jansen and Monte (1976).
[1] Percentage of *ad libitum* consumption.
[2] Mean ± standard error.

suggest a beneficial value of protein quality improvement of cereals consumed during pregnancy and lactation as well as during postweaning growth under conditions of inadequacy in dietary energy.

DISCUSSION

In considering the potential practical value of protein quality in improvement of cereals the two important issues previously mentioned are as follows. The first is whether there are situations occurring in real life where the protein quality of a cereal is a limiting factor in the overall nutritional value for humans of diets based on cereals. The second is the extent to which amino acid fortification of food staples is a viable alternative in protein improvement. Strongly related is the extent to which the protein needs of all segments of the population can be met by cereals alone or cereals in combination with small amounts of legumes and the extent to which a deficit in energy consumption reduces the expected benefit of protein quality improvement. These issues relate to all protein improvement programs, and are of interest especially in relation to protein quality improvement whether through plant breeding or amino acid fortification.

The extent to which lysine, lysine and threonine, or lysine and tryptophan are actually limiting nutritional factors in practical human diets is not known but is under active investigation in three large scale feasibility studies in Tunisia, Guatemala, and Thailand. In such studies it is important that a complete vitamin and mineral supplement be added with the amino acid(s). Field trials in which amino acid fortification is being evaluated that do not ensure an adequate intake of all required nutrients, such as zinc, may not show the expected nutritional benefit. It has been argued elsewhere that protein quality improvement of cereals would, in effect, put a floor under the protein value of cereal-based diets, below which the net protein value will not fall (Jansen 1973). In the past, considerations of the respective importance of lysine versus methionine have focused on amino acid needs for growth and maintenance (Jansen 1974). Recent work demonstrating the importance of dietary lipotrophic factors, including methionine, in promoting resistance to disease (Newberne and Wilson 1972) suggests that methionine intake could be more important than previously thought even when it is not the amino acid actually limiting growth.

The recent experiments reported in this paper dealt primarily with the protein-energy issue, particularly in relation to the two most vulnerable population groups of preschool children and pregnant/lactating women. The data obtained strongly support the conclusion that protein quality improvement of wheat fed to young growing rats improves growth and nitrogen utilization even when the supply of dietary food energy is clearly inadequate. In interpreting the relevance of rat growth data to the human situation, a major factor to consider is that the human infant grows at a slower rate than does the weanling rat. For the human infant Graham *et al.* (1971) have reported that lysine fortified wheat is comparable in protein quality to casein, while for the rat lysine and threonine addition is clearly needed (Jansen 1974). It seems likely that increasing the supply of usable protein in a cereal type diet fed to young children, whether through protein or amino acid fortification, or via plant breeding programs would be of as much value as was demonstrated to be the case for the more rapidly growing rat even if food consumed does not completely meet energy needs.

The present experiments also demonstrate very clearly the beneficial value of protein quality improvement of bread fed to pregnant or lactating rats under conditions of inadequacy in the supply of dietary energy. In this model, threonine addition along with the lysine was of considerable importance, more so than in the case of the postweaning rat. It would appear that more work should be carried out on the metabolism of threonine in the pregnant or lactating rat, especially in relation to brain development of the offspring. Based on the growth experiments in young children referred to earlier, threonine addition to wheat would not give any beneficial effects beyond those obtained with lysine. However, no data are available dealing with the effects of lysine and threonine fortification of wheat fed to women during pregnancy or lactation and so this question must remain unanswered at present.

A deficiency in total food supply in third and fourth world countries, compounded by high levels of population increases, shortages in energy, and shortages in fertilizer is probably the most crucial nutritional problem in the less developed world today. This does not mean, however, that protein improvement would be of no practical value under conditions of marginal energy deprivation. The data presented in this paper suggests that protein improvement programs including those directed toward protein quality improvement of cereals through plant breeding programs or fortification would likely be of value under these conditions. However, in order for a beneficial effect to actually result from protein improvement, it is necessary that steps be taken to ensure that the diet is adequate in all needed vitamins and minerals. The complexity of the practical situation should be recognized, especially in regard to the impact of cultural factors, including sanitation and breast feeding. It is often difficult to demonstrate in the field the advantages of nutritional intervention programs. For example, such a program in Guatemala in which nutritional supplements were given and which extended over a 5-yr period was reported to have little impact on growth of children and mortality and morbidity because of these supervening variables (Scrimshaw 1970). Mahloudji *et al.* (1975) recently reported that simultaneous fortification of bread with zinc and iron did not improve growth of Iranian boys in contrast to the positive growth effects that resulted from iron addition alone, even though the diets were known to be deficient in zinc and in fact, low plasma zinc levels in the subjects were observed. In order for significant progress to be made in the worldwide fight against malnutrition, many factors have to be altered simultaneously. Protein quality improvement of cereals may well be one, but only one, of these factors.

In considering the nature of diets in less developed countries in which protein-calorie malnutrition is a serious public health problem, it would appear that they may be arbitrarily divided into two types. These are situations in which most protein and energy is supplied by either cereals and legumes or root crops and legumes. In the former situation if enough legume protein is consumed together with cereals, the lysine deficiency in the cereal is balanced out and neither protein nor amino acid supplements are needed or will be beneficial. If not enough legume protein is consumed the diet will be limiting in lysine and will be low in utilizable protein. In this case cereal protein improvement, whether by protein or amino acid addition, through plant breeding programs, or any combination of the above should be desirable from a nutritional standpoint. Diets characterized by a high proportion of energy coming from root crops and legumes could conceivably benefit from methionine addition if the protein level of the overall diet is marginal or low. This would likely only occur in situations where large amounts of manioc are consumed.

SUMMARY

The literature dealing with the amino acid fortification of plant foods has been selectively reviewed and the results of new studies dealing with amino acid fortification during pregnancy and lactation and protein quality-energy relationships presented. Studies in experimental animals have demonstrated that legumes and cereals can be substantially improved in biological value by fortification with methionine and lysine, respectively. Experiments carried out in young infants have confirmed the results of the animal studies for methionine added to soy, lysine added to wheat and lysine and tryptophan added to corn. Human studies have not confirmed the value of lysine and threonine fortification of rice.

The potential value of protein quality improvement of cereals has been studied in rats during pregnancy and lactation and also under conditions of inadequacy in the supply of dietary energy. Bread was fortified with lysine or lysine and threonine and fed to rats either during pregnancy and lactation or for 28 days following weaning. Calorie levels ranged from 55% to *ad libitum* during postweaning growth and from 70% to *ad libitum* during pregnancy and lactation. Amino acid fortification of bread fed during pregnancy and lactation significantly increased weaning weight, brain weight, brain protein, and brain DNA in the offspring. When food intake was reduced during pregnancy and lactation or in the postweaning animal, the beneficial effects of amino acid fortification on growth, nitrogen utilization, and cellular development of the brain were clearly apparent. The results suggest that protein quality improvement programs, whether by plant breeding or amino acid fortification, may well be of practical value in human nutrition even if consumption of food calories does not fully meet the energy need provided that adequate vitamins and minerals are supplied.

BIBLIOGRAPHY

BARNES, R. H., FIALA, G., and KWONG, E. 1962. Methionine supplementation of processed soybeans in the rat. J. Nutr. 77, 278.

BARNESS, L. A., KAYE, R., and VALYASEVI, A. 1961. Lysine and potassium supplementation of wheat protein. Am. J. Clin. Nutr. 9, 331.

BENDER, A. E. 1958. Nutritive value of bread protein fortified with amino acids. Science 127, 874.

BORCHERS, R. (1962). Supplementary methionine requirement of weanling rats fed soybean oil meal rations. J. Nutr. 77, 309.

BRESSANI, R., and ELIAS, L. G. 1968. Processed Vegetable Protein Mixtures for Human Consumption in Developing Countries. In Advances in Food Research, Vol. 16, C. D. Chichester, E. M. Mrak, and G. F. Stewart (Editors). Academic Press, New York.

BRESSANI. R., and ELIAS, L. G. 1974 . Legume foods. In New Protein Foods, A. M. Altschul (Editor). Academic Press, New York.

BRESSANI, R., ELIAS, L. G., and BRAHAM, J. E. 1968. Supplementation of maize and tortilla with amino acids. Arch. Latinoamer. Nutricion. 18, 123.

BRESSANI, R., SCRIMSHAW, N. W., BEHAR, M., and VITERI, F. 1958. Supplementation of cereal proteins with amino acids. II. Effect of amino acid supplementation of corn-masa at intermediate levels of protein intake in the nitrogen retention of young children. J. Nutr. 66, 501.

BRESSANI, R., WILSON, D. L., BEHAR, M., and SCRIMSHAW, N. S. 1960. Supplementation of cereal proteins with amino acids. III. Effect of amino acid supplementation of wheat flour as measured by nitrogen retention of young children. J. Nutr. 70, 176.

BRESSANI, R., WILSON, D., BEHAR, M., CHUNG, M., and SCRIMSHAW, N. S. 1963A. Supplementation of cereal proteins with amino acids. IV. Lysine supplementation of wheat flour fed to young children at different levels of protein intake in the presence and absence of other amino acids. J. Nutr. 79, 333.

BRESSANI, R., WILSON, D., CHUNG, M., BEHAR, M., and SCRIMSHAW, N. S. 1963B. Supplementation of cereal proteins with amino acids. V. Effect of supplementing lime treated corn with different levels of lysine, typtophan and isoleucine on the nitrogen retention of young children. J. Nutr. 80, 80.

BRESSANI, R., WILSON, D. L., CHUNG, M., BEHAR, M., and SCRIMSHAW, N. S. 1963C. Supplementation of cereal proteins with amino acids. VI Effect of amino acid supplementation of rolled oats as measured by nitrogen retention of young children. J. Nutr. 81, 399–404.

BRESSANI, R., WILSON, D. M., VITERI, F., MOSOVICH, L., and ALVARADO, J. 1971. Effect of Amino Acid Supplementation of White Rice Fed to Children. Arch. Latinoamer. Nutr. 21, 347.

BRESSANI, R., and DE ZAGHI, S. 1970. Supplementation of casein and of vegetable mixtures based on soybean flour with methionine, methionine hydroxy analogue and vitamin B_6. Archiv. Latinoamer. Nutricion. 20, 179.

CHASE, H. P., and JANSEN, G. R. 1976. Effect of lysine and threonine fortification of bread during gestation and lactation on growth of brain. J. Nutr. 106, 41.

COMM. ON NUTR., AM. ACAD. OF PEDIAT. 1963. Appraisal of nutritional adequacy of infant formulas used as cow milk substitutes. Pediatrics 31, 329.

DANIEL, V. A., LEELA, R., DORAISWAMY, T. R., RAJALAKSHMI, D., RAO, S. V., SWAMINA-

THAN, M., and PARPIA, H. A. B. 1965. The effect of supplementing a poor Indian ragi diet with L-lysine and DL-threonine on the digestability coefficient, biological value and net utilization of the proteins and on nitrogen retention in children. J. Nutr. Dietet. India 2, 138.

DANIEL, V. A., LEELA, R., DORAISWAMY, T. R., RAJALAKSHMI, D., RAO, S. V., SWAMINA-THAN, M., and PARPIA, H. A. B. 1966. The effect of supplementing a poor kaffir corn (Sorghum Vulgare) diet with L-lysine and DL-threonine on the digestability coefficient, biological value and net utilization of proteins and retention of nitrogen in children. J. Nutr. Dietet. India 3, 10.

DORAISWAMY, T. R., SINGH, N., and DANIEL, V. A. 1969. Effects of supplementing ragi (Elusine Coracana) diets with lysine or leaf protein on the growth and nitrogen metabolism of children. Brit. J. Nutr. 23, 737.

DORAISWAMY, T. R., URS., T. S., RAO, S. V., SWAMINATHAN, M., and PARPIA, H. A. B. 1968. Effect of supplementation of poor kaffir corn diet (Sorghum Vulgare) with L-lysine on nitrogen retention and growth of school children. J. Nutr. Dietet. India 5, 191.

DREYER, J. J., and DU BRUYN, D. B. 1965. Supplementation of soya protein with L-methionine, DL-methionine hydroxy analog and certain natural sources of methionine. S. African J. Nutr. 1, 21.

FAO. 1970. Amino acid content of foods and biological data on proteins. Food Agr. Organ. U.N., FAO Nutr. Studies 24 (Rome).

FAO/WHO. 1973. Energy and protein requirements. Report of a Joint FAO/WHO Ad Hoc Expert Committee. World Health Organ. Tech. Rept. Ser. 522, (Geneva).

FOMON, S. J. 1959. Comparative Study of Human Milk and a Soya Bean Formula in Promoting Growth and Nitrogen Retention by Infants. Pediatrics 24, 577.

FOMON, S. J., THOMAS, L. N., FILER JR., L. J., ANDERSON, J. A., and BERGMANN, K. L. 1973. Requirements for protein and essential amino acids in early infancy. Acta Paediat. Scand. 62, 33.

GOMEZ, F., RAMOS GALVAN, CRAVIOTO, S. J., FRENK, S., DE LA PENA, C., MORENO, M. E., and VILLA, M. E. 1957. Protein metabolism in chronic severe malnutrition (Kwashiorkor). 2. Influence of amino acid supplements on the absorption and retention of nitrogen from a maize and beans diet. Acta. Paediat. 46, 286.

GRAHAM, G. G. 1971. Methionine or lysine fortification of dietary protein for infants and small children. In Amino Acid Fortification of Protein Foods, N. S. Scrimshaw, and A. M. Altschul (Editors). M.I.T. Press, Cambridge, Mass.

GRAHAM, G. G., MORALES, E., CORDANO, A., and PLACKO, R. P. 1971. Lysine enrichment of wheat flour: Prolonged feeding of infants. Am. J. Clin. Nutr. 24, 200.

GRAHAM, G. G., PLACKO, R. P., ACEVEDO, G., MORALES, E., and CORDANO, A. 1969. Lysine enrichment of wheat flour: Evaluation in infants. Am. J. Clin. Nutr. 22, 1459.

HANSEN, J. D. L. 1960. The effect of various forms of supplementation on the nutritive value of maize for children. S. African Med. J. 34, 855.

HARPER, A. E., PAYNE, P. R., and WATERLOW, J. C. 1973. Assessment of human protein needs. Am. J. Clin. Nutr. 26, 1168.

HEDAYAT, H., SHAHBAZI, H., PAYAN, R., and DONOSO, G. 1971. Lysine field trial in Iran. In Progress in Human Nutrition, Vol. 1, S. Margen (Editor). Avi Publishing Co., Westport, Conn.

HEGSTED, D. M. 1969. In Protein Enriched Cereal Foods for World Needs. M. Milner (Editor). American Association of Cereal Chemists, St. Paul, Minn.

HOWE, E. E. 1961. Summary of Progress on the use of purified amino acids in foods. In Progress in Meeting Protein Needs of Infants and Preschool Children. Publ. 843, Natl. Res. Council—Natl. Acad. Sci., Washington, D.C.

HOWE, E. E., GILFILLAN, E. W., and MILNER, M. 1965. Amino Acid Supplementation of Protein Concentrates as Related to the World Protein Supply. Am. J. Clin. Nutr. 16, 321.

HOWE, E. E., JANSEN, G. R., and ANSON, M. L. 1967. An approach toward the solution of the world food problem with special emphasis on protein supply. Am. J. Clin. Nutr. 20, 1134.

HUTCHINSON, J. B., MORAN, T., and PACE, J. 1959. The nutritive value of bread protein as influenced by the level of protein intake, the level of supplementation with L-lysine and L-threonine, and the addition of egg and milk proteins. Brit. J. Nutr. *13*, 151.

JANSEN, G. R. 1962. Lysine in human nutrition. J. Nutrition *76*, Suppl. 1, Part II, No. 2, 1.

JANSEN, G. R. 1969. Total protein value of protein—and amino acid—supplemented bread. Am. J. Clin. Nutr. *22*, 38.

JANSEN, G. R. 1973. Implications for maternal nutrition of protein quality improvement of cereals. Nutr. Rept. Intern. *7*, 555.

JANSEN, G. R. 1974. The amino acid fortification of cereals. *In* New Protein Foods, A. M. Altschul (Editor). Academic Press, New York. pp. 39–120.

JANSEN, G. R. 1975. Amino acid supplementation of common beans and other legumes. *In* Nutritional Aspects of Common Beans, and Other Legume Seeds as Animal and Human Foods, W. G. Jaffe (Editor). Arch. Latinamericanos de Nutricion, Caracas, Venezuela.

JANSEN, G. R., and CHASE, H. P. 1976. Effect of lysine and threonine fortification of bread during gestation and lactation on growth of the offspring. J. Nutr. *106*, 33.

JANSEN, G. R., and MONTE, W. C. 1976. Amino acid fortification of bread fed at varying energy levels during gestation and lactation. (Unpublished data.)

JANSEN, G. R., and VERBURG, D. T. 1976. Amino acid fortification of wheat at varying levels of energy intake. (Unpublished data.)

JENKINS, M. Y., MITCHELL, G. V., and ADKINS, J. S. 1975. Effect of sulfur amino acid fortification of a food grade soy protein concentrate. Nutr. Rept. Intern. *12*, 49.

KIES, C., and FOX, H. M. 1971. Comparison of the protein nutritional value of TVP, methionine-enriched TVP and beef at two levels of intake for human adults. J. Food Sci. *36*, 841.

KING, K. W., SEBRELL, W. H., SEVERINGHAUS, E. L., and STORVICK, W. O. 1963. Lysine fortification of wheat bread fed to Haitian school children. Am. J. Clin. Nutr. *12*, 36.

KNAPP, J., BARNESS, L. A., HILL, L. L., KAYE, R., BLATTNER, R. J., and SLOAN, J. M. 1973. Growth and nitrogen balance in infants fed cereal proteins. Am. J. Clin. Nutr. *26*, 586.

KORSLUND, M., KIES, C., and FOX, H. M. 1973. Comparison of the protein nutritional value of TVP, methionine-enriched TVP and beef for adolescent boys. J. Food Sci. *39*, 637.

KRUT, L. H., HANSEN, J. D. L., TRUSWELL, A. S., SCHENDEL, H. E., and BROCK, J. F. 1961. Controlled field trial of a bread diet supplemented with lysine for children in an institution. S. African J. Lab. Clin. Med. 7, 1.

LIENER, P. E. 1969. Toxic Constituents of Plant Foodstuffs. Academic Press, New York.

LONGENECKER, J. B., MARTIN, W. H., and SARETT, H. P. 1964. Improvement in the protein efficiency of soybean concentrates and isolates by heat treatment. J. Agr. Food Chem. *12*, 411.

MAHLOUDJI, M., REINHOLD, J. G., HAGHSHENASS, M., RONAGHY, H. A., SPIVEY FOX, M. R., and HALSTED, J. A. 1975. Combined zinc and iron compared with iron supplementation of diets of 6 to 12-year old village school children in southern Iran. Am. J. Clin. Nutr. *28*, 721.

MATTIL, K. F. 1974. Composition, nutritional and functional properties and quality criteria of soy protein concentrates and soy isolates. J. Am. Oil. Chem. Soc. *51*, 81A.

McLAREN, D. S. 1974. The great protein fiasco. Lancet *2*, 93.

McOSKER, D. E. 1962. The limiting amino acid sequence in raw and roasted peanut protein. J. Nutr. *76*, 453.

NEWBERNE, P. M., and WILSON, R. B. 1972. Prenatal malnutrition and postnatal responses to infection. Nutr. Rept. Intern. *5*, 151.

OSBORNE, T. B., and MENDEL, L. B. 1914. Amino acids in nutrition and growth. J. Biol. Chem. 17, 325–349.

PARTHASARATHY, H. N., DORAISWAMY, T. R., PANEMANGALORE, M., RAO, M. N., CHANDRASEKHAR, B. S., SWAMINATHAN, M., SREENIVASAN, A., and SUBRAHMANYAN, V. 1964A. The effect of fortification of processed soya flour with DL-methionine hydroxy analogue or DL-methionine on the digestibility, biological value and net protein utilization of the proteins as studied in children. Can. J. Biochem. *42*, 377.

PARTHASARATHY, H. N., JOSEPH, K., DANIEL, V. A., DORAISWAMY, T. R., SANKARAN, A.

N., RAO, M. N., SWAMINATHAN, M., SREENIVASAN, A., and SUBRAHMANYAN, V. 1964B. The effect of supplementing a rice diet with lysine, methionine and threonine on the digestibility coefficient, biological value and net protein utilization of the proteins and on the retention of nitrogen in children. Can. J. Biochem. 42, 385.

PARTHASARATHY, H. N., JOSEPH, K., RAO, M. N., SWAMINATHAN, M., SANKARAN, A. N., SREENIVASAN, A., and SUBRAHMANYAN, V. 1964C. The effect of supplementing processed soyabean meal proteins with DL-methionine hydroxy analogue (MHA) or DL-methionine on protein efficiency ratio and net protein utilization. J. Nutrition Dietet. India 1, 14.

PAYNE, P. R. 1975. Safe protein-calorie ratios in diets. The relative importance of protein and energy intake as causal factors in malnutrition. Am. J. Clin. Nutr. 28, 281.

PECORA, L. J., and HUNDLEY, J. M. 1951. Nutritional improvement of white polished rice by the addition of lysine and threonine. J. Nutr. 44, 101.

PEREIRA, S. M., BEGUM, A., JESUDIAN, G., and SUNDARARAJ, R. 1969. Lysine-supplemented wheat and growth of preschool children. Am. J. Clin. Nutr. 22, 606.

PEREIRA, S. M., JONES, S., JESUDIAN, G., and BEGUM, A. 1973. Feeding trials with lysine—and threonine—fortified rice. Brit. J. Nutr. 30, 241.

REDDY, V. 1971. Lysine supplementation of wheat and nitrogen retention in children. Am. J. Clin. Nutr. 24, 1246.

ROSENBERG, H. R. 1959. Amino acid supplementation of foods and feeds. In Protein and Amino Acid Nutrition, A. A. Albanese (Editor). Academic Press, New York.

ROSENBERG, H. R., CULIK, R., and ECKERT, R. E. 1959. Lysine and threonine supplementation of rice. J. Nutr. 69, 217.

ROSENBERG, H. R., and ROHDENBURG, E. L. 1952. The fortification of bread with lysine. II. The nutritional value of fortified bread. Arch. Biochem. Biophys. 37, 461.

ROSENBERG, H. R., ROHDENBURG, E. L., and ECKERT, R. E. 1960A. Multiple amino acid supplementation of white corn meal. J. Nutr. 72, 415.

ROSENBERG, H. R., ROHDENBURG, E. L., and ECKERT, R. E. 1960B. Supplementation of bread protein with lysine and threonine. J. Nutr. 72, 423.

SCHNEIDER, D. L., and SARETT, H. P. 1969. Growth of baby pigs fed infant soybean formulas. J. Nutr. 98, 279.

SCRIMSHAW, N. S. 1970. Synergism of malnutrition and infection. Evidence from field studies in Guatemala. J. Am. Med. Assoc. 212, 1685.

SCRIMSHAW, N. S., BRESSANI, R., BEHAR, M., and VITERI, F. 1958. Supplementation of cereal proteins with amino acids. I. Effect of amino acid supplementation of corn masa at high levels of protein intake on the nitrogen retention. J. Nutr. 66, 485.

SCRIMSHAW, N. S., and ALTSCHUL, A. M. 1972. Amino acid fortification of protein foods. M.I.T. Press, Cambridge, Mass.

SHURPALEKAR, S. R., CHANDRASEKHARA, M. R., LAHERY, N. L., SWAMINATHAN, M., INDIRAMMA, K., and SUBRAHMANYAN, V. 1961. Studies of milk substitutes of vegetable origin. 3. The nutritive value of spray dried soyabean milk fortified with DL-methionine and spray dried powder from a 2:1 blend of soyabean milk and peanut milk. Ann. Biochem. Expt. Med. 21, 143.

STEGINK, L. D., SCHMITT, J. L., MEYER, P. D., and KAIN, P. H. 1971. Effect of diets fortified with DL-methionine on urinary and plasma methionine levels in young adults. J. Pediatrics 79, 648.

STILLINGS, B. R., SIDWELL, V. D., and HAMMERLE, O. A. 1971. Nutritional quality of wheat flour and bread supplemented with either fish protein concentrate or lysine. Cereal Chem. 48, 292.

SWAMINATHAN 1967. Availability of plant proteins. In Newer Methods of Nutritonal Biochemistry Vol. III, A. A. Albanese (Editor). Academic Press, New York.

THEUER, R. C., and SARETT, H. P. 1970. Nutritional adequacy of soy isolate infant formulas in rats: choline. J. Agr. Food Chem. 18, 913.

VAGHEFI, S. B., MAKDANI, D. D., and MICKELSEN, O. 1974. Lysine supplementation of wheat proteins; a review. Am. J. Clin. Nutr. 27, 1231.

CHAPTER 10

R. Bressani

Protein Supplementation and Complementation

The efficiency of utilization of dietary protein for purposes related to cellular protein synthesis such as maintenance, repletion of protein depleted tissues, and growth of new cellular proteins, is a function of four variables. These are: (1) amino acid pattern provided by the protein in the diet; (2) the intake of nitrogen; (3) the intake of energy, and (4) the physiological state of the organism. For the purpose of this chapter, only the specific role of the essential amino acid pattern relative to the efficiency of protein utilization will be discussed.

The efficiency of protein utilization is dependent upon how well a minimum amount of a protein source provides the essential amino acids to the individual according to the specific needs required by a particular physiological state. Strictly speaking, therefore, the concept of the efficiency of protein utilization is not applicable to the many situations in which an excess of a protein source can provide the essential amino acid needs of the individual.

With only a very few exceptions, most protein sources do not have an essential amino acid pattern that meets amino acid needs when given in minimum physiological amounts for their efficient utilization. They have, therefore, specific essential amino acid deficiencies. On the other hand, most protein sources also have relative excesses of other specific essential amino acids with respect to the needs of the individual. These excesses also contribute in altering (decreasing) the efficiency of protein utilization. Little attention has been given to this aspect of the problem since it is usually assumed that there is no physiological cost paid by the individual in metabolizing such relative excesses.

Amino acid deficiencies can be corrected by at least three ways. One is by adding synthetic amino acids in amounts appropriate to bring the pattern to the level required by the individual. This approach does not consider the relative excesses of other essential amino acids in the protein. The second approach is by adding small amounts of protein which are a rich source in the deficient amino acid(s), providing, therefore, what is lacking in the deficient protein. This approach is known as protein supplementation. Finally, the third approach is to combine protein sources so that they will mutually balance each other's deficiencies or excesses. This is known as protein complementation.

The three approaches increase the efficiency of protein utilization, but probably not to the same degree. In the first case, amino acid fortification, the effect is caused only by an improvement of the essential amino acid pattern, which may then be limited by the relative excess of other amino acids. Protein supplementation also increases efficiency of protein utilization since it corrects amino acid deficiency; however, total protein is increased thereby possibly reducing the improved efficiency of utilization. Finally, protein complementation increases efficiency of utilization by improving the overall amino acid pattern even though in some cases the overall pattern may still not be the ideal pattern for meeting the amino acid needs of the individual. Since amino acid fortification has already been discussed, the present chapter will deal briefly with protein supplementation and will emphasize protein complementation.

PROTEIN SUPPLEMENTATION

As indicated in the introductory comments, the efficiency of protein utilization or protein quality can be increased by adding, to a deficient protein, small amounts of a protein which is a rich source of the amino acid(s) lacking in the deficient protein. The method usually followed consists in adding, to a fixed level of the deficient protein, increasing amounts of the supplemental protein. A typical example, for a deficient protein of low protein content, is shown in Fig. 10.1 for the supplementary effect of soybean flour to corn (Bressani 1975). The results show that there was an increase in protein quality which reached a maximum value when the addition of soybean flour to the diet was equal to about 8%. These diets contained a fixed level of corn of 70%. Adjusting these values to 100%, the ratio of soybean to corn flour would be 9:1. The improvement in protein quality is the result of the soybean flour protein compensating for the lysine deficiency in the corn protein. It is also due to a higher protein content, which increases as more soybean flour is added. However, beyond an optimum point of supplementation, this increase in protein content also causes a decrease in the estimated protein quality. This is due to the well known fact that maximum protein quality values are obtained in rat bioassays at about 10% protein in the diet and decrease as protein content is increased above the 10% level.

A second example in which both sources have a more concentrated level of protein is shown in Fig. 10.2. In this case, also a rat feeding study, cottonseed flour was supplemented with increasing levels of casein (Elías and Bressani 1971). At the same time, to be used as a reference, the cottonseed in the basal diet was supplemented with cottonseed flour added in amounts which would add equal quantities of protein as was added by the different levels of casein. The results in Fig. 10.2 show that 2% casein added to 20% cottonseed flour resulted in the maximum protein quality value, and a

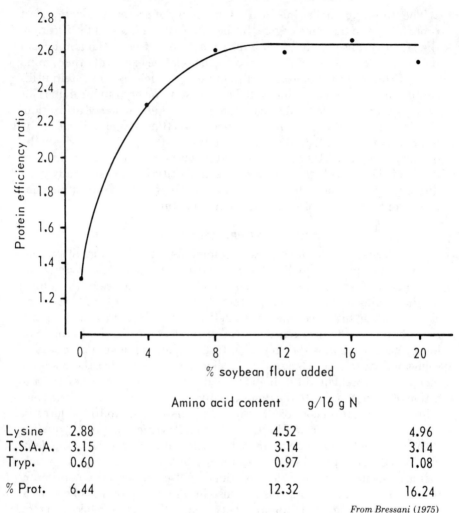

Amino acid content   g/16 g N

Lysine	2.88	4.52	4.96
T.S.A.A.	3.15	3.14	3.14
Tryp.	0.60	0.97	1.08
% Prot.	6.44	12.32	16.24

From Bressani (1975)

FIG. 10.1.   EFFECTS OF SUPPLEMENTATION OF CORN PROTEIN WITH SOYBEAN FLOUR
PROTEIN ON PROTEIN EFFICIENCY RATIO VALUES IN RAT FEEDING STUDIES

Levels of lysine, T.S.A.A. (total sulfur amino acids), Tryp. (tryptophan) and % protein are
listed for diets containing 0, 12 and 20% soybean flour; all diets contained 70% corn flour.

decrease was observed as more casein was added. On the other hand, the
addition of cottonseed flour, as shown in Fig. 10.2, to the basic level of 20%
caused a decrease. In all cases, the quality values resulting from the addition
of casein were higher than those resulting from the addition of equal
amounts of cottonseed flour protein. This example, therefore, shows the
improvement obtained as well as the effect of increasing protein content.

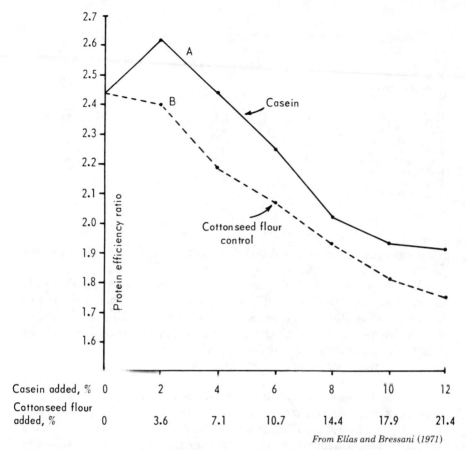

From Elías and Bressani (1971)

FIG. 10.2. EFFECTS ON PROTEIN EFFICIENCY RATIO VALUES OF SUPPLEMENTATION OF A DIET CONTAINING 20% COTTONSEED FLOUR WITH VARIOUS LEVELS OF CASEIN (CURVE A).

Effects of adding equivalent levels of protein from cottonseed flour are shown in curve B.

Consequently, on a 100% basis, the maximum quality value results when the weight ratio of cottonseed flour to casein is 9:1.

In both examples given, the corn-soybean flour study and the casein-cottonseed flour experiments, there is no doubt that improvement in protein quality resulted by the addition of the deficient amino acids in the protein being supplemented. In the first case, lysine which was deficient in the corn protein was provided by soybean flour, and in the second, lysine, deficient in the cottonseed protein, was provided by casein. However, other amino acids will be in a relative excess, particularly those present in high amounts in both protein sources. Secondly, total protein concentration,

TABLE 10.1

EFFECT OF PROTEIN SUPPLEMENTATION OF CORN

Protein Supplement	Optimum Amount Added (% of Diet)	Protein Efficiency Ratio
None	—	1.00
Egg protein	3.0	2.24
Casein	4.0	2.21
Dehydrated beef	4.0	2.34
Fish protein	2.5	2.44
Soybean protein	5.0	2.30
Soybean flour	8.0	2.25
Cottonseed flour	8.0	1.83
Torula yeast	2.5	1.97

Source: Bressani and Marenco (1963).

relative to the efficiency of utilization, is limited to a level that is controlled by the amount of supplement added.

Many other similar results have been published using mainly cereal grains, e.g., corn (Bressani and Marenco 1963), whole wheat (Jarquín et al. 1966), wheat flour (Jarquín et al. 1966), and rice (Elías et al, 1968). Results from rat studies in which corn was supplemented with proteins from vegetable and animal origin are shown in Table 10.1. The estimated optimum quantity varied from 2.5–8%. Depending upon the protein quality of the supplement itself, the efficiency of protein utilization of the corn protein was increased by up to 2.4 times. In these studies, a high correlation coefficient was observed between the improvement in quality obtained and the lysine content of the diet. Using the same approach, a high correlation ($r = 0.80$) was also found between lysine content and nitrogen balance in children fed corn proteins supplemented with various protein sources (Viteri et al. 1972). As indicated previously these high correlations are found because the protein supplements are providing various amounts of lysine, the most deficient amino acid in corn protein. By using the regression equation of lysine content to protein quality for other protein sources, it was possible to predict with a high degree of assurance the expected improvement in protein efficiency ratio. Tryptophan is the second most limiting amino acid in corn proteins and a high correlation was also found between tryptophan intake and protein quality. However, the correlation was not as high as that for lysine.

The results of similar studies carried out with experimental animals with protein supplementation of rice are shown in Table 10.2 (Elías et al. 1968). As with corn, the levels found to give maximum protein quality values varied for the various proteins used as supplements according to their own protein quality. Increases in the quality of the supplemental rice ranged

TABLE 10.2

EFFECT OF PROTEIN SUPPLEMENTATION OF RICE

Protein Supplement	Optimum Amount Added (% of Diet)	Additional Protein Added by Supplement (gm)	Protein Efficiency Ratio
None	—	—	1.73
Skim milk powder	12	4	3.16
Fish protein	8	4	2.88
Casein	6	5	3.22
Cottonseed flour	12	6	2.32
Soybean flour	8	4	2.88
Torula yeast	8	4	3.29
Torula yeast + soybean flour	5	5	2.81

Source: Elías et al. (1968).

TABLE 10.3

EFFECT OF PROTEIN SUPPLEMENTATION OF WHOLE WHEAT AND OF WHEAT FLOUR

Protein Supplement	Whole Wheat		Wheat Flour	
	Optimum Amount (% of Diet)	PER	Optimum Amount (% of Diet)	PER
None	—	1.62	—	0.80
Skim milk	6.0	1.98	10.0	2.19
Casein	4.0	2.54	6.0	2.62
Cottonseed flour	10.0	2.10	12.0	1.96
Soybean flour	6.0	1.89	10.0	2.01
Torula yeast	4.0	2.17	6.0	2.18

Source: Jarquín et al. (1966).

from 1.5–2.0 times that of rice alone. In this example, high correlation coefficients were reported between the lysine content of the supplemented diets and the index of protein quality. The optimum levels of supplementation found are higher than those for corn; this is due to the lower protein content in rice in comparison with corn.

An additional example for whole wheat and wheat flour is shown in Table 10.3. Using small quantities of protein supplements, increases in protein quality were highly significant in both cases. Again a high coefficient of correlation was found between the protein quality improvement and the lysine provided by the protein supplement.

One limitation in these studies concerns the selection of the optimum level of supplement to add. The level selected was the one previous to the first level in the plateau region of the protein quality response curve or, as

TABLE 10.4

NITROGEN BALANCE OF DOGS FED CORN DIETS SUPPLEMENTED
WITH MILK OR FISH PROTEIN

Diet	Nitrogen Balance			Absorbed (% of Intake)	Retained (% of Intake)
	Ingested	Feces	Urine		
	(mg/kg Body wt/Day)				
Corn	729	183	448	74.9	13.4
Corn + 5% skim milk	804	158	322	80.3	40.3
Corn	494	127	307	74.3	12.1
Corn + 4% fish protein concentrate	480	109	218	77.3	31.9

Source: Bressani and de Villarreal (1963).

it occurred in some cases, that level immediately before the level at which protein quality decreased. This decrease is due to the effect of protein content on protein efficiency ratio (Natl. Res. Council–Natl. Acad. Sci. 1963).

The supplementary effect, however, can also be shown by the use of other techniques which measure protein quality at constant levels of protein intake. An example is shown in Table 10.4 which summarizes results of nitrogen balance in young growing dogs fed on corn alone and corn supplemented with 5% and 4% skim milk and fish protein concentrate, respectively (Bressani and de Villarreal 1963). The results show that with 5% skim milk, nitrogen retention was 40.3% compared to 13.4% when protein intake was only from corn. The addition of 4% fish protein concentrate caused an increase in nitrogen retention from 12.1 to 31.9% of the ingested nitrogen.

Therefore, the quantities of supplementary protein needed to improve the quality of deficient proteins are small. In terms of practical applications or use of this type of information, it is important for such small quantities to be ingested with as high a frequency as possible relative to the ingestion of the protein being supplemented, in order to guarantee an efficient and continuous utilization of the ingested nutrients.

The observations shown in Table 10.5, obtained from studies with 21-day-old weanling rats fed human composite diets commonly consumed in rural areas of developing countries in Latin America, clearly reveal the effect of frequency (Braham *et al.* 1969; De Souza *et al.* 1970). The control group did not receive the supplementary protein used in the study which was milk. A second group of animals was fed daily with the basal diet and 3 gm of skim milk while the third group was offered the 3 gm of milk every other day. It is evident that the daily intake of milk caused increases in weight and

TABLE 10.5

EFFECT OF THE FREQUENCY OF SUPPLEMENTING CORN AND BEAN DIETS
(FED TO RATS) WITH SMALL QUANTITIES OF SKIM MILK

Frequency of Supplementation	Avg. wt.[1] (gm)	Serum Proteins (%)	Urea Nitrogen (mg)	Fat	
				Body (%)	Liver (%)
None	115	5.27	18.6	6.9	13.96
Daily (3 gm)	191	5.62	13.2	1.4	10.26
Every two days (3 gm)	154	5.32	25.4	1.3	13.22

Source: Braham *et al.* (1969).
[1] Initial weight: 52 gm.

serum proteins which surpassed the values for the control group and groups fed the milk supplement every other day. Although not shown, feed intake also increased; however, when the 3 gm of skim milk were offered every other day, the increases were not as large. Furthermore, daily intake of milk also reduced serum urea nitrogen and resulted in lower values for body and liver fat content.

PROTEIN QUALITY OF MIXTURES OF TWO OR MORE PROTEINS

Supplementation, as described in the previous paragraphs, increases both protein quality and content, particularly for cereal grains. Through a different experimental approach, protein quality alone is affected. This approach involves maintaining a constant protein content, usually at or slightly below 10% in rat feeding studies, by mixing two or more proteins in proportionate amounts. In the case of a study of two proteins, therefore, of the series of diets prepared, the proteins of two of the diets will be made up of each individual protein. In the remaining diets, the protein will be derived from the two sources to give a constant level of dietary protein. Therefore, the nitrogen from one of the proteins is progressively replaced by a compensating amount from the second one, in such a way, that all combinations have the same nitrogen content.

These series of diets properly supplemented with calories, vitamins and minerals are then subjected to biological assay, measuring the response by any of the techniques used to measure protein quality. To show the variety of responses obtained, various examples will be discussed.

In the first example (Fig. 10.3), the protein quality of combinations of peanut and corn proteins were evaluated. In these, common whole corn flour protein was progressively replaced by defatted peanut flour at a constant percentage of 8.5% protein in the diet. The results, using protein efficiency ratios, show that the quality of both protein sources individually is the same, as indicated by the values at the extremes. Furthermore, none of the mix-

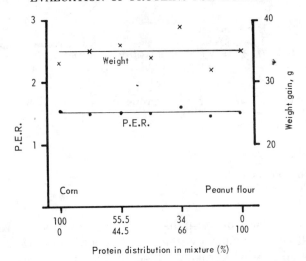

FIG. 10.3. EFFECTS OF FEEDING VARIOUS COMBINATIONS OF TWO PROTEINS ON PER (PROTEIN EFFICIENCY RATIO) VALUES

The two proteins do not have any supplementary or complementary effects.

tures give a better or a lower value, indicating that there was no change in protein quality. Therefore, these two proteins do not have supplementary or complementary effects. The reason for this is apparent from a consideration of the deficient amino acids in the two protein sources. Both are deficient in lysine; peanut protein is further deficient in total sulfur amino acids and threonine, while whole corn is also deficient in tryptophan. There is, therefore, no opportunity for either protein source to provide the amino acids which are deficient in the other protein. Higher protein content in such a mixture can be obtained by increasing the proportion of the protein source which is highest in nitrogen. In the example shown (Fig. 10.3), the protein content could be increased by feeding higher proportions and amounts of peanut flour (50% protein) and a lesser amount of corn (9% protein). The protein quality, however, will be the same for any mixture chosen.

A different type of response curve is observed in the example shown in Fig. 10.4. In this case whole corn flour was combined, at a constant dietary protein level, with cottonseed flour (Bressani and Scrimshaw 1961). As cottonseed flour protein was progressively replaced by corn protein, the quality of the cottonseed–corn protein mixture remained unaltered up through the mixture in which 30% of the protein was from corn. Increasing the proportion of corn protein beyond 30%, however, caused the protein quality of the mixture to decrease. In this case, the response is dependent

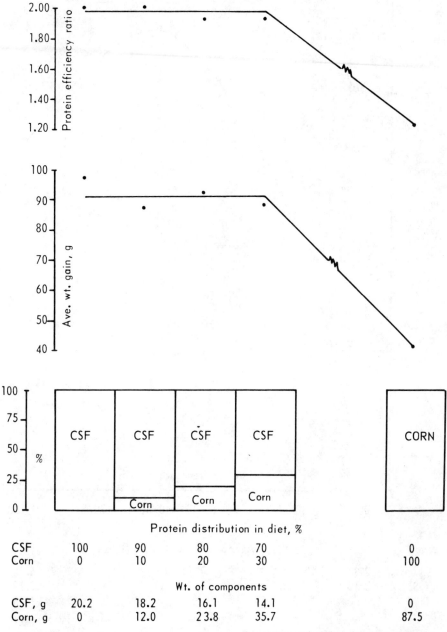

From Bressani and Scrimshaw (1961)

FIG. 10.4 EFFECTS OF FEEDING VARIOUS COMBINATIONS OF CSF (COTTONSEED FLOUR) PROTEIN AND CORN FLOUR PROTEIN AT A CONSTANT LEVEL OF TOTAL DIETARY PROTEIN

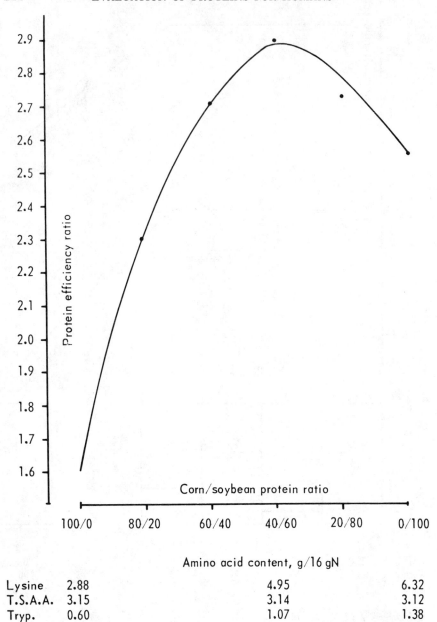

Amino acid content, g/16 gN		
Lysine 2.88	4.95	6.32
T.S.A.A. 3.15	3.14	3.12
Tryp. 0.60	1.07	1.38

From Bressani et al.(1974)

Fig. 10.5. Complementation Effects Observed in Rats Fed Various Combinations of Soybean Flour and Whole Corn Flour at a Constant Level of Total Dietary Protein

Levels of lysine, T.S.A.A. (total sulfur amino acids) and Tryp. (tryptophan) provided by only corn, only soybean or a 40/60 ratio of corn and soybean protein are listed.

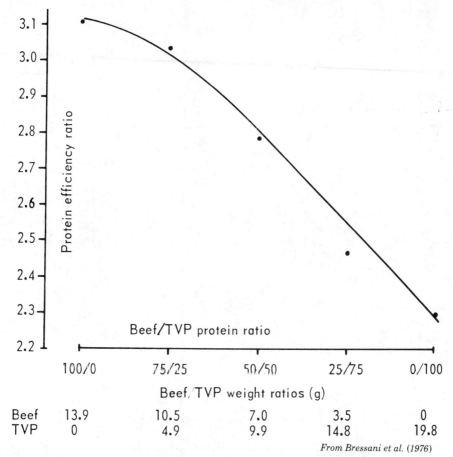

Beef/TVP protein ratio				
100/0	75/25	50/50	25/75	0/100
Beef/TVP weight ratios (g)				
Beef	13.9	10.5	7.0	3.5	0
TVP	0	4.9	9.9	14.8	19.8

From Bressani et al. (1976)

FIG. 10.6.   EFFECTS OF FEEDING RATS VARIOUS COMBINATIONS OF BEEF AND TVP
[TEXTURED VEGETABLE PROTEIN (SOYBEAN)]

upon the concentration of lysine and total sulfur amino acids. Lysine is limiting in corn and cottonseed, but significantly more so in corn. Sulfur amino acid content is essentially the same in both sources.

A different type of response is also observed from the results shown in Fig. 10.5, in which soy flour was combined with whole corn flour. In this case there is a maximum point of response above that of each individual component alone (Bressani et al. 1974). Again the response may be explained on the basis of the individual amino acid patterns of the components, and in this case, the high level of lysine in soybean protein is capable of balancing the lack of this amino acid in corn protein. In the combination with improved quality, the limiting amino acid is methionine followed closely by lysine and threonine.

Finally, Fig. 10.6 shows results from a study in which another different

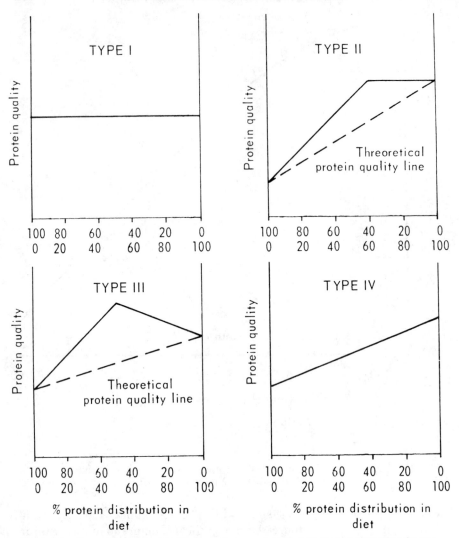

FIG. 10.7.   FOUR TYPES OF RESPONSES OBSERVED UPON FEEDING VARIOUS COMBI-
NATIONS OF TWO PROTEINS AT A CONSTANT LEVEL OF TOTAL DIETARY PROTEIN

Type I—No protein supplementary or complementary effects. Type II—Partially complementary (see text). Type III—True complementation. Type IV—Supplementation (but see
text).

type of quality response (Bressani *et al.* 1976), was obtained. For general
purposes this type of response is represented by a line going from a relatively high quality value to one of lower quality. In the specific example,
additions of increasing amounts of soybean protein (textured vegetable

TABLE 10.6

EXAMPLES OF TYPE II RESPONSES FROM COMBINATIONS OF TWO PROTEINS

Protein Sources	Optimum Combination Protein Distribution (%)	Protein Quality (PER)[1]		
		Component I	Optimum Combination	Component II
Opaque-2 corn/black beans	50/50	2.60	2.60	0.78
Wheat flour/casein	55/45	1.05	2.74	2.74
Wheat flour/soybean flour	50/50	1.03	1.98	1.98
Pea/wheat germ	50/50	0.95	2.00	1.25
Pea/corn germ	50/50	0.95	2.00	2.00

Source: Bressani and Elías (1969); De Groot and Van Stratum (1963); Dutra de Oliveira and De Souza (1972); Bressani (1975).
[1] Protein efficiency ratios.

protein) progressively decreased the protein quality of beef protein. The reason for the constant decrease is that methionine is the limiting amino acid in both protein sources, with soybeans having a greater deficit than beef. Both sources are rich in lysine.

PROTEIN COMPLEMENTATION

From the specific examples given in the previous section, the responses observed when two proteins are combined (as indicated and at a constant protein level) have been classified into four types, shown in Fig. 10.7.

Of the four types, Type I is the only case in which there is no protein supplementary or complementary effect. Generalizing, this type will result when the protein sources combined have a common essential amino acid deficiency of the same extent. The two proteins may also have other limiting amino acids.

Type II response is to be expected from combinations of two protein sources with a common amino acid deficiency; however, one of the two contains a higher concentration of the particular amino acid (in which both are deficient) than the other. This type may be considered to be partially complementary in nature. Other examples of a similar Type II response are given in Table 10.6. In each case, one of the proteins (beans, casein, soybean flour, wheat or corn germ) is a rich source of the essential amino acid, lysine. The same protein sources are also slightly deficient in the same amino acid, which is methionine. The other proteins (corn, wheat flour and peas) have lower concentrations of the same two amino acids (Bressani and Elías 1969; De Groot and Van Stratum 1963; Dutra de Oliveira and De Souza 1972; Bressani 1975).

The Type III response represents true complementation since there is a synergistic effect taking place when the two proteins are combined. The

TABLE 10.7

EXAMPLES OF TYPE III RESPONSES FROM COMBINATIONS OF TWO PROTEINS

Protein Sources	Optimum Combination Protein Distribution (%)	Protein Quality (PER)[1]		
		Component I	Optimum Combination	Component II
Opaque-2 corn/ soybean flour	40/60	2.20	2.82	2.20
Common corn/ soybean flour	40/60	1.53	2.76	2.45
Common corn/ black beans	50/50	1.13	2.00	0.30
Rice/black beans	80/20	2.25	2.63	0.00
Torula yeast/ sesame flour	60/40	1.30	2.70	1.75
Cowpea/cottonseed flour	40/60	1.75	2.60	2.32
Black beans/ cottonseed flour	30/70	1.18	2.30	1.95
Pigeon pea/ cottonseed flour	40/60	1.58	2.38	1.95
Common corn/ whole beans	35/65	0.69	2.54	2.03
Torula yeast/corn	40/60	1.00	2.40	0.92
Torula yeast/ cottonseed flour	20/80	1.41	2.58	2.32
Corn/milk	50/50	1.29	2.81	2.37
Opaque-2 corn/milk	66/34	2.21	2.74	2.44
Corn/cowpea	50/50	1.25	1.85	1.40

Source: Bressani et al. (1962); Bressani and Elías (1969); Bressani and Elías (1969); Bressani (1968); De Groot and Van Stratum (1963); Bressani (1975).
[1] Protein efficiency ratios.

effect is synergistic because the protein quality of the best combination is above that of each individual component. This type of response is to be expected when one of the protein sources has a definitely higher concentration of the most limiting amino acid than that of the second protein.

Table 10.7 shows examples of protein combinations which result in the Type III response. Because of the proteins which were studied, the amino acids involved are again lysine and methionine. One of the amino acids, lysine, is deficient in one protein source (in each combination) but present in higher concentration in the second protein. The other amino acid, methionine, is deficient in the protein in each combination which is rich in lysine but is present in relatively higher concentration in the lysine-deficient protein. In a way, the Type III response is similar to the one above (Type II), but with the difference that, in the Type III response, there is a synergistic effect between the two protein components in terms of nutritional quality (Bressani et al. 1962; Bressani and Elías 1969; Bressani and Elías 1966; Bressani 1968; De Groot and Van Stratum 1963; Bressani 1975).

TABLE 10.8

EXAMPLES OF COMBINATIONS OF TWO PROTEINS WHICH GIVE
TYPE IV RESPONSES

| | Protein Quality (PER)[1] | |
Protein Sources	Component I	Component II
Whole milk/soybean flour	3.10	2.00
Skim milk/full fat-soy flour	2.93	2.00
Beef/textured soy protein	3.12	2.30
Torula yeast/soybean flour	1.60	2.40
Brown beans/potato	35[2]	65[2]
Brown beans/veal	40[2]	78[2]
Brown beans/cod muscle	28[2]	78[2]

Source: Bressani (1968); De Groot and Van Stratum (1963); Kies and Fox
(1973); Bressani (1975).
[1] Protein efficiency ratios.
[2] NPU values from de Groot and Van Stratum (1963).

Finally, a Type IV response is observed when both protein sources have
a common amino acid deficiency, but to different extents, and are both rich
sources of the same amino acid, but again to different extents. The protein
component having the greatest effect is the one containing the higher
concentration of the deficient amino acid. Some examples of protein
combinations which result in a Type IV response are listed in Table 10.8.
Examination of the essential amino acids in the two sources of protein show
that they have a common amino acid deficiency although to a different
degree. For the examples shown, it is the sulfur-containing amino acids.
Because there is no combination giving a maximum protein quality value
as for the Type III response, the table only shows the protein quality of the
individual components (Bressani 1968; De Groot and Van Stratum 1963;
Kies and Fox 1973; Bressani 1975).

Although the responses have been explained on the basis of the limiting
amino acids in the combined protein sources, these deficiencies (or excess
concentrations for that matter), by themselves, do not explain in a completely satisfactory manner the responses observed. Other essential amino
acids and other factors, such as the digestibility of the protein, amino acid
availability and overall essential amino acid balance, are probably involved.

RESULTS FROM HUMAN STUDIES

There are only a few studies reported in the literature in which the protein quality of various mixtures of the same two components at the same
protein concentration have been evaluated in humans. Since various mixtures must be tested as well as the individual components, the cost of such

TABLE 10.9

MINIMUM AMOUNTS OF PROTEIN FROM MIXTURES RESULTING IN
NITROGEN EQUILIBRIUM IN HUMANS

Protein Sources	Optimum Combinations (%)[1]	Minimum Amount of Protein (gm/kg Body wt/Day)
Egg/beans	30/70	0.45
Egg/soybeans	60/40	0.41
Egg/corn	88/12	0.44
Egg/wheat	72/24	0.43
Egg/rice	62/38	0.46
Egg/potato	35/65	0.37
Milk/wheat	75/25	0.47
Egg	100	0.50

Source: Kofranyi and Jekat (1967).
[1] Percentage of protein in diet supplied by each protein source.

experiments, would be quite high. On the other hand, there is no reason to suspect that results might be different than those observed with rats.

In the results shown in Table 10.9, the mixtures of two foods (in proportions which are indicated in the middle column) gave what the authors called a "balance minimum" in human subjects. The protein intake levels in grams of protein per kilogram body weight at the "balance minimum" points are listed in the third column (Kofranyi and Jekat 1967). These values were called the minimum protein requirement when using mixtures of the two foods present, in the ratio shown in the middle column. The lowest protein intake of each mixture giving nitrogen equilibrium was defined as the "balance minimum." From this, therefore, it follows that the higher the protein quality or biological value of the protein in the mixture, the lower will be the amount of protein intake needed for a balance minimum or for nitrogen equilibrium. The balance minimum for whole egg was obtained from an intake of 0.5 gm protein per kg body wt. However, when egg protein was combined with certain other protein sources, even lower intakes of protein were required for the balance minimum level.

These results are difficult to explain since it is accepted that egg protein has a biological value of 100%. This implies that egg protein should give the balance minimum with the lowest intake in comparison with other sources of protein or mixtures of proteins. The results in Table 10.9 show, however, that the protein mixtures are better than egg protein alone since balance minima were obtained from intakes that varied from 0.37 gm per kg body wt per day for the 35/65 mixture of egg and potato, to 0.47 gm per kg body wt per day for milk and wheat in a ratio of 75:25. These results may be explained on the basis that: (1) the protein quality of the egg used was lower than expected because of processing damage; (2) that the values, with the exception of those from the egg/potato mixture are really not different from the value obtained by egg alone, representing a Type II response; (3) that the mixtures had a superior overall amino acid balance than egg and/or (4) that the subjects fed the mixtures were more protein depleted in comparison with the subjects that were fed whole egg.

The results, however, also show other information of interest. For example, it may be seen that less egg protein is needed for cereal grains of better protein quality (rice > wheat > corn). Furthermore, these same authors reported the optimum protein quality mixtures of corn and beans to be a mixture in which 55% of the protein was from beans and 35% from corn. This is not different from the optimum combination for these two protein sources observed in rat assays, as indicated previously in this chapter. In this respect, it is of interest to point out that children which were allowed to consume freely corn as tortillas, and cooked beans, chose a mixture which, on a protein basis, was calculated to be 49% of the protein intake from corn and 51% from beans (INCAP 1973). This confirmed results previously obtained in rats (Bressani et al. 1962; Bressani 1973). On the other hand, the mixture of egg/beans (Table 10.9) giving a balance minimum in humans was a 30/70 protein combination which is different from that of 50/50 reported from rat assays (De Groot and Van Stratum 1963). This apparent difference may be the result of the variety of beans used, since it is known that different varieties vary significantly in nutritive value.

There are other examples showing similar responses, in experimental animals and human subjects. The optimum mixture for rice and beans in rats was found to be 80/20 on a protein basis (Bressani and Valiente 1962). In children, a 76/24 mixture of rice and beans gave nitrogen balance values slightly below those obtained from feeding egg at the same level of protein intake (INCAP 1973).

Studies performed with young human subjects fed combinations of TVP (texturized vegetable protein) and beef using nitrogen balance techniques have been reported recently (Kies and Fox 1973). The results are presented in Fig. 10.8. They were obtained by feeding mixtures of beef and TVP, in protein ratios of 100/0, 75/25, 50/50, 25/75, and 0/100, at a constant level of nitrogen intake of 4 gm per day. Nitrogen retention decreased linearly as TVP replaced beef protein (a Type IV response). Various studies have shown that TVP is limiting in sulfur-containing amino acids (Bressani 1975; Kies and Fox 1971). The same is also true for beef protein; however, the concentration of sulfur-containing amino acids in beef is higher than that found in TVP. Therefore, mixtures of the two protein sources would be deficient in sulfur-containing amino acids. As previously discussed, a similar type of response was obtained with young growing rats.

In a study in which rice and chicken meat were fed to human subjects,

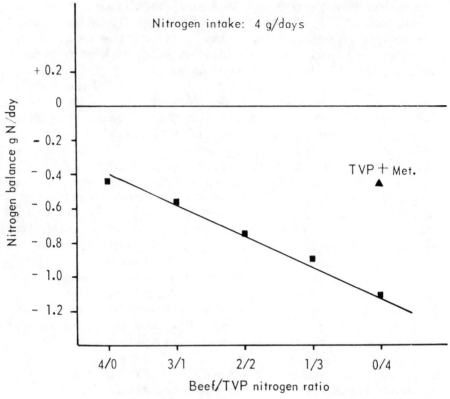

From Kies and Fox (1973)

FIG. 10.8. EFECTS ON NITROGEN BALANCE OF FEEDING VARIOUS COMBINATIONS OF BEEF PROTEIN AND TVP [TEXTURED VEGETABLE PROTEIN (SOYBEAN)]

Protein fed to young human subjects at a constant nitrogen intake of 4 gm per day.

it was found that an 85/15 combination of rice to chicken resulted in the highest nitrogen retention in comparison to 100% rice protein or a 70/30 mixture of rice and chicken meat protein. Since chicken meat was not fed alone, it is not possible to determine the type of response curve obtained. However, from the contents of lysine and methionine in both sources, it can be suggested that the Type IV response would be expected, i.e., a linear response from a low nitrogen balance with rice protein alone to much higher values with additions of increasing proportions of chicken meat (Lee *et al.* 1971).

From the results presented, even though limited in number, it may be concluded that in most cases results from nitrogen balance studies with humans will be similar to those from rat assays.

ANALYSIS OF THE PROTEIN QUALITY RESPONSE CURVES

The results discussed earlier, which permitted a classification of the protein quality response curves, have been explained on the basis of the limiting amino acids in the two protein sources which are mixed, as well as on the basis of the relative abundance of other essential amino acids in the two proteins. In general, the above explanations seem to be satisfactory. However, they are not completely satisfactory explanations for the protein quality response curves obtained in the Type III responses. In this case, other factors must be influencing the results, one of which may be overall amino acid balance. It is difficult, however, to estimate how much of the improvement is caused by this factor. Even though a higher protein quality is obtained, the mixture responds to amino acid supplementation (as will be discussed subsequently).

To be able to analyze the results presented for the Type III response curve, Fig. 10.9 is shown. It represents the results obtained when soybean flour is mixed with corn, maintaining the protein content at a constant level. The theoretical protein quality line of mixtures of corn and soybeans is represented by the line AC. However, there is a point (B) of maximum quality given by lines AB and CB. The extent of complementation is equal to line BD. Line AB represents, therefore, the increase in quality of corn protein (P1) by the contribution of amino acids, mainly the limiting amino acids in corn, that soybean protein (P2) provides. These amino acids are lysine and tryptophan. The line AB thus represents the supplementary effect of soybean protein on corn protein. On the other hand, line CB represents the converse, i.e., that corn proteins provide some amino acids in which soybean protein may be limiting (probably small amounts of sulfur-containing amino acids and of threonine). Thus, the line CB may be looked upon as the supplementary effect of corn on soybeans. These changes can also be deduced from the amino acid values listed.

The effects described are easily followed; however, there are other aspects which can not be explained. Point E (Fig. 10.9), for example, has the same quality as point C and, therefore, they should, in theory, have the same essential amino acid pattern. Examination of the amino acid values shows that this is not the case, except for the amino acids which are present in relatively low amounts in soybean protein (P2). From this analysis it may be inferred that the optimum quality mixture is limiting in those amino acids which do not change as the relative amounts of the two proteins change. Regression equations of amino acid content to protein quality show that tryptophan can predict the line AB, influenced by methionine which may provide the curvature. On the other hand, line CB is predicted by threonine and influenced by methionine. The best predictors for a single amino acid were either tryptophan or total sulfur amino acids. For two

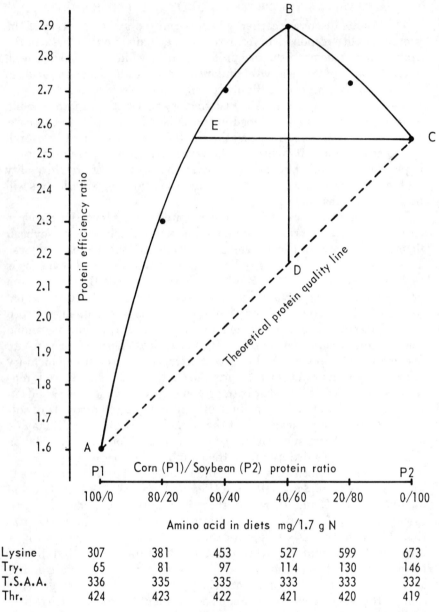

FIG. 10.9.   EFFECTS OF FEEDING VARIOUS COMBINATIONS OF CORN AND SOYBEAN
PROTEIN ON PROTEIN EFFICIENCY RATIOS

See text for explanation and discussion of the various points indicated on the curves. Levels of lysine, Try. (tryptophan), T.S.A.A. (total sulfur amino acids), and Thr. (threonine), as provided by the various protein combinations, are listed. Data from Bressani *et al.* (1974).

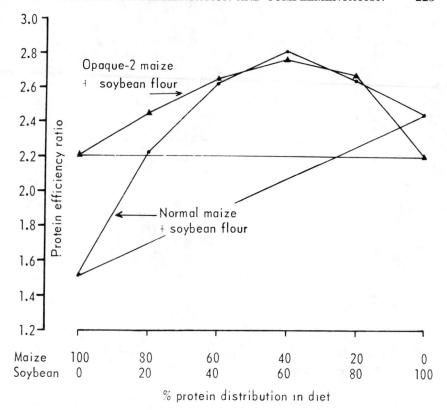

	Lys	Try.	T.S.A.A.
		mg/g N	
Normal maize	180	38	197
Opaque-2 maize	306	94	234
Soybean flour	395	86	195

From Bressani and Elías (1966, 1969)

FG. 10.10.   EFFECTS OF FEEDING RATS VARIOUS PROTEIN COMBINATIONS FROM NOR-
MAL MAIZE (CORN) OR OPAQUE-2 MAIZE (CORN) PROTEIN AND SOYBEAN FLOUR PRO-
TEIN

Lysine, Try. (tryptophan) and T.S.A.A. (total sulfur amino acids) concentrations are listed
for each of the protein sources used.

amino acids in the regression equations, the combinations giving best
predictions were: tryptophan-lysine, tryptophan-threonine, and trypto-
phan-sulfur amino acids. Little was gained when three or four amino acids
were incorporated in the regression equations.

TABLE 10.10

EFFECT OF AMINO ACID SUPPLEMENTATION OF 60/40 PROTEIN COMBINATION
OF SOYBEAN/OPAQUE-2 CORN AND SOYBEAN/COMMON CORN

Protein Combination	Amino Acids Added (%)	PER[1]
Soybean/Opaque-2 corn	None	2.30
	0.20% DL-Met	2.65
	0.20% DL-Met + 0.20% DL-Thr	2.95
	0.20% DL-Met + 0.20% DL-Thr + 0.20% L-Lys HCl	2.66
Soybean/Common corn	None	2.23
	0.20% DL-Met	2.81
	0.20% DL-Met + 0.20% DL-Thr	2.85
	0.20% DL-Met + 0.20% DL-Thr + 0.20% L-Lys HCl	3.06
Casein	—	2.65

Source: Bressani and Elías (1969).
[1] Protein efficiency ratios.

The effect of amino acid supplementation, together with protein complementation, are shown in Fig. 10.10. Mixtures of Opaque-2 corn and
soybeans, both high in lysine, were evaluated. Likewise, mixtures of common corn and soybeans were also assayed. In the latter case, lysine is deficient in only one of the two proteins (viz., common corn). The figure shows
a high protein quality value for both protein combinations when 40% of the
protein was provided by corn and 60% by soybeans (Bressani and Elías 1969;
Bressani and Elías 1966).

The mixtures were then supplemented with amino acids and the results
are shown in Table 10.10. Examining the results from feeding the Opaque-2
corn-soybean mixture, it is seen that its quality was improved by the addition of methionine, and even more so, by the addition of methionine and
threonine. The addition of lysine, together with methionine and threonine,
resulted in no additional improvement over the addition of methionine
alone. On the other hand, the mixture of common corn and soybeans was
improved in quality by methionine addition, but this improvement was not
increased further, as with the Opaque-2 corn-soybean mixture, by the addition of both methionine and threonine. However, the opposite was true
for the common corn-soybean mixture, when the three essential amino acids
were added together. These results, therefore, give some proof to the synergistic effect in protein quality observed in the Type III response (Bressani
and Elías 1969). However, up to the present time no way has been found

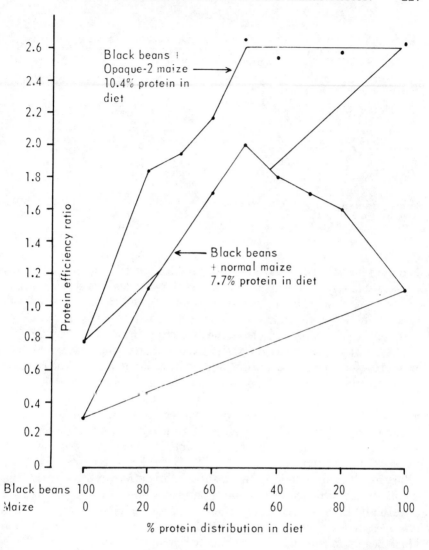

	Lys	Try.	T.S.A.A.
		mg/g N	
Normal maize	180	38	197
Opaque-2 maize	306	94	234
Black bean	464	58	125

From Bressani et al. (1962)

FIG. 10.11.   EFFECTS OF FEEDING RATS VARIOUS PROTEIN COMBINATIONS OF BLACK BEAN PROTEIN AND OPAQUE-2 MAIZE (CORN) OR NORMAL MAIZE (CORN) PROTEIN

TABLE 10.11

LIVER FAT CONTENT OF RATS FED SINGLE COMPONENTS AND OPTIMUM
PROTEIN QUALITY MIXTURES OF CORN AND BEANS AND EFFECT OF
AMINO ACID ADDITION

Protein Distribution in Diet

Lime Treated Corn (%)	Beans (%)	Amino Acids Added	Liver Fat[1] (%)
100	0	—	16.34
50	50	—	21.14
0	100	—	16.04
50	50	Lysine + methionine[2]	16.75

Source: Bressani and Valiente (1962).
[1] Dry weight basis.
[2] Lysine added at levels equivalent to 0.25%; methionine at 0.30%.

to permit a prediction as to whether or not a Type III response (or of any other type of response) will be obtained when two proteins are being mixed. Multiple regression equations based on amino acid data have been developed to predict protein quality of mixtures of foods (Alsmeyer et al 1974). Some of the equations were useful for predicting, in a reliable way, protein quality, particularly for a group of foods based on meat, poultry, yeast or grain. However, the contribution of meat proteins or yeast to the mixture had to be relatively high. These proteins have sulfur amino acid deficiencies in common. The equations failed to predict the protein quality of food mixtures which contained beans or other legumes. This suggests that, to be useful, equations must be developed for each family of foods which have common characteristics in terms of amino acid concentrations, relative excesses and deficiencies.

There are many other examples showing the effect of amino acid supplementation, which follow the same pattern as shown above for mixtures of corn and soybeans. However, there is an additional observation which it is of use to consider. As shown in Fig. 10.11, mixtures of common corn and black beans (Phaseolus vulgaris) and of Opaque-2 corn and black beans have a point of maximum quality when both protein sources contribute around 50% of the protein (Bressani et al. 1962). The amino acids which play a major role in this case are lysine and methionine and their addition increases the quality of the best mixture still further.

In the original studies of the protein quality of mixtures of corn and beans, besides weight gain and protein quality, the liver was analyzed for fat content. The results are shown in Table 10.11. It may be seen that the mixture giving the highest quality, also caused an increase in liver fat. The liver fat level decreased upon amino acid supplementation. The same was

TABLE 10.12

ESSENTIAL AMINO ACID PATTERNS (MG/GM NITROGEN)[1]

Amino Acid	Rat Studies				From Human Studies	FAO/WHO Provisional Scoring Pattern[2]
	PER (2.0–2.4)	PER (2.6–2.9)	Requirement Levels			
Lysine	322	342	335	351	378	340
Tryptophan	63	78	73	58	87	60
Total S.A.A.[3]	176	205	195	234	257	220
Threonine	234	247	243	195	280	250
Isoleucine	303	318	313	195	370	250
Leucine	510	508	508	312	525	440
Phenylalanine	340	316	324	351	335	380[4]
Valine	336	337	337	273	412	310
Arginine	436	424	428	78	362	—
Histidine	160	163	162	117	143	—
Total essential amino acids	2883	2938	2919	2164	3151	2250

[1] Calculated from mixtures giving Type III response curve.
[2] From FAO/WHO (1973).
[3] Total sulfur amino acids.
[4] Phenylalanine and tyrosine.

also observed in mixtures of rice and beans (*Phaseolus vulgaris*) (Bressani and Valiente 1962). High levels of hepatic fat have also been reported for low protein diets and diets with an amino acid imbalance (Elvehjem 1956). Although the first may be a factor in some of the studies carried out, the second seems to be more generally valid. However, additional studies must be carried out to obtain a clearer picture and explanation of the results obtained.

The implications of the results presented in terms of human nutrition are still not known. An additional point which is of interest is that the optimum quality mixture is obtained (in rat feeding studies) whether the animal consumes the ingredients mixed in a diet or is allowed to choose freely from the two foods (Bressani 1973).

USEFULNESS OF RESULTS

The results of the responses presented in this chapter have been useful in at least three practical applications.

Essential Amino Acid Patterns

The essential amino acid pattern of the optimum mixtures, representing Type III responses only, from both animal and human studies were calculated. These values are shown in Table 10.12, where amino acids are expressed as milligrams per gram nitrogen. The table also shows the rat requirements, the amino acid patterns calculated from the human studies and the FAO/WHO (1973) provisional amino acid pattern. The results with rats were divided into two groups, those having a PER value between 2.00 and 2.40 and those between 2.60 and 2.90.

One aspect of this analysis which was of interest is the fact that the essential amino acid pattern of the optimum mixtures resulting from human studies is also very similar to the experimentally derived pattern from the rat studies, although in general slightly higher. This was interpreted to mean that the rat pattern can be used to predict satisfactorily the protein quality of foods to be used in human nutrition. It was felt that the pattern from the human work gave higher values because most of the work was done with egg protein, a protein known to have a very high essential amino acid pattern. As would be expected, total essential amino acid content also was similar between rat and human work.

Finally, the overall amino acid pattern derived from protein mixtures which result in a Type III response curve (in feeding studies) agrees remarkably well with the Food and Agriculture Organization/World Health Organization (FAO/WHO 1973) provisional scoring pattern.

Preparation of High-protein Quality Foods

By choosing the mixture of optimum quality between two sources of protein, foods containing a high protein content and quality have been formulated (Bressani and Elías 1968). For example, a food product called "Maisoy" was recently developed and is being introduced in various Latin American countries. The results of various studies showed that the highest protein quality with mixtures of corn and whole soybeans resulted when 35% of the dietary protein came from corn and 65% from whole soybeans. The conversion of these figures to absolute values of each protein source, yielded a mixture of 72% corn and 28% whole soybeans. The resulting mixture contains 17.6% protein and about 10% fat. The protein quality is about 90% of the value of casein (Bressani et al. 1974).

Similar examples have been worked out for other combinations. These mixtures may be produced in a variety of forms, such as canned peas and corn (30/70), flours for use in bakery products, breakfast cereals and others.

Planning Agricultural Production

For developing countries where the availability of protein sources useful for protein supplementation (such as animal proteins) are relatively low, and socioeconomic conditions as well as food distribution and commercialization systems are far from ideal, better nutrition may be accomplished by promoting planned production of cereal grains and legume foods in the rural areas. Such planning should be in accordance with nutritional findings, as shown by the various examples of mixtures of staple foods such as corn and beans or rice and beans. The consumption of these foods, through increased availability and nutrition education, in adequate proportions to give optimum protein quality would provide a certain guarantee of good protein nutriture. Also, with this approach, if the population ingested smaller amounts of supplementary protein rather than only higher levels of cereals, a significant upgrading of their protein nutriture would result.

From the results of the studies discussed, it should be possible for governments at the national level to store reserves sufficient to provide the correct amounts of the two food components to those in need. This would ensure a certain degree of good nutrition for their people. That portion of a crop not set aside for reserves could be used in transformation industries or for export purposes.

BIBLIOGRAPHY

ALSMEYER, R. H., CUNNINGHAM, A. E., and HAPPICH, M. L.   1974.   Equations predict PER from amino acid analysis.   Food Technol. *28,* 34.

BRAHAM, J. E., FLORES, M., ELÍAS, L. G., DE ZAGHI, S., and BRESSANI, R. 1969. Mejoramiento del valor nutritivo de dietas de consumo humano. II. Supplementación con mezcla vegetal INCAP 9 y leche. Arch. Latinoam. Nutr. *19,* 253.

BRESSANI, R. 1968. Use of yeast in human foods. *In* Single-Cell Protein, R. I. Mateles, and S. R. Tannembaum (Editors). The MIT Press, Cambridge, Mass.

BRESSANI, R. 1973. Legumes in human diets and how they might be improved. *In* Nutritional Improvement of Food Legumes by Breeding, M. Milner (Editor). Protein Advisory Group, United Nations System, New York.

BRESSANI, R. 1975. Nutritional contribution of soy protein to food systems. J. Am. Oil Chem Soc. *52,* 254A.

BRESSANI, R., and ELÍAS, L. G.   1966.   All-vegetable protein mixtures for human feeding. The development of INCAP Vegetable Mixture 14 based on soybean flour.   J. Food Sci. *31,* 626.

BRESSANI, R., and ELÍAS, L. G. 1968. Processed vegetable protein mixtures for human consumption in developing countries. *In* Advances in Food Research Vol. 16, C. O. Chichester E. W. Mrak, and G. F. Stewart (Editors). Academic Press, New York.

BRESSANI, R., and ELÍAS, L. G. 1969. Studies on the use of Opaque-2 corn in vegetable protein-rich foods. J. Agr. Food Chem. *17,* 659.

BRESSANI, R., and MARENCO, E. 1963. The enrichment of lime-treated corn flour with proteins, lysine and tryptophan and vitamins. J. Agr. Food Chem. *11,* 517.

BRESSANI, R., and SCRIMSHAW, N. S. 1961. The development of INCAP Vegetable Mixtures. I. Basic animal studies. *In* Progress in Meeting Protein Needs of Infants and Preschool Children, Proceedings of an Intern. Conf., Washington, D.C. Aug. 21–24, 1960. Publ. *843,* Natl. Acad Sci.—Natl. Res. Council, Washington, D.C.

BRESSANI, R., and VALIENTE, A. T.   1962.   All-vegetable protein mixtures for human feeding. VII. Protein complementation between polished rice and cooked black beans.   J. Food Sci. *27,* 401.

BRESSANI, R., VALIENTE, A. T., and TEJADA, C. E. 1962. All-vegetable protein mixtures for human feeding. VI. The value of combinations of lime-treated corn and cooked black beans. J. Food Sci. *27,* 394.

BRESSANI, R., and DE VILLARREAL, E. M. 1963. Nitrogen balance of dogs fed lime-treated corn supplemented with proteins and amino acids. J. Food Sci. *28,* 611.

BRESSANI, R., MURILLO, B., and ELÍAS, L. G. 1974. Whole soybeans as a means of increasing protein and calories in maize-based diets. J. Food Sci. *39,* 577.

BRESSANI, R., NAVARRETE, D. A., and ELÍAS, L. G. 1976. Efecto de la substitución de la proteína de leche o de carne por harina de soya o proteina texturizada de soya sobre el valor proteínico. Arch. Latinoam. Nutr. (in press).

DE GROOT, A. P., and VAN STRATUM, P. G. C. 1963. Biological evaluation of legume proteins in combination with other plant protein sources. Qualitas Plant. Mater. Vegetabiles 10, 168.

DE SOUZA, N., ELÍAS, L. G., and BRESSANI, R. 1970. Estudios, en ratas, del efecto de una dieta básica del medio rural de Guatemala, suplementada con leche de vaca y una mezcla de proteínas. Arch. Lationam. Nutr. 20, 293.

DUTRA DE OLIVEIRA, J. E., and DE SOUZA, N. 1972. The nutritive value of maize milled products supplemented with amino acids and of mixtures of common or Opaque-2 maize. In Nutritional Improvement of Maize, R. Bressani, J. E. Braham, and M. Béhar, (Editors). Publ. L-4, INCAP, Guatemala.

ELÍAS, L. G., and BRESSANI, R. 1971. Amino acid and protein supplementation of defatted cottonseed flour. Arch. Latinoam. Nutr. 21, 149.

ELÍAS, L. G., JARQUÍN, R., BRESSANI, R., and ALBERTAZZI, C. 1968. Suplementación del arroz con concentrados proteínicos. Arch. Latinoam. Nutr. 18, 27.

ELVEHJEM, C. A. 1956. The effect of amino acid unbalance on maintenance and growth. In Some Aspects of Amino Acid Supplementation, W. H. Cole (Editor). Rutgers Univ. Press, New Brunswick, N.J.

FAO/WHO. 1973. Energy and Protein Requirements. Report of a joint FAO/WHO Ad Hoc Expert Committee, Rome, 22 Mar.–2 Apr., 1971, WHO Tech. Rept. Ser. 522, World Health Organ, Geneva, Switzerland.

INCAP. 1973. Unpublished data.

JARQUÍN, R., NORIEGA, P., and BRESSANI, R. 1966. Enriquecimiento de harinas de trigo, blanca e integral, con suplementos de origen animal y vegetal. Arch. Latinoam. Nutr. 16, 89.

KIES, C. V., and FOX, H. M. 1971. Comparison of the protein nutritional value of TVP, methionine enriched TVP and beef at two levels of intake for human adults. J. Food Sci. 36, 841.

KIES, C. V., and FOX, H. M. 1973. Effect of varying the ratio of beef and textured vegetable protein nitrogen on protein nutritive value for humans. J. Food Sci. 38, 1211.

KOFRANYI, E., and JEKAT, F. 1967. Zur Bestimmung der Biologischen Wetigkeit von Nahrungsproteinen, XII. Hoppe Seyler's. Z. Physiol. Chem. 348, 84.

LEE, C., HOWE, J. M., CARLSON, K., and CLARK, M. E. 1971. Nitrogen retention of young men fed rice with or without supplementary chicken. Am. J. Clin. Nutr. 24, 318.

NATL. ACAD. SCI.–NATL. RES. COUNCIL. 1963. Evaluation of Protein Quality, Publ. 1100 National Academy of Sciences, Washington, D.C.

VITERI, F. E., MARTÍNEZ, C., and BRESSANI, R. 1972. Evaluation of the protein quality of common maize, Opaque-2 maize and common maize supplemented with amino acids and other sources of protein. In Nutritional Improvement of Maize, R. Bressani, J. E. Braham, and M. Béhar (Editors). Publ. L-4, INCAP, Guatemala.

CHAPTER 11

R. E. Feeney | Chemical Changes in Food Proteins

Because of the unique properties of proteins, many different kinds of chemical changes can occur in the structures of proteins. Perhaps the most commonly encountered change is the scission of the peptide bonds of the protein backbone by hydrolysis. A quick look at the different side chains of the constituent amino acids, however, will immediately reveal that many of these side chains are also potential spots for chemical changes that may result in drastic changes in the properties of the protein molecule.

Food proteins are susceptible to many different types of chemical changes during processing and storage. Most of these changes are deleterious, but a few are beneficial. Some may even be caused on purpose by the addition of chemically reactive substances to give desirable characteristics in color, flavor, texture or functional properties. Losses in nutritive value of food constituents, in particular, vitamins, have been widely studied and found to occur in most all phases of the processing and utilization of foods.

DETERIORATIVE CHEMICAL CHANGES IN FOOD PROTEINS

The most studied chemical changes in food proteins are those resulting from deteriorative changes (Type I) caused by physical, chemical or enzymatic actions. These can occur during the many different steps encountered from the harvesting through the cooking of foods.

Deteriorative changes in food proteins are covered in many different publications. Recent general summaries, which emphasize the nutritional aspects, include those by Mauron (1972), Carpenter (1973), Finot (1973), and Ford (1973). Adverse effects of processing on the nutritive value of protein constituents are also covered in Chapter 12 of this volume.

CHEMICAL CHANGES IN FOOD PROTEINS PURPOSEFULLY ACCOMPLISHED

Chemical changes in food proteins may be purposefully accomplished in order to make a better food product (Type II). This type is largely in the developmental stage, but it is one which the author believes will be the cornerstone for the development of the important new and novel foods of the future.

There is a large and extensive literature on chemical changes caused by purposeful chemical modification. This literature has been primarily directed at fulfilling the rapidly developing needs in fundamental areas of

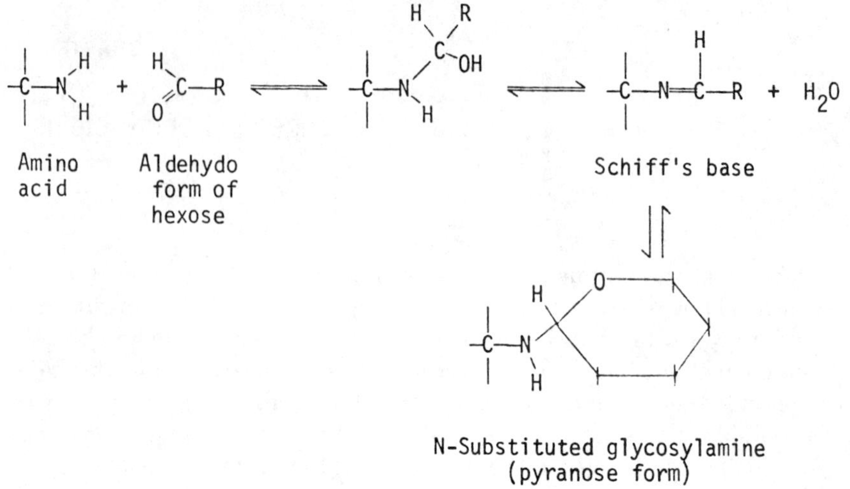

N-Substituted glycosylamine
(pyranose form)

Adapted from Gottschalk (1972)

FIG. 11.1. REACTION MECHANISM OF THE FORMATION OF *N*-SUBSTITUTED GLYCO-SYLAMINE

protein research. Publications are consequently nearly all directed at fundamental biochemistry and chemistry. A general textbook and research monograph on the subject is by Means and Feeney (1971). A recent monograph has also appeared (Glazer *et al.* 1975). The most extensive and detailed general coverage are in two different editions of *Methods in Enzymology* (Hirs 1967; Hirs and Timasheff 1972). Recent review articles include those by Heinrikson and Kramer (1974) and by Thomas (1974). Articles on specialized subjects by Knowles (1972), Rando (1975), Feeney *et al.* (1975), and Feeney and Osuga (1975) have also recently appeared. A symposium volume (Feeney and Whitaker, In Press), focused on the particular subject of the chemical and enzymatic improvement of foods, will soon be available.

DETERIORATIVE CHEMICAL MODIFICATIONS OCCURRING IN THE HANDLING, STORAGE AND PROCESSING OF FOODS (TYPE I)

The Nonenzymatic Browning or Maillard Reaction

The Maillard reaction is probably one of the best known deteriorative reactions occurring in the drying and storage of foods containing carbohydrates. The chemistry of this reaction has been recently reviewed (Feeney *et al.* 1975), so only a short description is necessary here.

The initial reaction is the carbonyl-amine reaction between the carbonyl group of the carbonyl compound (usually glucose, fructose, or pentose) and the amino groups of protein, predominantly the ϵ-amino groups of lysine (Fig. 11.1). Subsequent reactions involve rearrangements, and eventually scissions and multiple products. Proteins themselves may become insolubilized, and colored products and off-flavors produced. A loss of nutritive value occurs, but there is usually no gross toxicity in products still acceptable for consumption. The loss of nutritive value from the Maillard reaction has been the subject of numerous investigations (Carpenter 1973; Finot 1973). At least some of the Maillard derivatives of lysine in proteins are poorly digested and absorbed and are poorly utilized even if fed in the free form. In some instances, small amounts of the Maillard reaction impart to food products characteristics which are sought after rather than avoided.

The Maillard reaction can sometimes be the primary deteriorative chemical change occurring in foods. When shell eggs are stored, the reaction occurs in egg white before any other changes are seen (Feeney et al. 1964; Feeney and Allison 1969). The Maillard reaction causes the egg white proteins to give heterogeneous patterns on gel electrophoresis, a factor which causes confusion with naturally occurring multiple molecular forms ("isoproteins").

Amidation Between Gamma Carboxyl Groups of Aspartic Acid or Delta Carboxyl Groups of Glutamic Acid with Epsilon Amino Groups of Lysine

Cross-links between polypeptide chains via amide linkages are not normally found in proteins. It has often been suggested that damage to proteins during drying with severe heat, in the absence of carbohydrates, may be caused by the formation of such linkages by condensation between free acid groups and ϵ-NH_2 groups of lysine (Carpenter 1973; Asquith et al. 1974). However, Bjarnason and Carpenter (1970) suggested that the reactions probably proceeded through the amino group of asparagine and glutamine, with elimination of ammonia (Fig. 11.2).

There is a complication, however. Heated proteins in which the level of FDNB-reactive lysine has fallen show a drop in nutritive value and, in vitro, synthetic delta-glutamyl-ϵ-N-lysine is resistant to a range of proteolytic enzymes. But feeding experiments with rats indicate that the lysine in this glutamyl-lysine isopeptide is nutritionally available (Waibel and Carpenter 1972). It is thought that the dipeptide is absorbed as such and hydrolyzed by the kidney. The same cross linkages within a protein may, of course, prevent (or hinder) its digestion within the lumen of the gut. Such a fall in digestibility is in line with the observation that the availability of all amino acids seems to fall to a similar extent in severely heated animal proteins (Carpenter 1973).

Hayase et al. (1975A) have recently shown that amino acid residues in proteins and in synthetic peptides can racemize under roasting conditions. Dry heating was also found to cause irreversible changes in peptide bonds

A. By Amidation

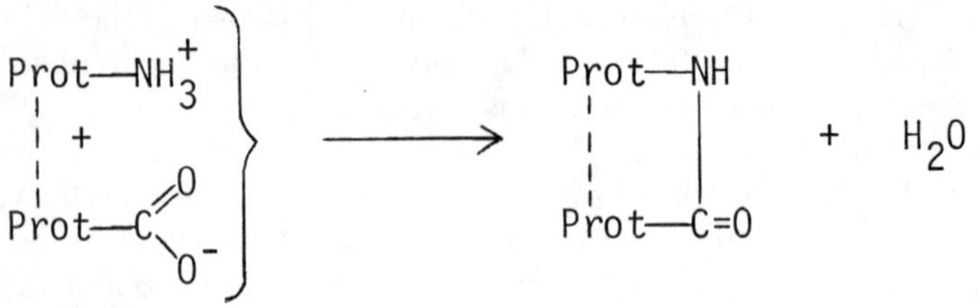

$$\left.\begin{array}{c} \text{Prot---NH}_3^+ \\ + \\ \text{Prot---C} \stackrel{O}{\underset{O^-}{\diagdown}} \end{array}\right\} \longrightarrow \begin{array}{c} \text{Prot---NH} \\ \vert \\ \text{Prot---C=O} \end{array} + \text{H}_2\text{O}$$

B. By Transamidation

$$\left.\begin{array}{c} \text{Prot---NH}_3^+ \\ + \\ \text{Prot---C} \stackrel{O}{\diagdown} \text{NH}_2 \end{array}\right\} \longrightarrow \begin{array}{c} \text{Prot---NH} \\ \vert \\ \text{Prot---C=O} \end{array} + \text{NH}_4^+$$

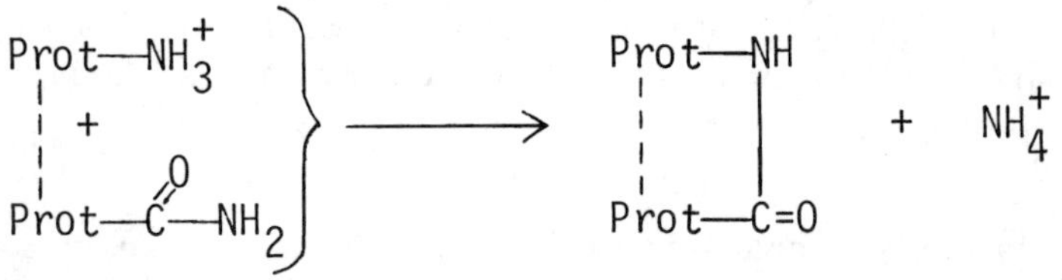

FIG. 11.2.   POSSIBLE ALTERNATIVE REACTIONS FOR FORMATION OF AMIDE CROSS-LINKAGES IN PROTEINS DURING HEATING

(Hayase *et al.* 1975B). The reactions with dry heating of proteins are therefore not simple and apparently still not adequately understood.

Oxidative or Reductive Deterioration

Oxidative or reductive deteriorations are frequently found in proteins which are dried as fluffy products, or which are stored in air. Many proteins are unaffected by this treatment; but some undergo changes, usually related to the sulfhydryl groups. Reductive changes are found in proteins heated with other proteins or with other substances which contribute reductive actions actually reducing the disulfide bond of proteins. Sulfhydryl-disulfide interchanges frequently occur and polymerization and insolubilization can ensue.

When lipids are present, chemical interactions between oxidized lipids and proteins can occur (Mauron 1972), apparently due to carbonylamine reactions between the oxidized lipid and the amino groups in the protein (Andrews *et al.* 1965; Feeney *et al.* 1975). Peroxy radicals may also lead to the destruction of most amino acids (Desai and Tappel 1963).

Changes Occurring During Dehydration

Many of the changes occurring during dehydration are changes caused, in part, by exposure to high temperature, and, in part, by the drying process itself. These can include a combination of denaturation with oxidation or reduction, as well as a formation of cross-links, and, in many instances, the ensuance of the Maillard reaction when reducing sugars are present. Most of these reactions are not caused by freeze-drying.

Extremes of Acidity or Alkalinity

Extremes of acidity and alkalinity have been commonly avoided in the food industry for products containing proteins. Mild acid conditions can, when together with heat, cause the scission of amide linkages and breakage of the peptide backbone by hydrolysis of the peptide bonds. N → O acyl shifts (transfer of the carbonyl group of a peptide bond to the hydroxyl group of serine or threonine) may also occur. These, of course, will cause extensive changes in the properties. For example, solutions of the egg white protein, lysozyme, bind only small amounts of normal heptane, but will bind over ten times as much at approximately pH 2 (Mohammadzadeh-K. *et al.* 1969). If this solution is heated to 80°C, partial acid hydrolysis is accompanied in 4 hr by an increase in binding of heptane to 100 times as much as the original solution. With further hydrolysis to smaller peptides, the binding decreases sharply.

Alkali treatment has been used for preserving and cooking foods for centuries (Katz *et al.* 1974). Apparently, entire Mexican and South American cultures may have survived because of the use of alkali for the treatment of corn. But such uses of alkali on foods were developed through many centuries of trial and error. Until relatively recently, the alkaline treatment of proteins by the food industry was more or less reserved for industrial purposes such as the manufacture of adhesives or the alkaline washing of wool fibers or for quick soakings of certain seeds. Wool chemists have known for a long time that these treatments produce strange amino acids. In fact, one is named after the Latin name for wool, lanthionine. In recent years, however, the texturization industry has used alkaline treatment. As a consequence, incidents have been reported in which deteriorative products have been found in food proteins (see Chapter 13). In addition to lanthionine, lysinoalanine has been reported (Fig. 11.3 and 11.4). Phosphoproteins also undergo similar β-eliminations (Taborsky 1974; Sen *et al.* 1975). The author's laboratory has also found lysino-α-aminobutyrate [made from lysine and threonine as a result of β-elimination of a sugar linkage with threonine in glycoproteins (Lee *et al.* 1975)]. The chemistry of these reactions will only be discussed briefly here, since they have been covered in detail elsewhere (Bohak 1964; Ziegler *et al.* 1967; Gross 1974; also see Feeney and Whitaker, in press).

Discrete studies on the β-elimination of sugars from O-glycosyl linkages have been made possible by the use of the fish blood antifreeze glycoprotein (Feeney 1974) available in our laboratory. This glycoprotein contains no

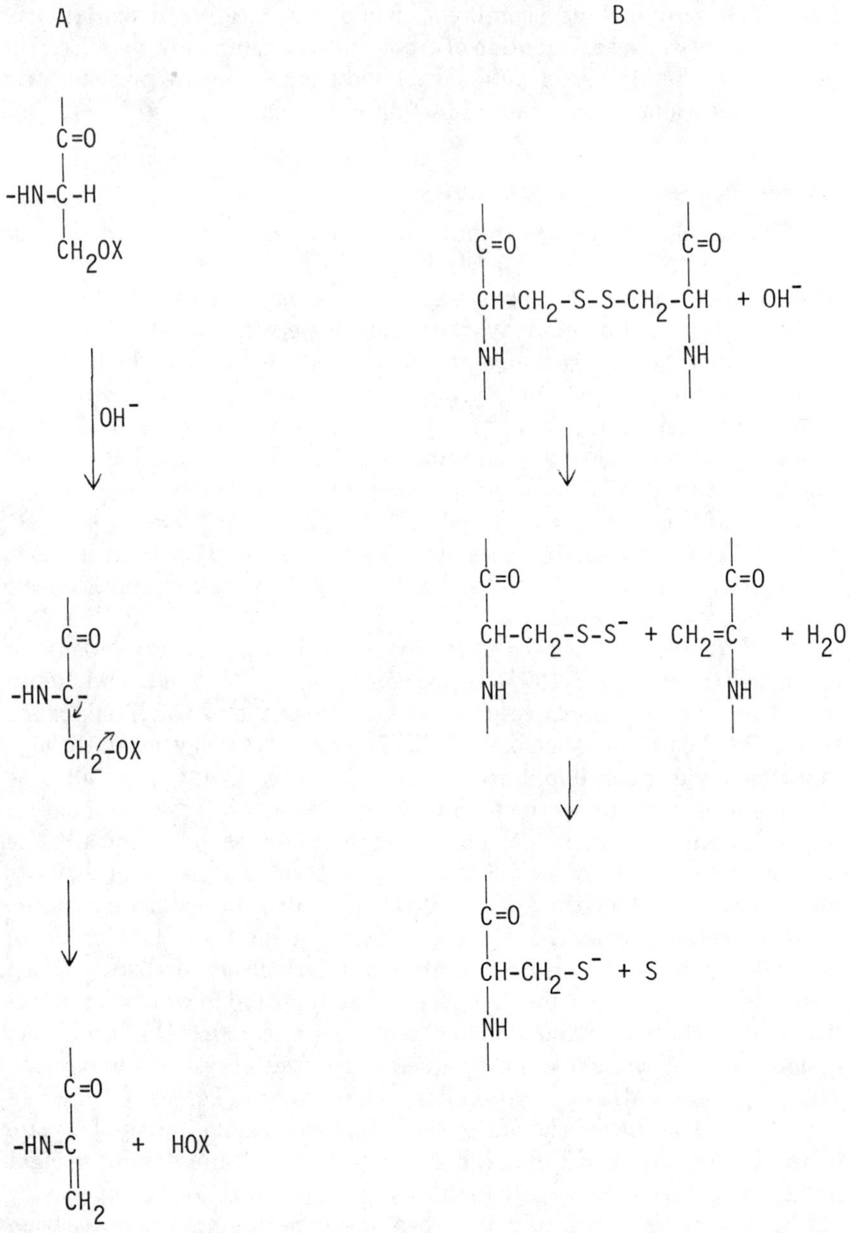

FIG. 11.3. PROPOSED REACTION FOR HYDROXIDE ION CATALYZED β-ELIMINATION FROM SUBSTITUTED SERINE OR THREONINE AND FROM DISULFIDE RESIDUES IN A PROTEIN

A—Serines and threonines. B—Cystines.

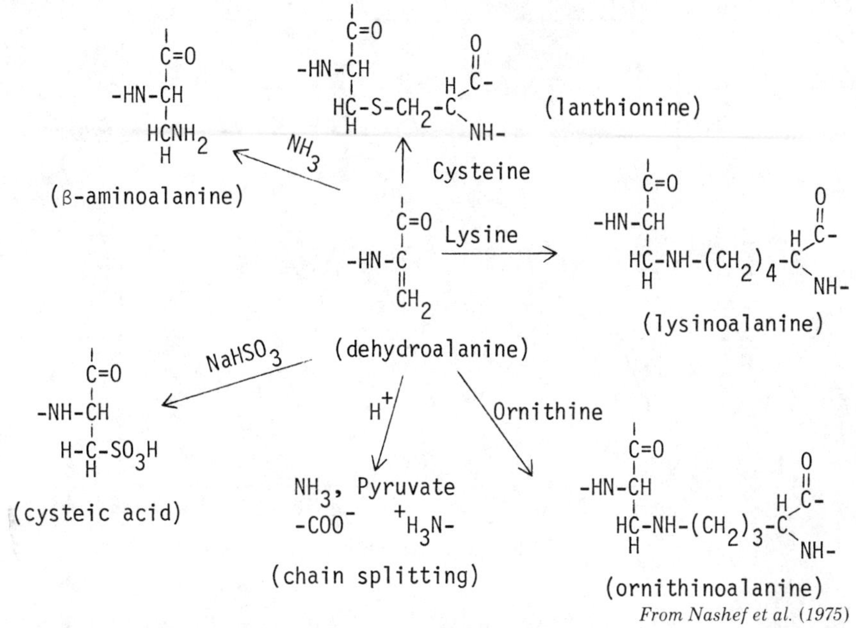

C=O
|
-HN-CH
|
HCNH$_2$
H
(β-aminoalanine)

C=O
|
-HN-CH
|
HC-S-CH$_2$-C
H   NH-
(lanthionine)

Cysteine

NH$_3$

C=O
|
-HN-C
‖
CH$_2$
(dehydroalanine)

Lysine

C=O
|
-HN-CH
|
HC-NH-(CH$_2$)$_4$-C
H   NH-
(lysinoalanine)

C=O
|
-NH-CH
|
H-C-SO$_3$H
H
(cysteic acid)

NaHSO$_3$

H$^+$

Ornithine

NH$_3$, Pyruvate
-COO$^-$ $^+$H$_3$N-
(chain splitting)

C=O
|
-HN-CH
|
HC-NH-(CH$_2$)$_3$-C
H   NH-
(ornithinoalanine)

From Nashef et al. (1975)

FIG. 11.4. THE ADDITION OF VARIOUS NUCLEOPHILES ACROSS THE DOUBLE BOND OF DEHYDROALANINE

TABLE 11.1

β-ELIMINATION: RELATIONSHIP OF LOSSES OF THREONINE TO ABSORBANCE AT 241 nm

Time (min)	$E_{241}^{0.1\%}$ [1]	Loss of Threonine (%)	Conversion Factor	Calculated β-Elimination (%)
15	0.48			4.8
45	1.16			11.5
75	1.95	20.9	10.72	19.4
90	2.72			27.0
330	5.25	49.5	9.42	52.3
540	7.03	68.2	9.70	70.0
720	8.04	80.0	9.95	80.0

Source: Ahmed et al. (1973).
[1] 0.1 mg of glycoprotein per ml of 0.1 N NaOH at 20°C.

disulfides, O-glycosyl linkages to only threonine, no lysines, and no amino acids absorbing light to any extent at the wavelength (241 nm) where the unsaturated product, 2-amino-2-butenoic acid, does absorb (Komatsu et al. 1970; Feeney 1974). Some of the results are seen in Table 11.1 and Fig.

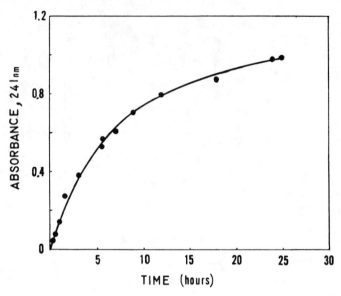

From Ahmed et al. (*1973*)

FIG. 11.5.   INCREASE IN ABSORBANCE AT 241 NM ON β-ELIMINATION OF CAR-
BOHYDRATE FROM ANTIFREEZE GLYCOPROTEIN

β-Elimination was done with glycoprotein concentrations of 0.1 mg per
ml in 0.1 N NaOH at 20°C for the times indicated.

11.5 and 11.6. Work in progress is now making kinetic interpretation possible (Lee *et al.* 1975).

   A strong note of caution in the use of alkali is necessary, however, because
the relative rates of these reactions are dependent not only upon the severity
of the conditions but also on the type of protein which is treated. The
process is very complicated (Fig. 11.4)! Thus, results which would not be
"severe" for one protein might be "severe" for another. Alkaline treatment
of food proteins presents a formidable problem in proper supervision of
plant practices, and in quality control. Such a factor as inadequate mixing
in some food plants during alkaline treatment might cause extensive formation of these compounds. The possibility of toxic products is under extensive investigation (Woodard and Short 1975; also see Chapter 13).
Kidney damage in rats has been reported on feeding rats either industrial
soy proteins or soy protein treated with alkali in the laboratory (Woodard
and Short 1973) or free lysinoalanine (Woodard and Short 1975). DeGroot
and Slump (1969), however, did not note such pathologies. The subject has
recently been reviewed by Woodard *et al.* (1975) (also see Chapter 13).

   In addition to the loss of several amino acids by this alkaline treatment,
and the possibility of toxic compounds being produced, alkaline (or acid)

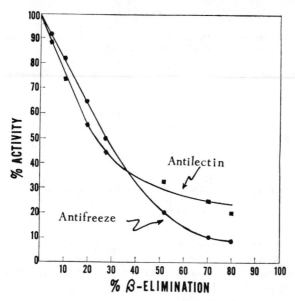

From Ahmed et al. (1973)

FIG. 11.6. INACTIVATION OF ANTIFREEZE AND ANTILECTIN ACTIVITIES OF ANTIFREEZE GLYCOPROTEIN BY β-ELIMINATION OF CARBOHYDRATE

Antilectin activity was determined by inhibition of Osage-orange lectin. Antifreeze activities were determined by measurements of freezing temperatures. β-Elimination was done with glycoprotein concentrations of 0.1 mg per ml in 0.1 N NaOH at 20°C. Extent of β-elimination was determined according to data of Fig. 11.5 and Table 11.1.

treatment may also cause racemization of amino acids (Neuberger 1948) as can also occur on roasting (Hayase *et al.* 1975A). There is great need here for nutritional investigations of such racemized products, as well as for fundamental studies on the racemizations of amino acids in different proteins under various conditions (Hayase *et al.* 1975A).

CHEMICAL MODIFICATIONS OF FOOD PROTEINS PURPOSEFULLY DONE (TYPE II)

The food industry has not intentionally chemically modified proteins to any great extent, as opposed to the modifications which occur when a reagent is used for another purpose, e.g., a bleaching agent. Undoubtedly, chemical modifications are frequently done intentionally when food materials are processed as mixtures according to "the art."

Immobilized enzymes have become very important to the food and pharmaceutical industry (Skinner 1975). The 1975 Food Technology Industrial Achievement Award was won for the use of the immobilized en-

TABLE 11.2

TOXIC COMPOUNDS PRODUCED IN FOODS AND FEEDS
BY CHEMICAL MODIFICATIONS

Chemical		Use	Product
Nitrogen trichloride (Agene)	NCl_3	Bleaching flour	Methionine sulfoximine $\quad\underset{\underset{\displaystyle NH}{\displaystyle\mid}}{\overset{\overset{\displaystyle C=O}{\displaystyle\mid}}{C}}\!\!-\!CH_2\!-\!CH_2\!-\!\overset{\overset{\displaystyle O}{\displaystyle\|}}{\underset{\underset{\displaystyle NH}{\displaystyle\|}}{S}}\!\!-\!CH_3$
Trichlor-ethylene	$ClCH{=}CCl_2$	Extraction of oil from soybean	Dichlorovinyl-cysteine $\quad\underset{\underset{\displaystyle NH}{\displaystyle\mid}}{\overset{\overset{\displaystyle C=O}{\displaystyle\mid}}{C}}\!\!-\!CH_2\!-\!S\!-\!CH{=}CCl_2$

zyme, glucose isomerase, to convert glucose to fructose (Mermelstein 1975). Many of the procedures for immobilizing enzymes incorporate a chemical modification step.

TOXIC COMPOUNDS PRODUCED BY TREATMENT OF PROTEINS WITH CHEMICALS

Chemical Used as a Bleaching Agent

Agenized flour is the most notorious example of the widespread use of a food product found to contain a toxic compound caused by chemical treatment. Agene, nitrogen trichloride, was added as a bleaching agent. When agenized flour was fed at relatively high levels (>20% of the diet) to dogs, the dogs developed the central nervous system disorder known as "running fits." The toxic product was identified as methionine sulfoximine (Table 11.2). Although there were no symptoms reported in man from eating agenized flour, the process was discontinued.

Chemicals Used as Solvents for Feeds and Foods

The use of trichloroethylene for the solvent extraction of soybeans is an example of the use of a chemical for its physical property only to encounter problems from its chemical reactivity. This product from reaction with the cysteine of the protein was dichlorovinyl-cysteine (Table 11.2), which caused toxicities in animals (Feeney and Hill 1960).

Chemicals Used as Sterilants

Chemisterilants, by the very nature of their proposed function, i.e., to kill organisms, should also be suspected of reacting with the constituents

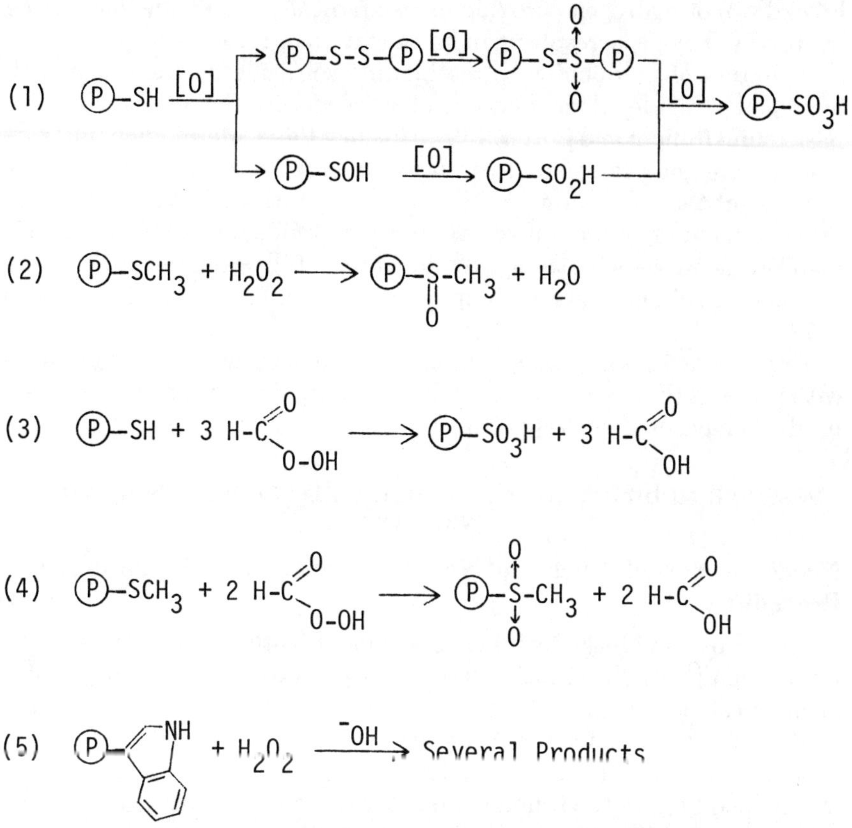

(1) (P)-SH $\xrightarrow{[0]}$

$\rightarrow$ (P)-S-S-(P) $\xrightarrow{[0]}$ (P)-S-$\overset{\overset{O}{\uparrow}}{\underset{\downarrow}{S}}$-(P) $\xrightarrow{[0]}$ (P)-SO$_3$H

$\rightarrow$ (P)-SOH $\xrightarrow{[0]}$ (P)-SO$_2$H

(2) (P)-SCH$_3$ + H$_2$O$_2$ $\longrightarrow$ (P)-$\overset{O}{\underset{\parallel}{S}}$-CH$_3$ + H$_2$O

(3) (P)-SH + 3 H-C$\overset{O}{\underset{O-OH}{}}$ $\longrightarrow$ (P)-SO$_3$H + 3 H-C$\overset{O}{\underset{OH}{}}$

(4) (P)-SCH$_3$ + 2 H-C$\overset{O}{\underset{O-OH}{}}$ $\longrightarrow$ (P)-$\overset{\overset{O}{\uparrow}}{\underset{\downarrow}{S}}$-CH$_3$ + 2 H-C$\overset{O}{\underset{OH}{}}$

(5) (P)$-$NH + H$_2$O$_2$ $\xrightarrow{^-OH}$ Several Products

From Means and Feeney (1971)

FIG. 11.7. OXIDATIONS OF AMINO ACIDS IN PROTEINS WITH PEROXIDE

of foods. Most of the chemisterilants which have been used contain reactive groups that actually participate in their chemical sterilization.

Ethylene oxide, one of the less reactive chemisterilants, is capable of forming esters with carboxyl groups of proteins. Hydrogen peroxide is a potent oxidant of many organic compounds (Means and Feeney 1971). It oxidizes methionine to the sulfoxide and sulfhydryls of cysteine to various stages of oxidation from the sulfinic to the sulfonic acids, depending upon the conditions. In the presence of certain metal ions, organic acids, or esters, hydrogen peroxide may also oxidize methionine to the sulfone and attack cystine, tryptophan, and tyrosine (Fig. 11.7).

Hydrogen peroxide reacts with certain organic acids to form corresponding acylperoxides or peracids (e.g., performic or peracetic, etc.), which are much more potent oxidants. Several heavy metal ions promote the breakdown of hydrogen peroxide to free radicals, and halide ions can be oxidized to halogens, resulting in halogenation of tyrosine rings.

Oxidation of methionine to methionine sulfoxide by treatment with hydrogen peroxide under conditions for the sterilization of egg white has been found (Snider and Cotterill 1972; Feeney 1968). Methionine sulfoxide residues are not released on hydrolysis of peroxide-treated casein by the enzyme pronase (Cuq et al. 1973), and young rats are initially unable to utilize fully methionine sulfoxide in proteins (Miller et al. 1970). But this inability decreases with the age of the rat until full utilization is achieved. Methionine sulfone, however, is apparently not utilized (Njaa 1962; Smith 1972).

Formaldehyde (without reduction) can produce a multitude of products with proteins (Feeney et al. 1975), but the nutritional properties of these products have not been reported.

POSSIBLE MODIFICATIONS FOR IMPROVED PROPERTIES OF FOOD PROTEINS

Needs for New Methods and New Reagents and for Examining Old Procedures

Procedures and reagents for chemical modification of proteins are currently almost entirely for nonfood uses. A large, extensive, and diverse field of chemical modification of proteins has been developed for fundamental studies of protein chemistry. A few reactions have been studied with food proteins, primarily in a superficial manner. Although much of the information acquired in the fundamental studies can be useful in developing reagents and methods for food proteins, and, in some cases, even used with but slight modification, the majority of them are useless for food proteins for a number of reasons.

The most important problem in many instances, is the absence of information on the effects of such modified proteins in the human diet or, for that matter, in the diet of any animal in the laboratory. Studies by a few investigators like Carpenter (1973) are in the extreme minority. Carpenter studied the nutritional availability, for rats, of the acetylated and propionylated ϵ-amino groups of lysines in test proteins. These are rather simple reagents in modifications compared to the many other reagents used in fundamental biochemistry.

Another important problem is the cost of many reagents which have been used on a laboratory scale. Many of these would be prohibitive on a commercial scale for food proteins. The toxicity of the reagents themselves presents still another problem. Although the products of the reaction with some of these reagents might be acceptable, either small traces of them left in the foodstuffs, or the attendant hazards in their use on a large scale in

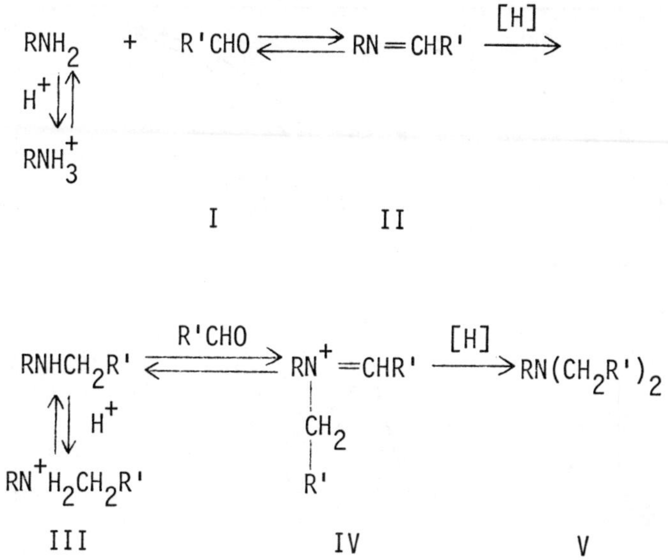

$$RNH_2 \quad + \quad R'CHO \rightleftharpoons RN{=}CHR' \xrightarrow{[H]}$$

$$H^+ \updownarrow$$

$$RNH_3^+$$

$$\text{I} \qquad\qquad \text{II}$$

$$RNHCH_2R' \underset{H^+}{\overset{R'CHO}{\rightleftharpoons}} RN^+{=}CHR' \xrightarrow{[H]} RN(CH_2R')_2$$

$$RN^+H_2CH_2R' \qquad\qquad \underset{R'}{\overset{CH_2}{|}}$$

$$\text{III} \qquad\qquad \text{IV} \qquad\qquad \text{V}$$

From Means and Feeney (1968)

FIG. 11.8. REDUCTIVE ALKYLATION OF AMINO GROUPS WITH CARBONYL
COMPOUNDS

food plants, would make their adoption difficult. Some of the chemicals
are carcinogens; others are inactivators or inhibitors of enzymes.

Testing of Reagents and Products Presently Used for Modification

Those reagents and modifications which have no apparent negative
factors attendant with their application to food proteins will still need to
be tested for their nutritional adequacy, and possibly for other physiological
or pharmacological effects when eaten. One such example is currently under
investigation in the author's laboratory. This is the modification of the
ϵ-amino groups by dimethylation with formaldehyde and reduction (Fig.
11.8), or by ethylation with acetaldehyde and reduction. This reductive
alkylation procedure leaves no detectable traces of formaldehyde in proteins
(Galembeck *et al.* 1976). Such modified food proteins would have many
advantages, because the ϵ-amino groups of lysine have nearly the same
charge as before modification, and there are very little changes in physical
properties in the protein (Fig. 11.8 and 11.9, Table 11.3). This would be
useful for food products in which no changes were desired. A desired effect,
however, would be that the amino groups could no longer undergo the
Maillard reaction because the groups are blocked. Similar derivatives of
proteins with dimethyl groups on the lysines are naturally existing in the
histones, proteins present in the genetic system of both plants and animals.

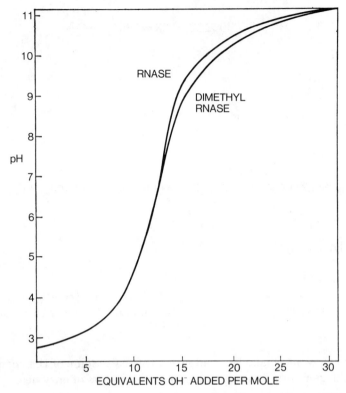

From Means and Feeney (1968)

FIG. 11.9. TITRATION OF RIBONUCLEASE AND DIMETHYL RIBONUCLEASE WITH
0.10 M KOH DONE IN 0.10 M KCl AT 20°C
No correction has been made for titration of the solvent.

In all of these cases, however, they comprise relatively small amounts of the total protein. ϵ-Methylaminolysines are apparently demethylated in the rat kidney (Neuberger and Sanger 1944). It would be necessary, however, to conduct feeding tests to see whether the lysines are demethylated sufficiently easily to be fed in more than small amounts, and whether they are actually used nutritionally. Ethylation might be more acceptable on an esthetic basis because ethyl alcohol rather than methyl alcohol is a by-product, even though the alcohol can be easily removed. ϵ-Ethylamino-lysines, however, are not normal constituents of some proteins as are ϵ-methylaminolysines. Careful study of these would therefore be necessary before they could be used in foods.

For sulfhydryl groups there are numerous blocking agents which would fall into the same class as the alkyl modification of ϵ-amino groups of lysine. Although they would appear to be innocuous, they might have a variety of

TABLE 11.3

VALUES FOR pK OF METHYLAMINES

Compound	pK
α-N-acetylysine	10.8
α-N-acetyl-ϵ-N,N-dimethyllysine	10.4
Alanine	9.8
α-N,N-Dimethylalanine	9.2

Source: Means and Feeney (1968).

detrimental properties when fed. Carboxymethylation of sulfhydryl groups is a commonly used technique and is an effective way of blocking their oxidations. The carboxymethylcystines apparently have not been fed either in free amino acid form or in peptide form.

This presents still a further problem, in that it would be necessary to feed the modified amino acids as part of the intact protein, as a free amino acid in the hydrolysate, or as a directly modified free amino acid. This would be necessary because the modified free amino acid might be easily absorbed and might be either metabolized or the substituent group removed and the regenerated amino acid nutritionally used as such. On the other hand, the same amino acid in a peptide or a protein might not be digested to the free amino acid state, but would remain as part of a small peptide. Whether these small peptides could be utilized, and whether such small peptides might have a toxicity, would need to be considered. In other words, enzymatic digestion of the proteins with these modified residues might produce toxic peptides, although the free amino acids would not be toxic. The opposite might also be the case.

Development of New Reagents

It is in this area that probably the greatest need exists. In general, the nutritional availability of the products, as well as the lack of toxicity as previously discussed, will be a primary factor in the choice of new reagents. Reagents that will need to be sought will be mainly of two types.

(1) The first type includes reagents which can be used for high-level modifications of amino acid side chains or for incorporation of a product into the diet at a high level. In these instances, close attention must be given to the nutritional availability of the modified residues as well as to the possible toxicities. This will be the case particularly when modified residues are essential and limiting amino acids in the diet.

(2) The second type includes reagents which can be used for modifying proteins or amino acids to products which will be used at a relatively low level in the diet (similar to an additive) for their functional or

other properties. In these cases, unavailability of essential amino acids could be trivial, but possible toxicity would still be important.

Particular side chains that it may be useful to modify are the carboxyls of aspartic and glutamic acids, the amino groups of lysines, the sulfhydryls of cysteines and the disulfides of the cystines, and the hydroxyl groups of serines and threonines.

Reversibility in chemically modified proteins could have extensive application. For example, the modification of the ϵ-amino groups of lysine by some reagents should be examined with the objective of removing the modifying group either by the proteolytic enzymes in the digestive tract or by such particular environmental conditions as the strong acidity of gastric juices. The amino groups of the original product would be blocked by the reagent so as to achieve the purpose of preventing the Maillard reaction or changing the physical properties. Then the removal of the modifying group after consumption of the food would make the lysine nutritionally available. The removed modifying agents should be nontoxic. In certain cases, they might even be of nutritional value.

Improving the Nutritional Value

The Covalent Binding of Important Nutrients to Proteins.—Such covalent binding of important nutrients to proteins could be a procedure for preventing the loss and waste of nutrients during the cooking and consumption of foods. Many nutritionally important additives are highly water soluble and can be lost in washing or in a preliminary soaking of a food product. However, if they were covalently attached, the loss would be greatly lessened. Such possible additives could be amino acids which are essential, such as methionine or lysine, or, in some cases, other proteins or peptides containing important or essential amino acids. An additional important aspect here is that these materials, in some cases, might have undesirable organoleptic characteristics when present without covalent attachment, but might be acceptable when covalently attached.

Increasing the Digestibility of Proteins.—Many proteins are poorly digestible, even after extensive and exotic practices. The well-known practice of extensively soaking legumes would fall into this category. Chemical modification can both increase and decrease digestibility (Lin et al. 1969A, 1969B; Galembeck et al. 1976). This is a poorly understood area of biochemical enzymology, but, in general, modifications that open cross-linkages, such as those in disulfides, result in increased digestibility. These are amenable for use in modifying food proteins.

Prevention of Deteriorative Reactions

The Maillard Reaction.—The Maillard is probably one of the best known deteriorative reactions involving proteins of foods (Feeney et al.

1975). The general procedure is to mask by modification the amino groups of proteins so as to prevent the carbonyl-amine reaction between the amino groups and the carbonyl groups of food sugars. Studies have indicated that N-acetylation of L-methionine leaves its nutritional value intact, while making it more resistant to Maillard damage. However, D-methionine loses its nutritional activity with acetylation (Boggs et al. 1975) and L-lysine has only 50% activity for rats after acetylation (Carpenter 1973). Carpenter (1973) has also shown that formation of internal ester bonds between carboxy groups and amino group side chains can occur. Thus, amide groups produced in the protein itself by appropriate handling, or by added amino acids or peptides, might be useful. Our laboratory has obtained results (Galembeck et al. 1976) indicating that dimethylation or ethylation may be of great potential.

Control of Undesirable Products on Exposure to Alkali.—The "lysinoalanine" problem has focused extensive attention in this area. Our laboratory (Lee et al. 1975; Nashef et al. 1975; Sen et al. 1975) has recently been interested in controlling the conditions of processing so as to lower the amounts of breakdown of the disulfides, cysteines, and the O-glycosyl or O-phosphoryl-threonine or serine derivatives, with the subsequent further condensation to make lysinoalanine, lanthionine, and other products (Fig. 11.3 and 11.4). We have been investigating the possibility of incorporating in the alkaline process other substances that would modify the alkaline-degraded products into substances which would be nontoxic and, in some cases, perhaps nutritionally available. Thus, deteriorations might be controlled not only by reducing the severity of the alkaline conditions, but also by different modifications of the intermediate unsaturated amino acids to prevent the formations of lysinoalanine and lanthionine.

Improving the Acceptability

Increasing the acceptability can include many different objectives. Some of the more obvious ones are those that directly affect the senses at the time of eating.

Increasing the Solubility.—Increasing the solubility of many protein products has been an objective for obtaining high-protein food supplements as beverages. With many proteins this has been a monumental problem, particularly because the products are sometimes under mildly acidic conditions wherein many of them are poorly soluble. Those with increased solubility have frequently been ones which caused some hydrolysis of protein, with consequent undesirable effects. A more logical approach to the problem would be through the covalent attachment of groups such as carbohydrates or by changes in the isoelectric point.

Decreasing the Solubility.—Decreasing the solubility of proteins is also sometimes desired for products such as breakfast cereals. Decreased solubility could be attained by the cross-linking used for texturization (see below), as well as by a change in isoelectric point. Also, polymerization of the proteins could cause aggregation or covalent attachment to other proteins and result in larger, more useful polymers.

Texturized Products.—Texturized products are currently in extensive use in the food industry. There are many possibilities here for chemical modification to produce products with desired degrees of structural change. Most of these methods involve cross-linkages, and can be done directly by chemical procedures rather than by present treatments which use heat, pressure, shear, alkali and acid. These can include cross-linkages of amides either with the side chains of the proteins themselves or with bifunctional carboxyl compounds. Certain carbohydrate cross-linkages have potential, but apparently have not been investigated.

Other.—The covalent attachment of certain materials which could impart flavor or color would be desirable. This would prevent their loss during food preparation.

Production of Desired Functional Properties

The imparting of certain functional characteristics to foods is an important and ancient art, as well as now, a science. There are many opportunities and needs for this category, both presently and in the future.

Whipping and Cake-baking.—There are now on the market many products that are present as additives for their desirable characteristics as whipping agents. Some of these are formed by partial hydrolysis of the protein and others by exposure to alkali. Perhaps better products can be made by modification of the protein side chains so as to change the surface characteristics and the conditions for denaturation. Addition of hydrophobic groups by such methods as acylations with fatty acids might be considered.

Cake-baking characteristics are related to the whipping and foaming qualities in many instances, but there are also distinct properties necessary for the maintenance of desirable cake volume, gas bubble stability, etc. There are many opportunities here for changing the denaturation of proteins or protein additives.

Bread Making.—Bread making has been one of the most important arts in food preparation throughout history. As previously discussed, science and technology have been used to make stable products, particularly for Western society. A great need, though, is in the incorporation of different protein products to make breads which fit ethnic and local areas of the world. The blending of chemically modified proteins into the types of products used in these areas should prove to be highly useful.

Other.—Many other food products used in the world require specific functional characteristics of the protein ingredients. Included here are products of the large macaroni, spaghetti and rice industries.

CHEMICAL MODIFICATION OF FOOD PROTEINS—BOON OR BANE

Increasing the health and well-being of people through scientific research, the development of technology from this research, and the application of this technology to world problems is a well-accepted series of events by most people of affluent nations. Dissenters to these events exist, but most of them eventually accept it, or at least become less vocal. The intentional chemical manipulation of foods would, therefore, seem to be a natural development under this broad umbrella. Doubtlessly there are many who would agree in this regard, but even the author, and those who do agree, can well understand that the exercise of this approach to foods requires very special considerations.

Perhaps the majority of food scientists agree with the author that the chemical approach could be a boon to relieving the pressure for inexpensive and more plentiful food in the future. The boon-bane dilemma, however, is considered by some to be a very real problem. A number of commercial researchers have expressed opinions that are generally favorable to the overall possibility of success in making better foods by the use of chemistry. In some instances, however, statements have been made to the effect that their organizations would not chance a heavy investment in research on products which might never reach the consumer because of the very large expense necessary in testing the product, much less the possibility that some products would actually prove to be unsuitable for human use.

Although many investigators believe that chemical treatment of foods can be used to make better foods, most would agree that adequate testing of chemically modified foods is essential before release for human use. The major difficulty, therefore, is the support and the pursuance of the research necessary to develop the products and to test them adequately. It is imperative that the research be done with Federal supports in university, private, and Federal laboratories, and by internationally supported food research centers which appear to be developing at this time (Feeney 1971; Feeney and Hill 1960).

ACKNOWLEDGEMENTS

Appreciation is due to Dr. Kenneth J. Carpenter and Dr. John R. Whitaker for their helpful suggestions, and also to Ms. Clara Robison for typing the manuscript and to Ms. Chris Howland for her editorial assistance. Background information for this article was supported by Food and Drug Administration grant FD 00568-02.

BIBLIOGRAPHY

AHMED, A. I., OSUGA, D. T., and FEENEY, R. E. 1973. Antifreeze glycoprotein from an Antarctic fish. Effects of chemical modifications of carbohydrate residues on antifreeze and antilectin activities. J. Biol. Chem. *248*, 8524.

ANDREWS, F., BJORKSTEN, J., TRENK, F. B., HENICK, A. S., and KOCH, R. B. 1965. The reaction of an autoxidized lipid with proteins. J. Am. Oil Chem. Soc. *42*, 779.

ASQUITH, R. S., OTTERBURN, M. S., and SINCLAIR, W. J. 1974. Isopeptide crosslinks—their occurrence and importance in protein structure. Angew. Chem. Internat. Edit. *13*, 514.

BJARNASON, J., and CARPENTER, K. J. 1970. Mechanisms of heat damage in proteins. 2. Chemical changes in pure proteins. Brit. J. Nutr. *24*, 313.

BOGGS, R. W., ROTRUCK, J. T., and DAMICO, R. A. 1975. Acetylmethionine as a source of methionine for the rat. J. Nutr. *105*, 326.

BOHAK, Z. 1964. N^ϵ-(DL-2-amino-2-carboxyethyl)-L-lysine, a new amino acid formed on alkaline treatment of proteins. J. Biol. Chem. *239*, 2878.

CARPENTER, K. J. 1973. Damage to lysine in food processing: its measurement and its significance. Nutr. Abstr. Rev. *43*, 423.

CUQ, J. L., PROVANSAL, M., GUILLEUX, F., and CHEFTEL, C. 1973. Oxidation of methionine residues of casein by hydrogen peroxide. Effects on in vitro digestibility. J. Food Sci. *38*, 11.

DEGROOT, A. P., and SLUMP, P. 1969. Effects of severe alkali treatment of proteins on amino acid composition and nutritive value. J. Nutr. *98*, 45.

DESAI, I. D., and TAPPEL, A. L. 1963. Damage to proteins by peroxidized lipids. J. Lipid Res. *4*, 204.

FEENEY, R. E. 1968. Identification and characterization of changes induced in egg components by potentially useful pasteurizing chemicals. Final Rept., USDA Contract 12-14-100-7715(74).

FEENEY, R. E. 1971. The world food supply. In The Social Responsibility of the Scientist, M. Brown (Editor). Free Press, New York.

FEENEY, R. E. 1974. A biological antifreeze. A glycoprotein in the blood of polar fishes lowers the freezing temperature. Am. Scientist *62*, 712.

FEENEY, R. E., and ALLISON, R. G. 1969. Evolutionary Biochemistry of Proteins: Homologous and Analogous Proteins from Avian Egg Whites, Blood Sera, Milk and Other Substances. John Wiley & Sons, New York.

FEENEY, R. E., BLANKENHORN, G., and DIXON, H. B. F. 1975. Carbonyl-amine reactions in protein chemistry. In Advances in Protein Chemistry, Vol. 29, C. B. Anfinsen, M. L. Anson, J. T. Edsall, and F. M. Richards (Editors). Academic Press, New York.

FEENEY, R. E., CLARY, J. J., and CLARK, J. R. 1964. A reaction between glucose and egg white proteins in incubated eggs. Nature *201*, 192.

FEENEY, R. E., and HILL, R. M. 1960. Protein chemistry and food research. In Advances in Food Research, Vol. 10, C. O. Chichester, E. M. Mrak, and G. F. Stewart (Editors). Academic Press, New York.

FEENEY, R. E., and OSUGA, D. T. 1975. Purification of chemically modified proteins. In Methods of Protein Separation Vol. 1, N. Catsimpoolas (Editor). Plenum Publishing Corp., New York.

FEENEY, R. E., and WHITAKER, J. R. In Press. Improvement of Food Proteins Through Chemical and Enzymatic Modifications. Adv. Chem. Ser., American Chemical Society, Washington, D.C.

FINOT, P. A. 1973. Non-enzymic browning. In Proteins in Human Nutrition, J. W. G. Porter, and B. A. Rolls (Editors). Academic Press, New York.

FORD, J. E. 1973. Some effects of processing on nutritive value. In Proteins in Human Nutrition, J. W. G. Porter, and B. A. Rolls (Editors). Academic Press, New York.

GALEMBECK, F., RYAN, D. S., WHITAKER, J. R., and FEENEY, R. E. 1976. Reaction of formaldehyde with proteins. Unpublished data.

GLAZER, A. N., DELANGE, R. J., and SIGMAN, D. S. 1975. Chemical Modification of Proteins. Selected Methods and Analytical Procedures. North-Holland, Amsterdam.

GOTTSCHALK, A. 1972. Interaction between reducing sugars and amino acids under neutral and acidic conditions. In Glycoproteins, Their Composition, Structure and Function, Vol. 5, A. Gottschalk (Editor). Elsevier Publishing Co., Amsterdam.

GROSS, E. 1974. α,β-Unsaturated amino acids in peptides and proteins: formation, chemistry and biological role. Abstr. *13* of paper presented at the 168th meeting of the Am. Chem. Soc. Div. Agr. Food Chem., Atlantic City, N.J., Sept. 9–13 (also see Feeney and Whitaker, In Press).

HAYASE, F., KATO, H., and FUJIMAKI, M. 1975A. Racemization of amino acid residues in proteins and poly(L-amino acids) during roasting. J. Agr. Food Chem. *23*, 491.

HAYASE, F., KATO, H., and FUJIMAKI, M. 1975B. Chemical investigation on the changes in lysozyme during heating. Agr. Biol. Chem. *39*, 1255.

HEINRIKSON, R. L., and KRAMER, K. J. 1974. Recent advances in the chemical modification and covalent structural analysis of proteins. *In* Progress in Bioorganic Chemistry, Vol. 3, E. T. Kaiser, and F. J. Kezdy (Editors). John Wiley & Sons, New York.

HIRS, C. H. W. 1967. Methods in Enzymology, Vol. XI, Enzyme Structure. Academic Press, New York.

HIRS, C. H. W., and TIMASHEFF, S. N. 1972. Methods in Enzymology, Vol. XXV, Enzyme Structure, Part B. Academic Press, New York.

KATZ, S. H., HEDIGER, M. L., and VALLEROY, L. A. 1974. Traditional maize processing techniques in the new world. Traditional alkali processing enhances the nutritional quality of maize. Science *184*, 765.

KNOWLES, J. R. 1972. Photogenerated reagents for biological receptor-site labeling. Accounts Chem. Res. *5*, 155.

KOMATSU, S. K., DeVRIES, A. L., and FEENEY, R. E. 1970. Studies of the structure of freezing point-depressing glycoproteins from Antarctic fishes. J. Biol. Chem. *245*, 2901.

LEE, H. S., OSUGA, D. T., NASHEF, A. S., AHMED, A. I., WHITAKER, J. R., and FEENEY, R. E. 1975. Unpublished data. Univ. California, Davis.

LIN, Y., MEANS, G. E., and FEENEY, R. E. 1969A. The action of proteolytic enzymes on N,N-dimethyl proteins. J. Biol. Chem. *244*, 789.

LIN, Y., MEANS, G. E., and FEENEY, R. E. 1969B. An assay for carboxypeptidases A and B on polypeptides from protein. Anal. Biochem. *32*, 436.

MAURON, J. 1972. Influence of industrial and household handling on food protein quality. *In* Protein and Amino Acid Functions, International Encyclopaedia of Food and Nutrition, Vol. 11, E. J. Bigwood (Editor). Pergamon Press, New York.

MEANS, G. E., and FEENEY, R. E. 1968. Reductive alkylation of amino groups in proteins. Biochemistry *7*, 2192.

MEANS, G. E., and FEENEY, R. E. 1971. Chemical Modification of Proteins. Holden-Day, San Francisco.

MERMELSTEIN, N. H. 1975. Immobilized enzymes produce high-fructose corn syrup. Food Technol. *29*, No. 6, 20.

MILLER, S. A., TANNENBAUM, S. R., and SEITZ, A. W. 1970. Utilization of L-methionine sulfoxide by the rat. J. Nutr. *100*, 909.

MOHAMMADZADEH-K. A., FEENEY, R. E., and SMITH, L. M. 1969. Hydrophobic binding of hydrocarbons by proteins. I. Relationship of hydrocarbon structure. Biochim. Biophys. Acta *194*, 246.

NASHEF, A. S., OSUGA, D. T., LEE, H. S., AHMED, A. I., WHITAKER, J. R., and FEENEY, R. E. 1975. Unpublished data. Univ. California, Davis.

NEUBERGER, A. 1948. Stereochemistry of amino acids. *In* Advances in Protein Chemistry, Vol. 4, M. L. Anson, and J. T. Edsall (Editors). Academic Press, New York.

NEUBERGER, A., and SANGER, F. 1944. The availability of ε-acetyl-d-lysine and ε-methyl-dl-lysine for growth. Biochem. J. *38*, 125.

NJAA, L. R. 1962. Utilization of methionine sulphoxide and methionine sulphone by the young rat. Br. J. Nutr. *16*, 571.

RANDO, R. R. 1975. Mechanisms of action of naturally occurring irreversible enzyme inhibitors. Accounts Chem. Res. *8*, 281.

SEN, L. C., GONZALEZ-FLORES, E., FEENEY, R. E., and WHITAKER, J. R. 1975. Unpublished data. Univ. California, Davis.

SKINNER, K. J. 1975. Enzymes technology. Chem. Eng. News *53*, No. 33, 22.

SMITH, R. C. 1972. Acetylation of methionine sulfoxide and methionine sulfone by the rat. Biochim. Biophys. Acta *261*, 304.

SNIDER, D. W., and COTTERILL, O. J. 1972. Hydrogen peroxide oxidation and coagulation of egg white. J. Food Sci. *37*, 558.

TABORSKY, G. 1974. Phosphoproteins. *In* Advances in Protein Chemistry, Vol. 28, C. B. Anfinsen, M. L. Anson, J. T. Edsall, and F. M. Richards (Editors). Academic Press, New York.

THOMAS, J. O.   1974.   Chemical modification of proteins. *In* Companion to Biochemistry. Selected Topics for Further Study, A. T. Bull, J. R. Lagnado, J. O. Thomas, and K. F. Tipton (Editors).   Longman Group Limited, London.

WAIBEL, P. E., and CARPENTER, K. J.   1972.   Mechanisms of heat damage in proteins. 3. Studies with ϵ-(γ-L-glutamyl)-L-lysine.   Brit. J. Nutr. *27*, 509.

WOODARD, J. C., and SHORT, D. D.   1973.   Toxicity of alkali-treated soyprotein in rats.   J. Nutr. *103*, 569.

WOODARD, J. C., and SHORT, D. D.   1975.   Renal toxicity of $N_x{}^\epsilon$-(DL-2-amino-2-carboxy-ethyl)-L-lysine (lysinoalanine) in rats.   Federation Proc. *34*, 929.

WOODARD, J. C., SHORT, D. D., ALVAREZ, M. R., and REYNIERS, J.   1975.   Biologic effects of $N_x{}^\epsilon$-(DL-2-amino-2-carboxyethyl)-L-lysine, lysinoalanine. *In* Protein Nutritional Quality of Foods and Feeds, Part 2, M. Friedman (Editor).   Marcel Dekker, New York.

ZIEGLER, K., MELCHERT, I., and LÜRKEN, C.   1967. N^δ-(2-amino-2-carboxyethyl)-ornithine, a new amino-acid from alkali-treated proteins.   Nature *214*, 404.

CHAPTER 12

D. A. Vaughan   # Processing Effects

Almost all of the foods we eat to obtain protein are processed in some way or other. Exceptions abound, of course, and one cannot overlook oysters on the half shell, sushi, steak tartare, unpasteurized milk, blood, and other animal protein delicacies eaten by people of diverse cultures. Plant proteins have their exceptions also in particular, many vegetables which provide small amounts of protein; but which are not considered primary sources of protein.

In contrast to treatment of animal proteins for human consumption (preservation and palatability), the major purpose of processing plant proteins is to increase digestibility by destroying inhibitory proteins and by releasing protein-rich fractions from poorly digested structural matrices. In the case of plant sources, milling and heating are the major vehicles for achieving increased digestibility.

Because there has been a tremendous amount of research done over many years on the effects of heat on the nutritive value of both animal and plant proteins, a comprehensive review will not be attempted. The reader is therefore referred to the excellent review by Mauron (1972) which appeared in E. J. Bigwood's volume on protein and amino acid functions. Mauron's review covers work done up to 1970, and the following are quotations of some of his major conclusions:

> Actual destruction of amino acids remains slight in food processing. The nutritive value of the proteins is often somewhat improved by moderate heating, especially in the case of vegetable proteins, whereas it is always impaired by intensive heat treatment. Enzymic release of amino acids is reduced in severely heat processed foods. The reduction is rather uniform for all the essential amino acids in foods low in carbohydrate such as meat, whilst it is very selective in foods rich in reducing carbohydrates, such as milk, in which lysine is most affected, followed by the sulphur amino acids. Heat damage to the protein may not become apparent in a biological test when the most damaged amino acid is not the limiting amino acid of the protein. High water content, such as in fluid foods, reduces heat damage, whereas low moisture content augments the latter. At a given temperature the damage is proportional to the time of heating.

The present report covers only some of the more recent reports on the effects of processing. Because of the increased importance of plant foods in providing protein for human consumption, this discussion is restricted for the most part to effects of heat processing on plant proteins as measured with animal assays.

Even when one narrows the overview of research on processing effects to this restricted focus, one is struck by the great diversity of heat treatments and protein sources studied and of the methods of nutritional evaluation used. For this reason, this brief review is organized from the standpoint of the type of nutritional information provided by the reports in terms of the proposed use of the proteins concerned. Let me expand briefly upon this proposition.

When we nutritionists are faced with the problem of determining whether the nutritional value of protein has been affected by a certain treatment, most of us think in terms of feeding that protein to rats or chicks or even humans as the sole source of protein and comparing it with its untreated counterpart or with some standard protein. We then interpret the results of this particular bioassay in terms of the protein as a whole. But actually, we have determined the effect of the treatment on the first limiting amino acid of that protein. Other essential amino acids may or may not have been affected.

Whether this is a critical drawback will depend upon the proposed use of this protein. If it is to be fed as a sole source of essential amino acids, an evaluation by sole source feeding should tell us all we need to know. However, if this protein is destined to be fed with other proteins, our evaluation of it by sole source feeding leaves much to be desired. At best it is a first approximation to a true evaluation of the protein's role in the total dietary mixture—the assumption being that what has or has not happened to the limiting amino acid has or has not also happened to the other essential amino acids in the protein.

Furthermore, the possibility that the protein's first limiting amino acid has been affected by processing may not really be of any great importance, because the protein may not have been expected to contribute that particular amino acid to the dietary mixture in any appreciable amount. On the other hand, essential amino acids which we expect this protein to contribute, may have been adversely affected by treatment, but because they are not limiting in this protein, any such effects would not be detected by the bioassay.

There are, of course, feeding techniques that can provide answers to the problem of the effects of processing on essential amino acids other than the most limiting one in a protein. Briefly stated, these methods involve either feeding the protein with supplemental amino acids in order to allow other essential amino acids to become limiting or feeding the protein with other proteins with which it is expected to be mixed as a final dietary combination.

Because of these considerations, recent results of processing experiments

TABLE 12.1

EFFECTS OF HEAT ON THE NUTRITIVE VALUES OF THE PROTEINS
OF BLACK GRAM AND GREEN GRAM

Treatment	BV	Digestibility	NPU	PER
Black gram				
Raw	62.1	83.6	51.9	1.27
Pressure cooking	70.2	81.0	56.9	2.31
Baking	63.2	81.7	51.6	1.59
Green gram				
Raw	50.5	82.0	41.4	0.87
Pressure cooking	60.6	80.1	45.7	1.96
Baking	58.9	80.1	47.2	0.89

Source: Data from Devadas *et al.* (1964).
BV = Biological value; NPU = net protein utilization; PER = protein efficiency ratio.

will be presented by grouping them into three broad areas according to the information they provide, i.e., (*1*) information about the limiting amino acid in the test protein, (*2*) information about nonlimiting essential amino acids in the test protein and (*3*) information about mixtures of proteins in a combination to be eaten "as is."

In addition to this information, many of the reports provide important information on the effects of processing on trypsin inhibitors, which is not directly related to the biological availability of specific essential amino acids.

SOLE SOURCE FEEDING: INFORMATION ABOUT LIMITING AMINO ACIDS

Devadas *et al.* (1964) compared the effects of pressure cooking and "baking" on several indices of protein quality of black gram and green gram flours. Pressure cooking was done at 15 lb per square inch for 15 min. The "baking" procedure consisted of spreading the flour $\frac{1}{4}$ in. thick and heating at 200°C for 10 min. The results are shown in Table 12.1. The effects of pressure cooking on the Protein Efficiency Ratios (PERs) and Biological Values (BVs) are attributed by the author to the destruction of trypsin and growth inhibitors. On the other hand, the baking procedure would seem to have been too severe, based on the evidence of the PER data although the Net Protein Utilization (NPU) and BV data are not as clear cut.

In another paper from India, Vijayalakshmi *et al.* (1972) report effects of boiling on the protein nutritive value of red gram. Their procedure was to boil dehusked split dhal for 1 hr, drying at 60°C, and finally grinding. Their results (Table 12.2) show that this treatment improved the PER and apparently destroyed trypsin inhibitors present in the red gram.

Amos *et al.* (1975) determined the effects of heat treatment on sunflower

TABLE 12.2

PROTEIN NUTRITIVE VALUE OF RAW AND COOKED RED GRAM

Treatment	PER	Trypsin Inhibitor (Units/100 mg)
Raw	0.68	10.8×10^{-3}
Cooked	1.43	Nil

Source: Data from Vijayalakshmi et al. (1972); PER = Protein efficiency ratio.

TABLE 12.3

EFFECT OF HEAT TREATMENT ON NUTRITIVE VALUE
OF SUNFLOWER MEAL IN RATS

	Results of Trials			
	Growth (gm)		Feed Efficiency (gm Feed/gm Gain)	
Treatment	I	II	I	II
Unheated	42.8	55.2	6.8	5.2
75°C	41.2	49.9	7.6	5.8
100°C	54.5	65.4	5.7	5.0
115°C	41.2	58.1	6.6	5.5
127°C	38.8	53.5	7.4	5.9

Source: Data from Amos et al. (1975).

meal, using growth of rats and food efficiency as the criteria. In the first trial, decorticated seeds were heated in a pressure cooker which was sealed and placed in a forced-air oven for 1 hr. In the second trial, decorticated seed was layered to a depth of 2.54 cm in trays and placed inside a steam-heated dryer. After heating, the seed was ground and oil-extracted.

Some of the results are shown in Table 12.3. The effects of heating were similar in that the optimum temperature appeared to be 100°C. The authors suggest that the improved response as heating temperature was raised to 100°C might be due to some heat sensitive material which is destroyed or inactivated by moderate heating. Destruction of chlorogenic acid—an effective trypsin inhibitor—is cited as a possibility. Above 100°C, a decrease in nutritive value occurs, but the data do not provide a specific explanation for these observations. However, because lysine is the limiting amino acid in sunflower meal, it is possible that changes in its bioavailability occurred at these temperatures.

In this country, a large amount of research has been carried out to determine effects of processing various soy products—the main problem being sufficient heat to destroy trypsin inhibitors and yet not adversely affect essential amino acid availability. Chicks, rats, and humans have been used to evaluate nutritive value. Arnold et al. (1971), working in Canada, have

TABLE 12.4

EFFECTS OF HEAT TREATMENT OF WHOLE SOYBEANS ON
PROTEIN NUTRITIVE VALUE FOR CHICKS

		10% H_2O		16% H_2O	
Time (min)	Temp (°C)	(gm Feed/ gm Gain)	P[1]	(gm Feed/ gm Gain)	P[1]
10	149	2.48	4.0	—	—
	160	2.50	3.7	2.92	4.0
	171	2.51	3.3	2.88	4.1
	182	2.66	3.4	2.87	3.9
	194	3.34	3.4	2.85	4.0
	204	poor	3.0	2.97	3.9
5	149	3.05	5.7	—	—
	160	2.65	4.6	6.98	6.6
	171	2.47	4.0	7.08	6.7
	182	2.37	3.3	3.33	4.8
	194	2.39	3.3	3.71	5.1
	204	2.48	3.1	3.11	4.6
Commercial meal		2.62	3.2	3.01	4.5
Raw		5.12	6.2	>5.00	>6.2
3	216	5.60	4.9	5.49	6.7
	227	4.10	4.5	5.60	5.2
	238	3.70	4.1	3.50	4.1
	246	3.10	3.5	3.00	3.1
Commercial meal		3.50	3.7	3.50	3.7

Source: Data from Arnold *et al.* (1971).
[1]Pancreas weight, mg/gm body wt.

investigated in some detail the effects of heat, as related to moisture content, on whole soybeans. The purpose of their work was to lay down guidelines for "on farm" processing, enabling the grower to use whole beans for livestock feeding. Their data may also be relevant to "village" economies, where large scale processing and oil extraction are not economically feasible. Arnold *et al.* (1971) used chicks as the test animal, the criteria being food efficiency and relative pancreas weight to determine protein bioavailability and trypsin inhibitor activity. Heat treatment was carried out on whole soybeans, after which they were ground for incorporation into the diets. The data (Table 12.4) show that, as the moisture content of the beans rises, higher temperatures are required to inactivate trypsin inhibitors. Furthermore, there is an optimum range of temperature (depending also on moisture content) for optimum feed efficiency. In fact, this range shifts somewhat toward high temperatures as the moisture content increases.

Rackis and McGhee (1975) examined the relationship of trypsin inhibitor activity to nutritive value as affected by heat treatment of soy flour. Heat treatment consisted of live steam at atmospheric pressure for various periods of time. Rats were used to determine PERs and the response of pancreas weight to presence of trypsin inhibitors. The results, summarized in

TABLE 12.5

COMPARISON OF TRYPSIN INHIBITOR (TI) ACTIVITY AND PROTEIN
NUTRITIVE VALUE IN PROCESSED SOY FLOUR

Heat Treatment (min)	TI[1] (mg/ 100 gm Diet)	PER	Pancreas Weight (gm/100 gm Body wt)
Trial I			
0	887	1.19	0.70
2	532	1.77	0.58
4	282	2.07	0.50
7	157	2.22	0.49
10	119	2.30	0.47
20	71	2.26	0.45
Trial II			
0	1001	1.13	0.68
1	774	1.35	0.58
3	464	1.75	0.51
6	288	2.07	0.52
9	212	2.19	0.48
20	104	2.08	0.49

Source: Data from Rackis and McGhee (1975); PER = protein efficiency ratios corrected to 2.50 for casein.
[1] Method of Kakade et al. (1974).

Table 12.5, show that pancreatic hypertrophy did not occur in these rats when as much as 46% of trypsin inhibitor [by the method of Kakade et al. (1974)] remained (following heat treatment for 3 min), but that 79% of the trypsin inhibitors had to be destroyed (by heat treatment for 9 min) before maximum PERs were observed. The upper limits of heat treatment which could be used prior to causing a decrease in nutritive value were not determined.

The first limiting amino acid in soy and the Indian grams is methionine and we can assume that the evaluations of them discussed thus far provide qualitative information about the availability of methionine as affected by heat treatment.

In a recent report, Longenecker and Lo (1974) have attempted to make a quantitative estimate of the bioavailability of methionine in a soy product which was heated rather severely, i.e., with live steam for 8 hr in an autoclave. The experiments were carried out with rats and one human subject. Results are given in Table 12.6. The essential technique of these experiments was to add L-methionine to the diets in order to bring the biological criteria back to the level of the unheated soy concentrate. In rats, the criterion was the PER. In the human subject, the criterion was the difference between the average postprandial plasma methionine and fasting plasma methionine. In either case, Longenecker and Lo estimated the methionine availability in the heated soy concentrate to be 54% of that in the unheated product.

TABLE 12.6

PROTEIN NUTRITIVE VALUE OF HEATED SOY CONCENTRATE

Treatment	Unheated	Heated	Heated	Heated
Methionine, gm/ 16 gm N	1.30	1.11	1.11	1.11
Methionine added after heating	—	—	0.30	0.60
PER	2.10	1.13	1.61	2.24
		Human Subject		
Plasma methionine				
Avg. postprandial	0.88	0.64	0.81	0.96
Fasting	0.59	0.56	0.66	0.60
Difference	0.29	0.08	0.15	0.36
Estimated methionine availability: $\dfrac{1.30-0.60}{1.30} \times 100 = 54\%$				

Source: Data from Longenecker and Lo (1974).

SOLE SOURCE FEEDING: INFORMATION ABOUT NONLIMITING AMINO ACIDS

As stated in the introductory remarks, we are often interested in information about the availability of nonlimiting essential amino acids which products, especially high protein products such as legumes, might contribute to diets. Let us now, therefore, look at some reports which give us that additional insight into the effects of processing on nutritive value of protein.

One technique which has been used to estimate the availability of nonlimiting amino acids is by feeding the limiting amino acid as a supplement to the processed products. Kon et al. (1974) have prepared legume powders, from California small white (CSW) beans and pinto beans, which would be used as extenders to many cereal products. Their data on the nutritive value of these powders are shown in Table 12.7. The short acid treatment (cooking for 15 min in boiling acidified water) did not adversely affect the PERs of the subsequently dried powders. The PER values of the methionine-supplemented powders indicate that there were no gross effects on the nonlimiting amino acids, but also that the low PERs of the pinto bean products were not due solely to a low content of the limiting amino acid methionine.

The same approach was used by Erbersdobler et al. (1972) to evaluate the effect of heating for 24 hr on a soy isolate. Results are shown in Table 12.8. The heat-treated samples were all supplemented with methionine and fed at 12% protein levels in the diets. According to the authors, the lower PERs observed with the most severe heat treatments were caused by reduced availability of essential amino acids other than methionine.

To elucidate these effects further, Erbersdobler et al. (1972) showed that

TABLE 12.7

PROTEIN NUTRITIVE VALUE OF PROCESSED BEANS (*PHASEOLUS VULGARIS*)

Treatment	PER		N Digestibility	
CSW[1] Bean Products				
Cooked whole	1.39	(2.45)[2]	74	(77)[2]
Regular powder	1.44	(2.51)	78	(79)
Acid powder	1.47	(2.49)	81	(81)
Pinto Bean Products				
Cooked whole	0.77	(2.10)	78	(79)
Regular powder	0.83	(1.99)	77	(78)
Acid powder				
Cooked 15 min	1.04	(1.95)	80	(79)
Cooked 30 min	0.98	(1.87)	77	(80)
Cooked 60 min	0.91	(1.92)	78	(76)

Source: Data from Kon *et al.* (1974); PER = protein efficiency ratio.
[1] California Small White.
[2] Values in parentheses: 0.6% methionine added.

TABLE 12.8

PROTEIN EFFICIENCY RATIOS (PER) AND FEED EFFICIENCY RATIOS
OF RATS FED HEATED SOY ISOLATE[1]

Heat Treatment	G Feed/gm Gain	PER
95°C + 105°C	2.45	3.26
115°C + 125°C	2.56	3.22
138°C + 146°C	3.12	2.55

Source: Data from Erbersdobler *et al.* (1972).
[1] All diets supplemented with 0.15% DL-methionine.

"available" lysine was reduced by 27% at these temperatures and at even higher temperatures (160°C) was reduced 60%. Furthermore, they carried out experiments feeding test meals of the isolate to rats followed by measurements of the free amino acids in the portal blood. Results are shown in Table 12.9. The appearance of free lysine in the portal blood was markedly reduced following the meal of the soy isolate heated at 138–146°C. Erbersdobler *et al.* therefore suggested that the nonlimiting amino acid most severely affected was lysine.

Wing and Alexander (1971) have evaluated the effects of microwave heating on "available" lysine, PERs, and trypsin inhibitor activity of hexane extracted soybeans. Their data concerning optimum duration of microwave heat processing (using a frequency of 2450 megaherz and an output of 1250 watts) are shown in Table 12.10. The results show that trypsin inhibitor activity, as reflected by chick pancreas weights, is minimal after 1.5 min of microwave heating and that heating as long as 5.0 min sharply reduced the nutritive value of the soymeal as estimated by the PER method. A

TABLE 12.9

FREE AMINO ACIDS IN PORTAL PLASMA OF RATS FOLLOWING MEALS
OF HEATED SOY ISOLATE

Amino Acid	Plasma Level (% of 95°C)		
	95°C	138°C + 146°C	160°C
Lysine	100	42	0
Methionine	100	72	28
Threonine	100	58	10
Valine	100	68	12
Isoleucine	100	73	11
Leucine	100	78	9
Phenylalanine	100	94	19
Tyrosine	100	83	14
Arginine	100	82	14
Histidine	100	61	12
Alanine[1]	100	75	13

Source: Data from Erbersdobler *et al.* (1972).
[1] Similar values were observed for other nonessential amino acids.

TABLE 12.10

EFFECTS OF MICROWAVE HEATING ON PROTEIN NUTRITIVE
VALUE OF SOY MEAL

Treatment (min)	PER (Rats)	Pancreas weight[1] (Chicks)	Assessment
0.5	0.76	461	Underheated
1.5	1.74	422	Correctly heated
2.0	1.66		Correctly heated
2.5	1.86	363	Correctly heated
3.0	1.70		Correctly heated
4.0	1.92		Correctly heated
5.0	0.97		Overheated

Source: Data from Wing and Alexander (1971); PER = protein efficiency ratio.
[1] Mg/100 gm body wt.

comparison of this type of heating with other processing methods, i.e., dry heat (120 min. at 120°C), autoclaving (30 min at 15 lb) and no heat is shown in Table 12.11. In addition, effects on "available" lysine are given. According to the authors, the dry-heated meal was underheated and there was some "browning" in the autoclaved meal to which they related the reduction in "available" lysine.

An additional point to be drawn from these data is that PERs, determined with sole source feeding of a protein designed to be used as a supplement, do not give us sufficient information about the essential amino acid we want the supplement to provide, i.e., the PER values are quite unrelated to the "available" lysine values.

TABLE 12.11

COMPARISON OF THE EFFECTS OF HEATING METHODS ON
PROTEIN NUTRITIVE VALUE OF SOY MEAL

Treatment	PER	Available Lysine %
Unheated	0.63	58
Dry heat	1.00	53
Autoclave	1.75	46
Microwave	1.86	58

Source: Data from Wing and Alexander (1971); PER = protein efficiency ratio.

TABLE 12.12

PER (MODIFIED) FOR CASEIN AND FOR BOILED BEANS, CANNED BEANS
AND CANNED REFRIED PINTO BEANS

Protein Source	PER (Modified)
Casein	3.40 ± 0.10[1]
Boiled beans	2.65 ± 0.07[2]
Canned beans	2.49 ± 0.06[2]
Canned refried beans	1.91 ± 0.10[2,3]

Source: Data from Womack et al. (1975); PER = protein efficiency ratio.
[1] Standard error.
[2] Significantly lower than casein.
[3] Significantly lower than boiled beans and canned beans.

The development of a new soy-lipid protein concentrate (LPC) for beverages by Mustakas (1974) is an example of a process which is designed to fill a need and which has been evaluated from that standpoint. LPC was isolated from full-fat soy flour by using an isoelectric acid wash at pH 3.5. This was followed by acid cooking, removal of the whey fraction, cooking at pH 9.0, wet-milling and homogenizing to give a product which suspended well in water or could be spray-dried to a reconstitutable powder. Mustakas evaluated this product and found 100% inactivation of trypsin inhibitor and 6.6 gm "available" lysine per 100 gm protein, the latter value indicating little or no heat damage. If the product is to be used as a supplement, the determination of lysine availability provides valuable information. If it is to be used as a sole protein source (as in infant feeding), methionine supplementation would probably be required.

In an attempt to determine the effects of processing on commonly used foods, Womack et al. (1975) carried out animal feeding studies with boiled beans, canned beans and canned refried pinto beans. Because of the extremely low content of methionine and cystine, these products would not be eaten to provide sulfur amino acids. They would be used to provide other essential amino acids, such as lysine, threonine and tryptophan, in sup-

TABLE 12.13

PER (MODIFIED) OF BOILED AND CANNED REFRIED PINTO BEANS[1]

	Boiled Beans	Canned Refried Beans
Control	3.62	3.18
Lysine test	2.96[2]	2.67[2]
Threonine test	2.39[2]	1.40[2,3]
Tryptophan test	2.28[2]	1.42[2,3]

Source: Data from Womack *et al.* (1975); PER = protein efficiency ratio.
[1] Added free amino acids = critical levels except for amino acid under test.
[2] Significantly lower than value for the control diet.
[3] Significantly lower than values for boiled beans.

TABLE 12.14

PROTEIN NUTRITIVE VALUES OF PASTAS DRIED AT DIFFERENT TEMPERATURES

Temperature	Wheat Only		Wheat with Eggs	
	PER	NPU	PER	NPU
20°C	1.07	52.0	2.44	62.3
60°C (50°C)[1]	1.01	51.6	2.39	60.6
80°C	0.96	46.6	2.10	53.3

Source: Data from Cubadda *et al.* (1970, 1971); PER = protein efficiency ratio;
NPU = net protein utilization (rats).
[1] Temperature used for egg pasta.

plementing marginal diets containing poor quality grain proteins. In the first experiment, the diets were adjusted so that the rats received at least 100% of the "critical" level of each essential amino acid. (Critical level is the percentage of an essential amino acid in the diet, which, when reduced by 20%, causes a significant reduction in PER.) The results in Table 12.12. show that the nutritive value of these bean products (especially canned refried beans) compared poorly with casein. This was true even when the analytical values for the essential amino acids in the products were taken into account and used to adjust the diets to "critical" levels by adding free amino acids. Table 12.13 shows the results of a further feeding trial in which the rats were obliged to obtain the test amino acid solely from the bean products, with the remaining essential amino acids being furnished at "critical" levels. The authors' interpretation is that the bioavailability of lysine is essentially the same in the two products, but that the bioavailabilities of threonine and tryptophan are much lower in the canned refried beans.

The foregoing studies represent attempts, consciously or not, to provide the user of these variously processed foods with some clues as to what nutritional deficits these foods can fill.

TABLE 12.15

EFFECT OF BAKING ON PROTEIN NUTRITIVE VALUE OF
SUPPLEMENTED WHEAT FLOUR

Supplement	PER	
Fish Protein Conc. (%)	As Flour	As Bread
0	1.04	1.13
5	2.32	2.04
10	2.97	2.53
15	3.41	2.86
20	3.35	3.04
25	3.43	3.35

Source: Data from Stillings *et al.* (1971); PER = protein efficiency ratio.

MIXED PROTEIN FEEDING

Perhaps the most effective way to evaluate processed proteins is by feeding them with the foods they are designed to supplement or complement, or, in other words, to evaluate final complete mixtures of proteins as they would be eaten.

Cubadda *et al.* (1970, 1971) evaluated the protein availability of pastas dried at different temperatures. Results are shown in Table 12.14. As one would expect, PERs of the pasta prepared from wheat only were very low. Even so, an adverse effect on PER and net protein utilization (NPU) was observed as drying temperatures increased. The effects were more dramatic when the heat treatments were carried out on egg-enriched pasta. Decreases were observed in PERs and NPUs from what were, at ambient temperature drying, quite respectable values. The authors attribute these changes to losses in "available" lysine of up to 30% in the egg-enriched pasta when dried at 80°C.

Stillings *et al.* (1971) determined the supplemental value of fish protein concentrate (FPC) and lysine when added to wheat flour and the effects of baking thereupon, i.e., as bread. The data in Table 12.15 show that baking affects the nutritive value of the FPC-supplemented flour. The PERs of the bread are lower than those of the flour at levels below 25% FPC. The authors suggest that these effects may be caused by losses in availability of essential amino acids other than lysine. The rationale for this conclusion is that, in a parallel experiment, the authors determined PERs on lysine-supplemented bread and found no adverse effect of baking even though their analytical data indicated a lysine loss of 6–16%. This is in contrast to the observations of Jansen *et al.* (1964). In any case, the effects of baking on FPC-supplemented wheat flour seem to be clearcut.

Another type of processing was evaluated by Prasannappa *et al.* (1972) on a "complete" food. These authors studied the effect of extrusion cooking on two Indian blended foods, Bal-Ahar and Indian Multipurpose Food. The

TABLE 12.16

PROTEIN NUTRITIVE VALUES OF EXTRUSION COOKED BAL-AHAR
AND INDIAN MULTIPURPOSE FOOD (IMPF)

| | PER | |
Treatment	Bal-Ahar	IMPF
Raw	1.9	1.8
Extrusion cooked	2.3	2.0
Composition (%)[1]		
Wheat flour	75.0	—
Groundnut flour	20.0	75.0
Bengal gram flour	5.0	25.0

Source: Data from Prasannappa et al. (1972); PER = protein efficiency ratio.
[1] Vitamins and minerals added.

TABLE 12.17

EFFECTS OF MICROWAVE HEATING ON PROTEIN NUTRITIVE
VALUE OF SOYBEANS IN CHICKS

Protein-energy Source	Change in Body Weight (gm)	gm Feed/ gm Gain	Pancreas Weight (% of Body wt)
SB meal + SB oil	652	1.708	0.257
SB meal + animal fat	648	1.661	0.272
Soybeans − microwave	575	1.850	0.285
Soybeans − raw	342	2.320	0.602

Source: Data from Gustafson et al. (1971).

purpose of precooking these blends would be to prevent development of rancidity and infestation during storage and to increase convenience to the staff involved in feeding these blends. Their results are shown in Table 12.16. Extrusion was carried out with a Wenger extruder X-25. Strands were collected, dried in hot air and powdered for the rat diets. The blends were formulated before extrusion cooking according to the composition percentages shown in Table 12.16. Extrusion cooking slightly improved the PERs of both products. Furthermore, physical characteristics and taste were improved—certainly a practical advantage for human nutrition.

Gustafson et al. (1971) have also evaluated the nutritive value of soybeans treated in a microwave oven (frequency of 2450 megahertz and an output of 0.8 kilowatts) for a total heating time of 20 min (Table 12.17). After the heat treatment, the beans were ground, dried and extracted. Quoting the authors' summary, "The feed conversion and pancreas weight of chicks fed the microwave-heated soybeans was comparable to that of the control soybean meal diets and better than chicks fed the raw soybean diet." The diets fed to the chicks contained corn, alfalfa meal, fish meal, dried whey, and corn distillers' dried solubles in addition to the soybean meal, so that the data on feed efficiency are applicable to the microwave-treated soybeans as they are intended to be used in a final mixture of proteins.

CONCLUSIONS

It seems quite evident that research efforts on processing effects continue unabated. It is difficult to summarize these recent papers except to say that the conclusions of Mauron cited at the outset are certainly applicable in a general way to protein-containing foods designed or proposed for human consumption. The effects of heat treatment depend on the product treated and upon the length and intensity of the applied heat. Moist heat is generally less damaging than dry heat. Microwave treatment would seem to have definite possibilities for destroying inhibitors without endangering amino acid availability.

When a processed food is evaluated for use in human diets, I believe it is important to consider the essential amino acids which that food is expected to contribute to the final dietary combination. If the food is intended to be the sole source of protein, an evaluation of the effects of processing on its limiting amino acid(s) is necessary and can be achieved by a variety of techniques, depending on the investigator's preference. When a protein source is intended to supplement another food protein (probably of lower "quality"), the evaluation would be more useful if it were carried out on the final mixture. Thus, the supplementary value of the essential amino acids, which the protein source is to provide, would be estimated and the complementary effects of the protein source and the "poor" quality food protein would be allowed full play. If, however, this type of evaluation is not possible, it would be desirable to measure the bioavailability of the nonlimiting essential amino acids which the protein source could supply to a hypothetical dietary mixture. Various approaches have been made in this direction, but none have as yet been completely successful.

BIBLIOGRAPHY

AMOS, H. E., BURDICK, D., and SEERLEY, R. W. 1975. Effect of processing temperature and L-lysine supplementation on utilization of sunflower meal by the growing rat. J. Animal Sci. 40, 90.

ARNOLD, J. B., SUMMERS, J. D., and BILANSKI, W. K. 1971. Nutritional value of heat treated whole soybeans. Can. J. Anim. Sci. 51, 57.

CUBADDA, R., FRATONI, A., and QUATTRUCCI, E. 1970. Valutazione del valore nutritivo di paste alimentari essiccate a varie temperature. Nota I. Prove biologiche con paste di sola semola. Quad. Nutr. 30, 134.

CUBADDA, R., FRATONI, A., and QUATTRUCCI, E. 1971. Valutazione del valore nutritivo di paste alimentari essiccate a varie temperature. Nota II. Prove chimiche e biologiche con paste all'uovo. Quad. Nutr. 31, 101.

DEVADAS, R. P., LEELA, R., and CHANDRASEKARAN, K. N. 1964. Effect of cooking on the digestibility and nutritive value of the proteins of black gram (Phaseolus mungo) and green gram (Phaseolus radiatus). J. Nutr. Dietet. 1, 84.

ERBERSDOBLER, H., WEBER, G., and GUNSSER, I. 1972. Untersuchungen zur analytischen und physiologischen charakterisierung der aminosäurenschädigung. Z. Tierphysiol. Tierernaehr. Futtermittelk. 29, 325.

GUSTAFSON, M. A., JR., FLEGAL, C. J., and SCHAIBLE, P. J. 1971. The effects of microwave heating on the properties of raw unextracted soybeans for utilization by the chick. Poultry Sci. 50, 358.

JANSEN, G. R., EHLE, S. R., and HAUSE, N. L. 1964. Studies of the nutritive loss of supplemental lysine in baking. I. Loss in a standard white bread containing 4% nonfat dry milk. Food Technol. 18, 109.

KAKADE, M. L., RACKIS, J. J., MCGHEE, J. E., and PUSKI, G. A. 1974. Determination of trypsin inhibitor activity of soy products: A collaborative analysis of an improved procedure. Cereal Chem. 51, 376.

KON, S., WAGNER, J. R., and BOOTH, A. N. 1974. Legume powders: preparation and some nutritional and physicochemical properties. J. Food Sci. 39, 897.

LONGENECKER, J. D., and LO, G. S. 1974. Protein digestibility and amino acid availability—assessed by concentration changes of plasma amino acids. In Nutrients in Processed Foods, Proteins, P. L. White, and D. C. Fletcher (Editors). Publishing Sciences Group, Acton, Mass.

MAURON, J. 1972. Influence of industrial and household handling on food protein quality. In Protein and Amino Acid Functions, E. J. Bigwood (Editor). Pergamon Press, New York.

MUSTAKAS, G. C. 1974. A new soy lipid-protein concentrate for beverages. Cereal Sci. Today 19, 62.

PRASANNAPPA, G., CHANDRASEKHARA, H. N., VYAS, K., SRINIVASAN, K. S., GOWRI, V., MURTHY, I. A. S., and CHANDRASEKHARA, M. R. 1972. Precooked Bal-Ahar and Indian Multipurpose Food. J. Food Sci. Technol. (India) 9, 174.

RACKIS, J. J., and MCGHEE, J. E. 1975. Biological threshold levels of soybean trypsin inhibitors by rat bioassay. Cereal Chem. 52, 85.

STILLINGS, B. R., SIDWELL, V. D., and HAMMERLE, O. A. 1971. Nutritive quality of wheat flour and bread supplemented with either fish protein concentrate or lysine. Cereal Chem. 48, 292.

VIJAYALAKSHMI, D., KURIEN, S., NARAYANASWAMY, D., VENKAT RAO, S., and SWAMINATHAN, M. 1972. Blood amino acid studies in the weanling rat on diets containing raw and cooked red gram. Indian J. Nutr. Dietet. 9, 129.

WING, R. W., and ALEXANDER, J. C. 1971. The heating of soybean meals by microwave radiations. Nutr. Rept. Intern. 4, 387.

WOMACK, M., VAUGHAN, D. A., and BODWELL, C. E. 1975. A modified PER method for estimating changes in the bioavailability of individual essential amino acids. In Protein Nutritional Quality. Part I. Assay Methods-Biological, Biochemical, and Chemical. M. Friedman (Editor). Marcel Dekker, New York.

A. P. de Groot
P. Slump
L. van Beek
and V. J. Feron

CHAPTER 13

Severe Alkali Treatment of Proteins

Alkali treatment has been practiced as a food processing technique for many centuries. The best known example is undoubtedly the cooking of corn in solutions of lime, woodash, or lye as applied in many societies of the Western Hemisphere, a treatment credited with making possible the rise of Mesoamerican civilizations (Katz *et al.* 1974). The purpose of this process seems to be primarily softening of the tough outer layer of the corn kernel, thus rendering critical nutrients available.

Modern food technology applies alkali treatment for a wide variety of purposes, e.g., to solubilize and to isolate proteins (Sullivan 1943; Tannenbaum *et al.* 1970; Betschart 1974; Lindblom 1974), to improve foaming and emulsifying properties (Circle and Smith 1972; Hermansson *et al.* 1971; Lindblom 1974), and to obtain protein solutions suitable for spinning fibers (Anon. 1967; Wipf 1972).

In addition to the favorable technological properties imparted to foods by treatment with alkali, undesirable chemical changes may occur varying in type and degree with the intensity of the treatment, viz. the degree of alkalinity, temperature and duration of exposure. The main types of change are racemization of amino acids, destruction of amino acids, splitting of peptide bonds, and formation of new amino acids. The latter includes lysinoalanine (Patchornik and Sokolovsky 1964; Bohak 1964), lanthionine (Horn *et al.* 1941; Hupf and Springer 1971), and ornithinoalanine (Ziegler *et al.* 1967). Of these three, lysinoalanine has received the most attention in recent years probably because of its relatively easy detection and frequent presence in several types of treated proteins. Lysinoalanine (N^ϵ-[DL-2-amino-2-carboxyethyl]-L-lysine), further designated as LAL, is probably formed through the addition of a lysyl residue to the double bond of a dehydroalanyl residue formed by a β-elimination reaction from serine or cystine (Bohak 1964).

NUTRITIONAL ASPECTS

Drastic Treatments

There is no doubt that several of the changes which occur in proteins under drastic conditions of treatment may lead to a reduction in protein quality. This effect is illustrated with results of our studies with isolated

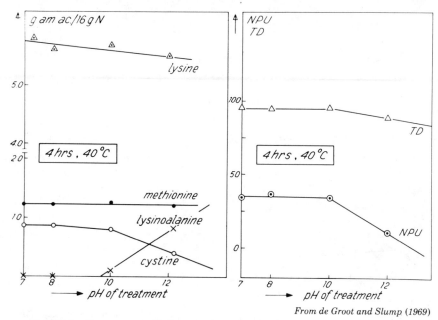

From de Groot and Slump (1969)

FIG. 13.1. EFFECTS OF PH, DURING ALKALINE TREATMENT OF SOY PROTEIN

On levels of lysine, methionine, cystine and lysinoalanine and on nutritive value as estimated by net protein utilization (NPU) and true digestibility (TD) in rats; "g am. ac./16 g N" equals gm amino acid per 16 gm nitrogen.

soy protein (ISP, Promine D) after alkali treatment under different conditions of pH, temperature and duration. The treated protein was precipitated at pH 4.5, and examined by amino acid analysis and by protein quality assays in rats (de Groot and Slump 1969). Figures 13.1, 13.2, and 13.3 show the changes in the contents of the three major amino acids (lysine, cystine, and methionine) and the contents of lysinoalanine, together with the net protein utilization (NPU) and true digestibility (TD).

Treatment at 40°C for 4 hr, at increasing pH levels, did not result in significant changes in the parameters examined up to pH 10. The presence of LAL was, however, detectable (Fig. 13.1). A further increase of pH up to 12 resulted in a marked loss of cystine accompanied by a sharp decline in NPU and a considerable increase of LAL. Lysine tended to decrease and the *in vivo* digestibility was slightly lowered.

Treatment at pH 12.2 for 4 hr, at increasing temperature levels, resulted in gradual changes of each of the parameters examined at all temperatures above 20°C. (Fig. 13.2). Lysine decreased to an extent comparable to the increase of LAL. In addition to a slight decrease of cystine, there was a distinct loss of serine at 60 and 80°C. The slight, but consistent, increase

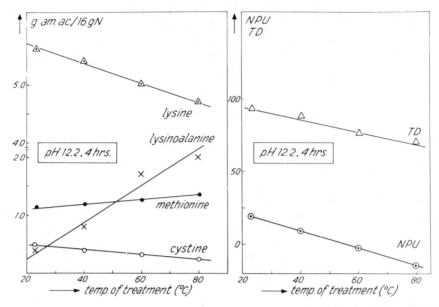

From de Groot and Slump (1969)

FIG. 13.2.   EFFECTS OF TEMPERATURE, DURING ALKALINE TREATMENT OF SOY PRO-
TEIN

On levels of specific amino acids and nutritive value; see legend to Fig. 13.1 for explanation
of abbreviations.

in methionine might be a relative change, caused by losses of other amino
acids.

Treatment at pH 12.2 and 40°C for increasing periods of time was accompanied by a rapid initial loss of cystine and a rapid increase in LAL
content within the first hour (Fig. 13.3). Upon lengthening the treatment
period, the cystine level remained constant, but lysine showed a further
decrease with time and LAL increased accordingly. The decrease in NPU
was most marked in the first hour of the treatment period and declined
gradually thereafter.

When summarizing the results obtained with soy protein it appears that:
(1) with increasing alkalinity, little or no change was noticeable up to pH
10; (2) any increase in temperature above 20°C was accompanied by a
gradual alteration of all parameters examined; (3) under drastic conditions,
the changes were most pronounced in the initial phase of the treatment
period.

Apart from losses in amino acids, alkali treatment of proteins may result
in decreased digestibility and intestinal absorption of some amino acids
as was observed with the everted sac technique (de Groot and Slump 1969).

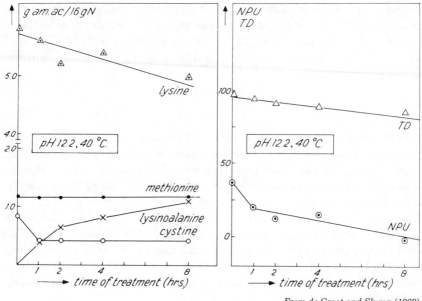

From de Groot and Slump (1969)

FIG. 13.3.   EFFECTS OF DURATION OF ALKALINE TREATMENT OF SOY PROTEIN ON
LEVELS OF SPECIFIC AMINO ACIDS AND NUTRITIVE VALUE

See legend to Fig. 13.1 for explanation of abbreviations.

Decreased intestinal absorption of amino acids might be caused by racemization or by the occurrence of cross-links in the protein.

A progressive decrease of *in vitro* digestion with pepsin and trypsin has
been observed with milk protein, treated at pH 12 for 30 min, by increasing
the temperature from 30°C to 90°C (Krause and Schmidt 1974).

Considerable losses of cystine have been found in fish protein treated
with heat and alkali to remove the oil. After treatment of herring with 2–3%
NaOH and heating to 70–90°C for 10–30 min, about 75% of the cystine was
lost. The products were found to be of poor nutritive value if fed at low
dietary levels and to be toxic if fed at high levels (Carpenter and Duckworth
1950).

Severe alkaline conditions are applied in processing corn for tortillas.
The dried kernels are usually heated to 80–90°C in about two volumes of
a 1–5% aqueous solution of lime (CaO) for about ½ hr and allowed to stand
overnight. The pH of the mixture will be between 12 and 13 depending, e.g.,
upon the lime concentration used. After decanting, washing and draining,
the kernels are ground to a dough and cooked in a thin layer on a hot plate
for several minutes.

While this lime treatment decreases the contents of many nutrients, improvements have been observed in the balance of essential amino acids, the availability of niacin and the rate of enzymatic release of amino acids *in vitro*. Such changes may explain why rats and pigs gain faster when fed on tortilla diets than on raw corn diets (Bressani *et al.* 1958; Bressani and Scrimshaw 1958).

Mild Treatments

Mild alkali treatment is generally applied in the production of protein fiber ingredients used in the manufacture of analogs of common foods possessing the fibrous, chewy texture of meat. The protein used as a starting material is kept in aqueous suspension at pH 10.5–12.0 and room temperature for several minutes to obtain the desired properties prior to being forced through spinnerettes into a coagulating bath which contains acid and salt to neutralize and precipitate the protein fibers (Anon. 1967; Wipf 1972). Although the limited degree of alkali treatment does not suggest any important chemical changes in the protein, several of these products have been examined for nutritive value and safety in studies with both animals and humans.

A beef analog made from a mixture of soy protein fibrils, egg albumin and wheat gluten was found to possess a protein quality for rats and dogs comparable to that of beef dehydrated at 70°C. For children, the protein quality was 80% of that of milk (Bressani *et al.* 1967). Also, a similar meat analog (based on a 2:1 ratio of spun-fiber soy protein with egg albumin) has been tested in eight young human volunteers at dietary levels up to 80% of the daily protein intake for five weeks. Because positive nitrogen balances were observed at intake levels of 0.4 gm of protein per kg body wt per day, it was concluded that the test product contained a high quality protein (Turk *et al.* 1973).

The wholesomeness of a spun soy isolate, not containing any protein additives, has been examined recently in our Institute by feeding rats on semipurified diets containing the alkali-treated material at levels of 5, 10, or 20% crude protein in a 90-day safety evaluation study. All groups fed the test protein showed the same growth rate and food efficiencies as did the two control groups which contained comparable levels of protein from either soy isolate or casein. It should be mentioned that the level of amino acids containing sulfur was equalized in the various diets. These results indicate that in spite of the alkali treatment applied, the spun product is fully capable of supporting normal growth and food efficiency when fed to rats as the sole dietary source of protein if the natural deficiency of sulfur amino acid in soy protein is replenished by a supplement of methionine (van Beek *et al.* 1974).

SAFETY ASPECTS

In view of the multitude of chemical changes that may take place in proteins upon drastic treatment with alkali, it is desirable to consider the safety aspects.

Alkali hydrolysates of casein obtained by autoclaving with barium hydroxide were found to be toxic when fed to rats at a level of 20% in the diet. The presence of toxic reaction products was considered as a possible cause (Ramasarma et al. 1949).

Deleterious effects have been observed in rats and chickens fed an alkali-reduction meal from herring (obtained as a by-product from herring-oil extraction). The process, which involves storage and heating of the herring in an equal weight of 3% aqueous sodium hydroxide, destroyed vitamin B-12 and cystine, but the addition of these nutrients did not restore the nutritive value (Carpenter and Duckworth 1950; Carpenter et al. 1952).

Effects of Alpha Protein

More recently, feeding studies in rats have been conducted with a nonfood protein very severely treated with alkali to obtain the physical properties necessary for certain industrial applications. The product, known as Alpha Protein, has been used as the sole source of protein in semipurified diets, which, not unexpectedly, were found to be inadequate for normal growth. Moreover histological changes in the kidneys were observed (Newberne and Young 1966; Woodard and Alvarez 1967; Woodard 1969). The renal abnormality consisted of degenerative changes in the pars recta of the proximal tubules, characterized by enlarged nuclei and increased cytoplasmic portions of the epithelial cells. The phenomenon, designated as renal cytomegalia, was attributed to LAL, which was present at a dietary level of 0.12% (Woodard and Short 1973).

Feeding studies with alkali-treated, edible soy protein and casein conducted in our Institute, however, failed to reveal cytomegalia or any abnormalities in growth, hematology, clinical chemistry or pathology, although the dietary levels of LAL were comparable to those fed in the previously mentioned studies (de Groot and Slump 1969; van Beek et al. 1974).

Based on the assumption that these divergent results could be caused by differences in strain sensitivity, short-term tests (up to 12 weeks) were conducted in rats from two different Wistar derived strains and in Sprague Dawley rats. Alpha Protein was used as a source of LAL (0.34% of the product) and incorporated into diets of different composition at levels of 20% and 35% to provide 0.07% and 0.12% LAL, respectively. Each of the diets was fed to groups of 10 weanling male rats. Five of them were sacrificed for kidney examination after 4 weeks, the remaining 5 after 12 weeks. Diets containing 20% Alpha Protein afforded poor growth and low food efficiency

TABLE 13.1

EFFECTS OF FEEDING FREE LAL (LYSINOALANINE) TO RATS[1]

Parameters Examined	% LAL in Stock Diet			
	0	0.1	0.3	1.0
Gain in body weight (gm/rat)	89	68[5]	69[5]	55[6]
Food intake (gm/rat)	277	237	229	207
Food efficiency (gm gain/ gm food consumed)	0.32	0.28	0.30	0.27
UGOT (R-F units)[2]	33.2	33.1	33.8	56.6
SG of urine[3]	1.078	1.074	1.069	1.058[5]
% Phenolred excretion (1 hr)	68	70	51	71
Kidney weight (g/100 g)[4]	0.88	0.85	0.85	0.86
Micr. tubular nephrosis	—	+	+	+
Micr. cytomegalia	—	+	+	+

[1] Mean values of groups of five male weanling rats after four weeks.
[2] UGOT = Glutamic oxalacetic transaminase activity of urine.
[3] SG = Specific gravity of urine.
[4] gm/100 gm of body weight.
[5] $P < 0.05$.
[6] $P < 0.001$.
— absent; + present.

and induced diarrhea. Results improved considerably by increasing the level of Alpha Protein to 35%, which does not support the idea of a toxic factor in the product. Microscopically, no indications of renal cytomegalia were detectable in any of the rats, either after 4 or after 12 weeks of feeding.

Observations with Synthesized LAL

In order to study the biological properties of LAL, the compound was synthesized by the Organic Synthesis section of our Institute, from lysine according to a modified method of Okuda and Zahn (1965). The resulting crystalline LAL.2HCl, contained 0.8% lysine as its main impurity.

The compound was fed as a dietary supplement to several species of laboratory animals in short-term studies. The main results, obtained in male rats fed stock diet supplemented with 0.1, 0.3, or 1.0% free LAL for 4 weeks, are shown in Table 13.1. Distinct growth depression and decreased food efficiency occurred in the high-dose group only. Urine samples of this group (collected after 16 hr of deprivation of food and water) showed a decreased specific gravity and an increased activity of glutamic oxalacetic transaminase (UGOT). These findings indicate kidney damage, but the phenolred excretion did not reveal impaired renal function. Upon microscopical examination severe tubular nephrosis was observed in all rats in each group fed the test compound. The lesion, which was located mainly in the inner zone of the renal cortex, consisted of necrosis, regeneration, and cytomegalia of epithelial cells of the straight portion of the proximal tubules. The cytomegalia was characterized by enlarged cells with gigantic vesicular nuclei which often contained multiple nucleoli and showed a reticulate chromatin pattern. Upon electron microscopy, megalocytes often showed vacuolated cytoplasma and loss of the normally present deep foldings of the plasma membrane at the basal side of the cells. The nuclei were ultrastructurally unremarkable.

There were no abnormalities in hematologic indices or in the activities of serum enzymes (glutamic oxalacetic transaminase, glutamic pyruvic transaminase, alkaline phosphatase). Apart from UGOT activity and specific gravity of the urine none of the other urinary findings were abnormal. No treatment-related changes occurred in the organ-to-body weight ratios of the heart, liver, kidneys, and spleen, or in the microscopical structure of the 16 organs examined, except for the renal cytomegalia.

Upon examination of LAL at lower feeding levels, the only effect observed consisted of nephrocytomegalia at 100 ppm, whereas none of the parameters examined was affected at 30 ppm. These findings indicate that the no-effect level of free LAL is between 30 and 100 ppm in the diet, or between 3.0 and 10.0 mg per kg body wt per day.

A limited number of observations have been made on the effects of LAL in species other than the rat. No cytomegalia or other microscopic evidence of renal changes were observed in two beagle dogs fed 700 ppm LAL in a normal diet for 4 and 9 weeks, respectively. Likewise, young male mice, Syrian Golden hamsters, and Rhesus monkeys and newly hatched, male and female Japanese quail failed to show any relevant renal changes when they were fed 1000 ppm LAL in their diets for 8 weeks (de Groot et al. 1976).

Studies on the metabolism of LAL in rats are at present being conducted in our Institute with the compound labeled with carbon-14 in the alanine moiety, viz. N^ϵ-(2-amino-2-carboxy-[1-^{14}C]ethyl)-L-lysine. When administered in a single oral dose of 8–9 mg per kg body wt, the compound was found to be partly degraded to carbon dioxide and partly excreted after biotransformation in the feces and urine. Only a minor proportion of the dose administered was excreted as unchanged LAL (Leegwater 1975). Comparative metabolism studies in different species may provide valuable information to explain the differences in susceptibility to LAL-induced renal changes.

Observations with Protein-bound LAL

The occurrence of renal abnormalities in rats fed 0.01% free, synthetic LAL and their absence upon feeding alkali-treated proteins at levels providing up to 0.24% LAL, led to the hypothesis that LAL in a free form is

TABLE 13.2

INFLUENCE OF ACID HYDROLYSIS OF ALKALI-TREATED PROTEIN ON VARIOUS
PARAMETERS WHEN FED TO RATS

Dietary Protein	Weight Gain (gm/rat)	Food eaten (gm/rat)	gm of Gain ─────── gm of Food	Organ Weight as % of Body wt		Cyto-megalia
				Liver	Kidneys	
ISP (control)[2]	73	255	0.29	3.67	0.77	−
ISPH[2]	55	192	0.29	3.68	1.13[4]	−
ISPA[2]	68	218	0.31	3.34	0.87[3]	−
ISPAH[2]	43[3]	166	0.26	3.53	1.08[4]	+
ISP + LAL 0.02%	67	254	0.26	3.64	0.79	+
ISP + LAL 0.06%	67	247	0.27	3.66	0.81	+
ISP + LAL 0.18%	49[3]	226	0.22	3.60	0.86[1]	+

[1] Mean values of groups of 5 male rats after 4 weeks.
[2] ISP = isolated soy protein; ISPH = ISP acid-hydrolyzed; ISPA = ISP alkali-treated (0.96 gm LAL/16 gm N); ISPAH = ISPA acid-hydrolyzed; LAL = lysino-alanine.
[3] $P < 0.05$.
[4] $P < 0.001$.
− absent; + present.

much more active in terms of inducing kidney changes than is protein-bound LAL (as present in alkali-treated proteins). This hypothesis was supported by the results of a subsequent experiment in which the activity of alkali-treated isolated soy protein (ISP) was compared before and after complete acid hydrolysis. Portions of treated and untreated protein were completely hydrolyzed by refluxing with 6 N HCl for 22 hr. The HCl was largely removed and the hydrolysate was purified by filtration and treatment with charcoal. The proteins and hydrolysates were incorporated into a semipurified diet as the only source of amino acids (at levels equivalent to 20% crude protein and supplemented with 0.5% methionine). In addition, a supplement of 0.2% tryptophan was added to the diets containing the acid hydrolysates to correct for losses during hydrolysis. For comparison, three diets were included each containing 20% protein from untreated ISP and pure LAL added at dietary levels of 0.02, 0.06, and 0.18%, respectively. The highest level was comparable to that of the diet containing the severely alkali treated ISP. Each of these diets was fed to five male weanling rats for 4 weeks. Then the rats were sacrificed for examination of the liver and kidneys. Table 13.2 shows a summary of the results.

Growth rate and food intake were diminished in rats fed the two hydrolyzed proteins and in those fed the highest level of free, synthetic LAL. Food efficiency was decreased in the latter group only. There were no increases in the liver-to-body weight ratios but the kidney ratios were markedly increased in the two groups fed acid-hydrolyzed proteins. All rats fed synthetic LAL and all rats fed the protein subjected both to alkali treatment and acid hydrolysis (ISPAH), revealed severe tubular nephrosis including cytomegalic changes. These renal lesions did not occur in any of the rats fed the other diets. However, the diet containing the acid-hydrolyzed, but not alkali-treated, protein (ISPH) induced a slightly swollen tubular epithelium in the outer renal cortex (de Groot *et al.* 1976).

The most significant finding in this study is undoubtedly the presence of renal changes in rats fed ISPAH and their absence in rats fed the same protein which, however, had not been submitted to acid hydrolysis. Since the same type of changes are induced by free, synthetic LAL, it is obvious to attribute their occurrence to free LAL as present in the ISP subjected both to alkali treatment and acid hydrolysis. The fact that these changes were not observed with the same alkali-treated protein that had not been submitted to acid hydrolysis indicates that free LAL is considerably more active in terms of inducing renal changes than is protein bound LAL. Recently, Woodard and Short (1975) arrived at a similar conclusion.

The absence of any noticeable activity of bound LAL as present in alkali-treated protein may be caused by poor intestinal absorption. Supporting evidence for this assumption was obtained from tentative observations on absorption and excretion of free and bound LAL. In an experiment with diets containing either bound or free LAL (0.24 or 0.17% respectively), only about ½ of the ingested amounts were recovered in the hydrolyzed urine and feces. The urinary excretion predominated when free LAL was administered, whereas excretion with the feces was found to be the major route when protein bound LAL was fed.

The absence of renal activity in proteins severely treated with alkali and the induction of renal changes upon feeding the same protein after acid hydrolysis has been established not only with ISP, but also with casein. A commercial acid-precipitated casein was treated with alkali in a way which resulted in a LAL content of more than 5%. After precipitation and centrifugation the residue was added to normal stock diet in an amount which provided 0.6% LAL. No renal changes were noticed microscopically after four weeks of feeding. In contrast, distinct abnormalities were induced by the alkali-treated and completely acid-hydrolyzed casein in the same basal diet in a concentration which provided only 120 ppm LAL. The type and degree of these changes were similar to those observed upon feeding stock diet supplemented with 125 ppm free, synthetic LAL (de Groot *et al.* 1976).

These observations with treated casein not only confirm those obtained with ISP, but they also indicate the lack of activity of very high levels of LAL bound in proteins. Since renal changes are induced by free LAL at a level as low as 100 ppm, whereas a 60 times higher level fed as alkali-treated acid precipitated protein did not produce this effect, it seems justified to conclude that LAL bound in protein is not nephrotoxic in rats. This would indicate that even very drastic alkali treatment of proteins does not impart any nephrotoxic potential to protein provided that the content of free LAL is reduced to a minimum, either by preventing its occurrence or by its removal in a subsequent purification treatment. Further feeding studies with different proteins for prolonged periods of time are desirable for substantiating this conclusion.

Significance of LAL in Peptides

The nephrotoxic properties of free LAL and the lack of activity observed with protein-bound LAL inevitably leads to the question about the significance of LAL in poly- and oligopeptides which may be formed upon severe alkali treatment of proteins.

A diet containing a commercially available, partially degraded and alkali-treated food protein at a level providing a total of 0.55% LAL (40% of which was poorly soluble and 60% highly soluble in water at pH 3.5) evoked a slight cytomegalic response in rat kidneys although the dietary free LAL concentration was only 4 ppm. Since the lowest level of free LAL showing renal activity in similar studies was found to be 100 ppm, whereas protein-bound LAL even at 0.6% was inactive, the above findings suggest that peptide-linked LAL in smaller protein fragments may exert effects qualitatively similar to those of free LAL. Supporting evidence for this assumption was obtained from the differences in the blood serum levels of free LAL found between rats fed LAL either in the free form, or as intact or partially acid-hydrolyzed, alkali-treated protein.

DISCUSSION AND CONCLUSIONS

From the available evidence, it appears that severe alkali treatment of proteins induces chemical changes which may affect both the nutritive value and the safety of the product. These undesirable alterations are minimized by lowering the pH and the temperature of treatment, and by shortening the duration of exposure. Little or no change was found with soy protein at pH values below 10 at room temperature. With more drastic conditions of treatment, the most marked effects are lowering of protein digestibility and utilization, decreasing levels of cystine and lysine, and increasing levels of LAL. Cystine is a sensitive indicator of losses in nutritive value, while the safety is connected with the contents of LAL.

The occurrence of LAL in proteins is not necessarily caused by the addition of alkaline agents. According to Gross et al. (1975), LAL is a natural constituent of cinnamycin and duramycin, two peptides present in certain Streptomyces species. Recently, we obtained evidence for the presence of small amounts of LAL in the whites of commercially available hen's eggs, the level increasing considerably by simply boiling the eggs in water. Analyses of newly laid eggs were negative. In addition LAL has been detected in a variety of foods and food ingredients (infant milk formula, products from corn, milk, meat and eggs, hydrolyzed vegetable protein and whipping agents) at levels usually ranging from 100–1000 ppm (Sternberg et al. 1975).

It has been reported that alkali treatment of soy proteins induces nephrotoxic properties which are correlated with the appearance of LAL (Woodard and Short 1973). The results of our studies, however, failed to show renal alterations or any other indications of toxicity when rats were fed very high dietary levels of bound LAL as provided by alkali-treated casein or soy protein. In contrast, typical renal changes occurred by feeding relatively low levels of free LAL, either as the organically synthesized compound, or as alkali treated and subsequently acid-hydrolyzed proteins. These findings suggest that alkali treatment does not impart any nephrotoxic properties to proteins, provided that the LAL formed remains protein bound.

In addition to free and protein bound, LAL may occur in oligo- and polypeptides. Indications have been obtained that renal changes may be induced not only by free LAL but also by peptide-linked LAL in small protein fragments. Although the renal activity of the latter type of compounds is probably less than that of free LAL it is desirable to assume provisionally that all LAL not bound in acid precipitable protein is potentially active material. Further studies are desirable to establish possible renal activity of LAL in peptides of varying molecular weight ranges.

The lowest level of free LAL which was found to induce renal cytomegalia was 100 mg per kg diet, which is equivalent to 10 mg per kg body wt of young rats. With increasing levels, growth depression was not observed until 1000 ppm, and a further 10-fold increase was necessary before clinical signs of kidney damage became manifest, viz. increased UGOT activity and decreased concentrating ability. From the short-term studies, it would appear that renal cytomegalia has little clinical implications. Its toxicological significance, however, has to be established in long-term studies. The absence of any renal changes in the other species so far examined (dog, mouse, hamster, monkey, quail), suggests that the LAL-induced lesion may be species specific.

ACKNOWLEDGEMENTS

Thanks are due to Dr. R. J. C. Kleipool and Dr. A. C. Tas for synthesizing lysinoalanine, Mr. B. J. Spit for electron microscopy, and to Dr. D. C. Leegwater for reading the manuscript. Studies supported, in part, by Miles Laboratories, Inc.

BIBLIOGRAPHY

ANON. 1967. Soy fibers; a new approach to vegetable protein acceptability. Nutr. Rev. 25, 305.

282   EVALUATION OF PROTEINS FOR HUMANS

BEEK, L. VAN, FERON, V. J., and GROOT, A. P. DE. 1974. Nutritional effects of alkali-treated soyprotein in rats. J. Nutr. *104*, 1630.

BETSCHART, A. A. 1974. Nitrogen solubility of alfalfa protein concentrate as influenced by various factors. J. Food Sci. *39*, 1110.

BOHAK, Z. 1964. N^{ϵ}-(DL-2-amino-2-carboxyethyl)-L-lysine, a new amino acid formed on alkaline treatment of proteins. J. Biol. Chem. *239*, 2878.

BRESSANI, R., PAZ Y PAZ, R., and SCRIMSHAW, N. S. 1958. Chemical changes in corn during preparation of tortillas. Agr. Food Chem. *6*, 770.

BRESSANI, R., and SCRIMSHAW, N. S. 1958. Effect of lime treatment on in vitro availability of essential amino acids and solubility of protein fractions in corn. Agr. Food Chem. *6*, 774.

BRESSANI, R., VITERI, F., ELIAS, L. G., ZAGHI, S. DE, ALVARADO, J., and ODELL, A. D. 1967. Protein quality of a soybean protein textured food in experimental animals and children. J. Nutr. *93*, 349.

CARPENTER, K. J., and DUCKWORTH, J. 1950. The nutritive value of herring "alkali-reduction" meal for chicks. J. Agr. Sci. *40*, 44.

CARPENTER, K. J., DUCKWORTH, J., ELLINGER, G. M., and SHRIMPTON, D. H. 1952. The nutritional evaluation of protein concentrates obtained from the alkali digestion of herrings. J. Sci. Food Agr. *3*, 278.

CIRCLE, S. J., and SMITH, A. K. 1972. Processing soy flours, protein concentrates, and protein isolates. *In* Soybeans: Chemistry and Technology, Vol. 1. A. K. Smith, and S. J. Circle (Editors). Avi Publishing Co., Westport, Conn.

GROOT, A. P. DE, SLUMP, P., FERON, V. J. and BEEK, L. VAN. Effects of alkali-treated proteins. Feeding studies with free and protein-bound lysinoalanine in rats and other animals. J. Nutr. *106*, 1527.

GROOT, A. P. DE, and SLUMP, P. 1969. Effects of severe alkali treatment of proteins on amino acid composition and nutritive value. J. Nutr. *98*, 45.

GROSS, E., CHEN, H. C., and BROWN, J. H. 1975. Peptides with α,β-unsaturated amino acids and lanthionines: Biological properties and studies to elucidate the structure of cinnamycin and duramycin. Federation Proc. *34*, 819.

HERMANSSON, A. M., SIVIK, B., and SKJÖLDEBRAND, C. 1971. Functional properties of proteins for foods. Factors affecting solubility, foaming and swelling of fish protein concentrate. Lebensm. Wiss. Technol. *4*, 201.

HORN, M. J., JONES, D. B., and RINGEL, S. J. 1941. Isolation of a new sulphur-containing amino acid (lanthionine) from sodium carbonate-treated wool. J. Biol. Chem. *138*, 141.

HUPF, H., and SPRINGER, R. 1971. Bildung von Lanthionin in Nahrungsproteinen. Z. Lebensm. Untersuch. Forsch. *146*, 138.

KATZ, S. H., HEDIGER, M. L., and VALLEROY, L. A. 1974. Traditional maize processing techniques in the new world. Science *184*, 765.

KRAUSE, W., and SCHMIDT, K. 1974. Untersuchungen zur enzymatischen Hydrolyse von alkalibehandelten Milchproteinen. Nahrung *18*, 833.

LEEGWATER, D. C. 1975. Unpublished data. Centr. Inst. Nutr. Food Res. CIVO-TNO, Zeist, Netherlands.

LINDBLOM, M. 1974. Alkali treatment of a yeast protein concentrate. Lebensm. Wiss. Technol. *7*, 295.

NEWBERNE, P. M., and YOUNG, V. R. 1966. Effect of diets marginal in methionine and choline with and without vitamin B_{12} on rat liver and kidney. J. Nutr. *89*, 69.

OKUDA, T., and ZAHN, H. 1965. Synthese von N^{ϵ}-(2-amino-2-carboxy-äthyl)-L-lysin, einer neuen Aminosäure aus alkalibehandelter Wolle. Chem. Ber. *98*, 1164.

PATCHORNIK, A., and SOKOLOVSKY, M. 1964. Chemical interactions between lysine and dehydroalanine in modified bovine pancreatic ribonuclease. J. Am. Chem. Soc. *86*, 1860.

RAMASARMA, G. B., HENDERSON, L. M., and ELVEHJEM, C. A. 1949. Purified amino acids as a source of nitrogen for the growing rat. J. Nutr. *38*, 177.

STERNBERG, M. L., KIM, C. Y., and SCHWENDE, F. J. 1975. Lysinoalanine: presence in foods and food ingredients. Science, *190*, 992.

SULLIVAN, J. T. 1943. Protein concentrates from grasses. Science *98*, 363.

TANNENBAUM, S. R., BATES, R. P., and BRODFELD, L. 1970. Solubilization of fish protein concentrate. 2. Utilization of the alkaline-process product. Food Technol. *24*, 607.

TURK, R. E., CORNWELL, P. E., BROOKS, M. D., and BUTTERWORTH, C. E. 1973. Adequacy of spun-soy protein containing egg albumin for human nutrition. J. Am. Dietet. Assoc. *63*, 519.

WIPF, V. K. 1972. Structured foods. Activities Rept. Res. Develop. Assoc. Mil. Food Package Systems *24*, 125.

WOODARD, J. C., and ALVAREZ, M. R. 1967. Renal lesions in rats fed diets containing alpha protein. Arch. Pathol. *84*, 153.

WOODARD, J. C. 1969. On the pathogenesis of alpha protein-induced nephrocytomegalia. Lab. Invest. *20*, 9.

WOODARD, J. C., and SHORT, D. D. 1973. Toxicity of alkali-treated soy protein in the rat. J. Nutr. *103*, 569.

WOODARD, J. C., and SHORT, D. D. 1975. Renal toxicity of N^ϵ-(DL-2-amino-2-carboxyethyl)-L-lysine (lysinoalanine) in rats. Federation Proc. *34*, 929.

ZIEGLER, K., MELCHERT, I., and LÜRKEN, C. 1967. N^δ-(2-amino-2-carboxyethyl)—ornithine, a new amino acid from alkali-treated proteins. Nature *214*, 404.

CHAPTER 14

I. E. Liener | # Protease Inhibitors and Hemagglutinins of Legumes

Although it is accepted as a general premise in nutrition that the nutritional value of a protein is determined by its amino acid composition and the availability of these amino acids, the legumes constitute a valuable source of protein which does not always follow this rule. This deviation arises from the fact that the legumes are known to contain a variety of factors which, in one way or another, may exhibit deleterious effects when ingested in the diet. In this chapter, two of the most important of these factors, namely the protease inhibitors and hemagglutinins, are discussed and an attempt is made to assess their possible significance in the human diet.

PROTEASE INHIBITORS

Historical Background

The fact that protease inhibitors are found in the legumes which contribute an important source of dietary protein for many segments of the world's population has served to stimulate a vast amount of research regarding their possible nutritional significance [see review by Liener and Kakade (1969)]. Because of the important role which the soybean plays as a source of protein in animal feedstuffs, and potentially for human nutrition as well, it is the soybean protease inhibitor which has received the most attention. Therefore, much of this discussion will deal with this particular inhibitor. Anyone who has attempted to delve very deeply into this subject is soon frustrated by the inconsistencies and claims and counterclaims which are found in the literature. Nevertheless, I will attempt to assemble our existing information on the subject into what I hope will be a coherent picture of the role which protease inhibitors might play in the nutrition of animals and man.

It was not long after soybeans were introduced into the United States, primarily as a source of oil, that Osborne and Mendel (1917) made the significant observation that soybeans had to be heated in order to support the growth of rats. Kunitz (1945) subsequently isolated from raw soybeans a protein which had the unique property of combining with trypsin to form an inactive complex. Purified soybean fractions high in antitryptic activity were capable of inhibiting the growth of chicks (Ham *et al.* 1965), rats

(Klose *et al.* 1946), and mice (Westfall and Hauge 1948), an effect which was generally accompanied by a decrease in protein digestibility (Evans and McGinnis 1948; Kwong *et al.* 1962). On the basis of this evidence it seemed reasonable to assume at the time that the trypsin inhibitor was responsible for the poor nutritive value of unheated soybeans, presumably by virtue of its ability to inhibit intestinal proteolysis. The fact also that methionine markedly enhanced the nutritive value of raw soybeans (Hayward and Hafner 1941) was taken to indicate that the trypsin inhibitor somehow interfered with the availability or utilization of methionine from the raw bean.

Melnick *et al.* (1946) noted that, during the *in vitro* digestion of raw soybean protein by pancreatin, methionine was released at a slower rate than the other essential amino acids. This led them to postulate that during the intestinal digestion of raw soybean protein the release and subsequent absorption of methionine is delayed to the point where it is no longer available for the mutual supplementation of the other essential amino acids. Attractive as this hypothesis was, it did not explain why trypsin inhibitor preparations were capable of inhibiting growth even when incorporated into diets containing predigested protein or free amino acids (Desikachar and De 1947; Khayambashi and Lyman 1966). Such experiments obviously rule out an inhibition of proteolysis as the sole factor responsible for growth inhibition and served to focus attention on some alternative mode of action of the trypsin inhibitor.

Mode of Action

Perhaps the most significant observation which has ultimately led to a better understanding of the mode of action of the soybean inhibitor was the finding that animals fed raw soybeans developed marked hypertrophy of the pancreas (Chernick *et al.* 1948; Booth *et al.* 1960) which is accompanied by an increased rate of synthesis of proteolytic enzymes (Konijn and Guggenheim 1967). The same effect can be produced by feeding highly purified preparations of the Kunitz inhibitor (Nesheim *et al.* 1962). Histological and biochemical examination of the enlarged pancreas reveals true hyperplasia which is characterized by an increase in the number of cells in the pancreatic tissue (Applegarth *et al.* 1964) but which at the same time shows evidence that the zymogen granules have been depleted (Salman *et al.* 1967).

These findings led Lyman and Lepkovsky (1957) to suggest that the growth depression caused by the soybean inhibitor might be the result of an endogenous loss of protein produced by a hyperactive pancreas. Being of pancreatic origin, this protein consists largely of such enzymes as trypsin, chymotrypsin, and amylase which are known to be rich in cystine. Since much of the cystine required for the biosynthesis of these proteins is presumably derived from methionine, an accelerated rate of synthesis of these enzymes in the pancreas would in effect deplete the rest of the body tissues of methionine. This increased need for methionine would be rendered even more acute in the case of soybean protein which is notoriously deficient in the sulfur-containing amino acids. It is not surprising therefore that methionine supplementation will effectively counteract most of the growth depression caused by the inhibitor despite the persistence of pancreatic hypertrophy (Khayambashi and Lyman 1966; Booth *et al.* 1960).

The mechanism whereby the trypsin inhibitor leads to pancreatic enlargement with its attendant intensification of enzyme synthesis is not well understood. It has been recently reported (Green and Lyman 1972; Niess *et al.* 1972) that it is the level of active trypsin in the intestines which controls the amount of enzymes secreted by the pancreas. When the level of trypsin in the intestinal tract drops below its normal levels, such as would be the case in the presence of trypsin inhibitor, the pancreas responds by producing more enzyme. Whether this effect is mediated through the action of pancreozymin is not known.

It is evident from the foregoing observations that an inhibition of intestinal proteolysis need not be invoked to explain the growth inhibition produced by the soybean inhibitor. On the other hand, neither do I believe that we can ignore the possibility than an inhibition of intestinal proteolysis may play a significant role in the overall nutritive properties of the soybean protein. For example, if the amount of trypsin produced by the pancreas is not sufficient to neutralize all of the inhibitor present in the intestinal tract, the proteolysis of intact protein will be obviously depressed. Thus, the increase in fecal nitrogen, which is generally observed in animals receiving diets containing the inhibitor (Lyman and Lepkovsky 1957; Alumot and Nitsan 1961) may be of dietary as well as of endogenous origin (from the pancreas). Experimentally it may prove very difficult to differentiate between these two effects.

Effect of Processing

It is the relative ease with which the deleterious components of legumes, including the trypsin inhibitor, can be destroyed by heat which has permitted their universal use as an important dietary component. The soybean inhibitor again has received the most study in this respect, and, in general, the extent to which the inhibitor is destroyed is a function of the temperature, duration of heating, moisture conditions, particle size, etc.—variables which are closely controlled in the commercial processing of soybeans in order to produce a product having maximum nutritive value. An example of how heat affects the nutritive properties of soybean protein in relation to trypsin inhibitor activity is shown in Fig. 14.1. Not shown in this figure, however, is the fact that excessive heat treatment may damage the nutritive

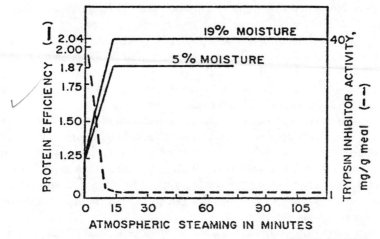

From Rackis (1965)

FIG. 14.1. EFFECT OF AUTOCLAVING ON PROTEIN EFFICIENCY
AND TRYPSIN INHIBITOR ACTIVITY OF RAW SOYBEAN MEAL
Conditions: live steam at atmospheric pressure, 100°C with 5% or 19%
moisture prior to autoclaving.

TABLE 14.1

EFFECT OF SOY FLOUR CONTAINING VARIOUS LEVELS OF TRYPSIN
INHIBITOR (TI) ON GROWTH AND PANCREATIC SIZE OF RATS

TI Content		Body Weight (gm)	PER	Pancreas Weight (gm/100 gm Body wt)
mg/100 gm Diet	% Destruction			
887	0	79	1.59	0.70
532	40	111	2.37	0.56
282	68	121	2.78	0.50
157	82	134	2.97	0.49
119	87	148	3.08	0.47
71	92	142	3.03	0.45
Casein	—	145	3.35	0.55

Source: Rackis et al. (1975).   see Table 12.5.

value of the protein so that the absence of inhibitor activity is not always
a guarantee of a product having optimal nutritional quality.

Rackis et al. (1975) have recently determined the biological threshold
level in rats of trypsin inhibitory activity in soybean meals having different
levels of trypsin inhibitor activity. Data taken from their paper are shown
in Table 14.1. Maximum body weight and protein efficiency values were
obtained with rats fed soy samples in which about 80% of the inhibitor was

inactivated. No pancreatic hypertrophy occurred in rats fed soyflour in which 50–60% of the inhibitor activity had been destroyed.

The trypsin inhibitor activity which may be present in soymilk can be effectively eliminated by sterilization of the liquid product or by spray drying (Hackler et al. 1965). It is of significance to note that properly processed soybean milk has a nutritional quality which is essentially equivalent to that of cow's milk (Shurpalikar et al. 1961).

Food dishes derived from soybeans have been used in the Orient for centuries without any apparent deleterious effect. The biological value of soybean curd ("tofu") is equivalent to that of properly processed soybean meal (Pian 1930) or casein (Standal 1963). Since the preparation of tofu involves the cooking or steaming of the beans prior to extraction with water, tofu is believed to be free of the inhibitor (Dean 1958) although no specific data on this point are available.

Fermented soybean products such as "tempeh" and "natto" are readily digested (Van Veen and Schaeffer 1950) which would indicate that the inhibitor present in the original raw bean had been inactivated. This conclusion is consistent with the observation that there is no prancreatic enlargement in rats fed diets containing tempeh (Smith et al. 1964). The inhibitor is presumably destroyed by the heat treatment involved in the preparation of tempeh in which the beans are boiled for at least 30 min prior to the fermentation.

More recently, considerable attention has been given to the nutritional properties of soybean isolates and the textured meat analogues fabricated therefrom. Although the nutritive quality of these textured food products has been reported to be essentially equivalent to casein or beef, the protein efficiency of the original protein isolate was very low and could be improved by heat treatment (Bressani et al. 1967). These results would indicate the possible presence of residual growth inhibitors in the protein isolate which were inactivated during the process of converting the isolate into fiber. We have had occasion to examine a number of these textured products for antitryptic activity. As the data in Table 14.2 show, the soybean isolate and fiber are surprisingly rich in trypsin inhibitor activity. The processed meat analogues have a reduced but measurable level of antitryptic activity.

Other Considerations

Since there would appear to be little doubt that the trypsin inhibitors can produce adverse physiological effects in animals, the question naturally arises as to whether these are of any physiological significance to man. The only report on man indicates that raw soyflour can support positive nitrogen balance, but not as efficiently as autoclaved flour (Lewis and Taylor, 1947). Earlier reports from two different laboratories (Feeney et al. 1969; Travis and Roberts 1969; Coan and Travis 1971) had indicated that the cationic

TABLE 14.2

TRYPSIN INHIBITOR CONTENT OF VARIOUS SOYBEAN PRODUCTS
AND THEIR INTERMEDIATES

Product	Antitrypsin Activity	
	(TIU/gm Dry Solids) $\times 10^{-3}$ [1]	% of Soy Flour
Soy flour (unheated)	86.4	100
Soybean isolate	25.5	30
Soybean fiber	12.3	14
Chicken analog	6.9	8
Ham analog	10.2	12
Beef analog	6.5	7

[1] TIU = trypsin inhibitor units as defined by Kakade et al. (1972).

form of human trypsin was only weakly inhibited by the soybean inhibitor. More recently, however, Mallory and Travis (1973) and Figarella et al. (1975) isolated and characterized an anionic form of human trypsin which could be fully inactivated by the soybean inhibitor. It is important to note, however, that the human trypsin which fails to be inhibited by the soybean trypsin inhibitor represents the major part (65%) of the potential trypsin activity of the whole juice (Figarella et al. 1969). Regardless of whether human trypsin is affected by the soybean inhibitor or not, it would be reasonably safe to conclude that the low levels of residual activity in most soybean products intended for human consumption are far below the biological threshold value, albeit established with rats.

Another question which may be logically posed is—to what extent is the poor nutritive value actually caused by the trypsin inhibitor itself? Our first indication that the trypsin inhibitor may not be the only factor responsible for the poor growth response one obtains on raw legumes are from a study which we made on the trypsin inhibitor content of over 100 different varieties of soybeans. From this initial survey, 26 varieties representing low, medium, and high levels of trypsin inhibitor activity were also assayed for their ability to support the growth of rats as measured by PER. Figure 14.2 shows a scatter diagram of trypsin inhibitor activity in relation to PER. The absence of any correlation between inhibitor activity and PER is obvious. Since pancreatic hypertrophy has been shown to be a characteristic response of the rat to the trypsin inhibitor, we also recorded in our study the weights of the pancreas fed the various soybean diets (Fig. 14.3). Much to our surprise, we now observed a significant level of correlation (negative) between the weights of the pancreas and PER.

It is apparent from these studies that an in vitro measurement of trypsin inhibitor activity does not provide a true reflection of the nutritive properties of soybean protein in its unheated state. On the other hand, growth

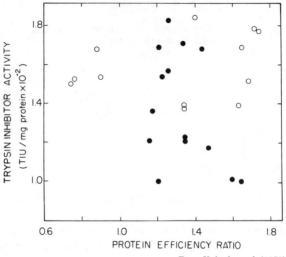

From Kakade et al. (1972)

FIG. 14.2.   SCATTER DIAGRAM RELATING TRYPSIN INHIBITOR
ACTIVITY TO PER OF VARIOUS SOYBEAN SAMPLES

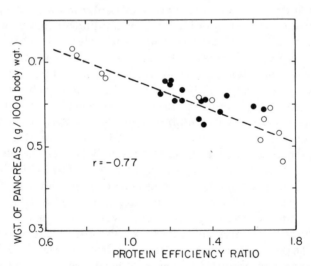

From Kakade et al. (1972)

FIG. 14.3.   RELATIONSHIP OF WEIGHTS OF PANCREAS TO PER OF
VARIOUS SOYBEAN SAMPLES
The coefficient of correlation, r, is significant at a level of $P < 0.05$.

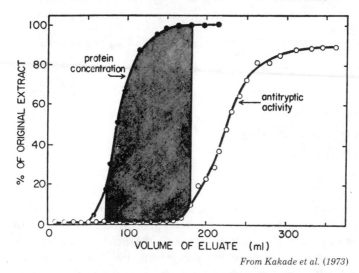

From Kakade et al. (1973)

FIG. 14.4.   REMOVAL OF TRYPSIN INHIBITORS FROM SOYBEAN EX-
TRACT BY AFFINITY CHROMATOGRAPHY ON SEPHAROSE-TRYPSIN
Shaded area between the two curves denotes those tubes which were
pooled to give extract-free of trypsin inhibitor.

response and pancreatic hypertrophy appear to be closely associated effects.
The corollary to these conclusions is that there must be present in raw
soybeans some other factor, which is totally unrelated to the trypsin in
hibitor, which is also capable of causing pancreatic enlargement and an
inhibition of growth.

In order to obtain a more definitive answer to this problem, we chose a
somewhat different approach to this problem, one which involved feeding
unheated soybean protein from which the inhibitor had been selectively
removed by affinity chromatography using immobilized trypsin. By comparing the growth response of rats fed the unheated soybean protein from
which the inhibitor had been removed with the original protein still containing the inhibitor, it should be possible to assess the nutritional significance of the inhibitor itself. Another control group fed the heated soybean
protein should then make it possible to evaluate the effect produced by heat
treatment *per se* (Kakade *et al.* 1973).

A crude extract of unheated soybeans, containing about 90% of the total
protein of the original bean, was passed through a column of Sepharose-
bound trypsin (Fig. 14.4). Those tubes which were devoid of antitryptic
activity were pooled and incorporated into diets at a level of 10% protein.
Also fed to rats were diets containing the original extract from which the
inhibitor had not been removed, as well as an extract which had been

TABLE 14.3

EFFECT OF REMOVAL OF TRYPSIN INHIBITORS FROM SOYBEAN EXTRACT
ON PER AND PANCREAS

Source of Protein in Diet	PER	Weight of Pancreas (gm/100 gm Body wt)
Soybean extract, unheated	1.4	0.74
Soybean extract, heated	2.7	0.52
Soybean extract minus inhibitor	1.9	0.65
Soybean flour, unheated	1.5	0.71
Soybean flour, heated	2.8	0.57

Source: Kakade et al. (1973).

subjected to the usual heat treatment one gives soybeans. Referring to the data shown in Table 14.3, it may be noted that, although the removal of the inhibitor increased the PER from 1.4 to 1.9, heat treatment effected a greater increase to 2.7. The latter effect is comparable to what one gets with soy flour itself. It may be calculated from these data that approximately 40% of the difference in PER between raw and heated soybean protein may be attributed to the trypsin inhibitor. Also included in this study were measurements of the size of the pancreas. Although removal of the inhibitor served to decrease the size of the pancreas, this reduction was again only about 40% of the decrease produced by heat treatment.

These results made us consider the possibility that the fact that the protein itself had not been heated might be responsible for the poor growth and pancreatic hypertrophy not accounted for by the inhibitor. Accordingly, the protein extract from which the inhibitor had been removed was subjected to in vitro digestion by trypsin. Comparisons were made with the original extract, before and after heat treatment. From the results shown in Fig. 14.5, it is evident that although the absence of the inhibitor serves to enhance the susceptibility of the protein to proteolytic attack by trypsin, heating nevertheless causes a further increase in digestibility. Again, about 40% of the difference in digestibility between the raw and heated soybean extract can be attributed to the inhibitor.

These results have led us to conclude that the principal cause of growth inhibition in raw soybeans is a combination of the effects of the trypsin inhibitor and the fact that the soybean protein is in an undenatured state. In both cases, however, a common mechanism may be invoked, namely, they both lead to hypersecretion by the pancreas. As pointed out earlier the level of pancreatic secretion is controlled by the level of trypsin in the intestine by feed-back inhibition. Thus the presence of trypsin inhibitors or undigested protein serves to overcome this feed-back inhibition by reducing the effective level of active trypsin in the intestinal tract, thereby leading to hypersecretion by the pancreas.

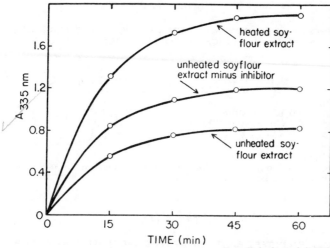

From Kakade et al. (1973)

FIG. 14.5. *IN VITRO* DIGESTIBILITY BY TRYPSIN OF SOYBEAN
EXTRACT FROM WHICH TRYPSIN INHIBITORS HAD BEEN
REMOVED
Compared with the original extract before and after heat treatment.
Progress of digestion was followed by measuring absorbance at 355 nm
using trinitrobenzene sulfonic acid as reagent for free amino groups
according to Habeeb (1966).

The Role of Trypsin Inhibitors in Other Legumes

To what extent the trypsin inhibitor accounts for the poor digestibility
of other legumes is not certain at the present time. The situation with other
legumes is particularly puzzling since there does not appear to be any
clear-cut correlation between the trypsin inhibitor content of various legumes and the beneficial effect of heat treatment (Borchers and Ackerson
1950). The presence of other growth inhibitors such as the phytohemagglutinins (see below) no doubt tends to obscure whatever detrimental
effects the trypsin inhibitor *per se* may have on growth. Nevertheless, it
may be significant to note that the trypsin inhibitors of such legumes as
navy beans and kidney beans are quite rich in cystine; although they
comprise only 2.5% of the total bean protein, they account for about 30–40%
of the total cystine content of the bean protein (Kakade *et al.* 1969). It is
conceivable, therefore, that a dietary loss of cystine from the inhibitor itself
could contribute in a significant fashion to the poor quality of these legumes.
The results of experiments (with chicks) designed to test this hypothesis
are shown in Table 14.4. It is evident from these data that the cystine of
the unheated navy bean inhibitor is much less available to the chick than
the cystine provided by the heat-inactivated inhibitor. *In vitro* digestibility
data (Table 14.5) suggest that the unavailability of cystine from the un-

TABLE 14.4

EFFECT OF FEEDING NAVY BEAN TRYPSIN INHIBITOR (NBTI)
ON GROWTH OF CHICKS AND AVAILABILITY OF CYSTINE

Diet	Weight Gain (gm/Day)	% Availability of Cystine[1]
Basal diet[2]	−1.0	
Basal diet + 0.15% cystine	4.6	
Basal diet + 2% unheated NBTI	−1.8	44.5
Basal diet + 2% heated NBTI	3.3	76.3

Source: Kakade et al. (1969).
[1] Percentage of cystine ingested which was not excreted in the feces.
[2] Amino acid mixture deficient in cystine.

TABLE 14.5

IN VITRO DIGESTIBILITY OF NATIVE AND HEATED NAVY BEAN
TRYPSIN INHIBITOR (NBTI)

Enzyme Tested	Extent of Proteolysis[1]	
	Unheated NBTI	Heated NBTI
Trypsin	0.050	0.320
Chymotrypsin	0.050	0.420
Pronase	0.680	0.910

Source: Kakade et al. (1969).
[1] Increase in absorbance at 280 nm of deproteinized filtrate.

heated inhibitor is most likely the consequence of its resistance to enzymatic attack. Thus the trypsin inhibitors of legumes may be a doubled-edged sword; they not only reduce the digestibility of the protein but may also "lock-in" a significant fraction of the total cystine of the bean protein which is already in short supply.

THE PHYTOHEMAGGLUTININS

It should be appreciated that the trypsin inhibitors are but one of a number of factors which have from time-to-time been postulated to exert an antinutritional effect in legumes (Liener 1973). Among those which have received prominent attention are the so-called phytohemagglutinins or lectins which are present in most edible legumes (Liener 1974).

Soybeans

In our laboratory, we have attempted to evaluate the nutritional significance of the phytohemagglutinin in soybeans by selectively removing those substances from crude extracts of the soybean using affinity chromatog-

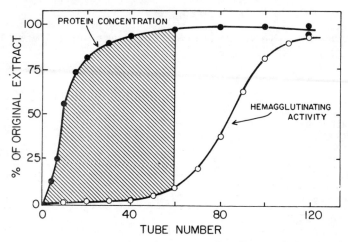

From Turner and Liener (1975)

FIG. 14.6. REMOVAL OF HEMAGGLUTININ FROM CRUDE SOYBEAN EXTRACT BY AFFINITY CHROMATOGRAPHY ON SEPHAROSE-BOUND CONCANAVALIN-A

Shaded area between the two curves denotes those tubes which were pooled to give extract free of the hemagglutinins.

TABLE 14.6

EFFECT OF REMOVING SOYBEAN HEMAGGLUTININ (SBH) ON THE GROWTH-PROMOTING ACTIVITY OF RAW SOYBEANS

Protein Component of Diet	Hemagglutinating Activity (units/gm protein) $\times 10^{-3}$	PER
Original soybean extract	324	0.91
Original extract minus SBH[1]	29	1.13
Original extract, heated	6	2.25
Raw soy flour	330	1.01
Heated soy flour	13	2.30

Source: Turner et al. (1975).
[1] SBH removed by affinity chromatography on Sepharose-bound concanavalin-A.

raphy on Sepharose-bound concanavalin-A. The latter had been previously shown by Bessler and Goldstein (1973) to have a high affinity for mannose-containing glycoproteins such as the soybean hemagglutinin. Crude extracts of a soybean flour which had received a minimum amount of heat treatment was passed through a column of Sepharose-bound concanavalin-A with the results shown in Fig. 14.6. Fractions devoid of hemagglutinating activity were pooled and fed to rats, comparisons being made with groups receiving the original crude extract before and after heat treatment.

TABLE 14.7

EFFECT OF HEAT ON NUTRITIVE VALUE OF SOME LEGUMES

Source of Protein	Gain in Weight Raw (gm/Day)	Heated (gm/Day)
Phaseolus vulgaris		
Black bean	−1.94 (4−5)[1]	+1.61
Kidney bean	−1.04 (11−13)[1]	+1.48
Cicer arietinum		
Bengal gram	+1.25	+1.16
Cajanus cajan		
Red gram	+1.33	+1.74
Phaseolus aureus		
Mung bean	+1.05	+1.07

Source: Honavar *et al.* (1962).
[1] 100% mortality observed during period (in days) shown in parentheses.

From the results of this experiment, summarized in Table 14.6, it may be concluded that the removal of soybean hemagglutinin from a crude extract of soyflour had little effect on the PER of rats and produced essentially the same poor growth as raw soyflour itself. It may also be mentioned in passing that the elimination of soybean hemagglutinin did not reduce the pancreatic hypertrophy characteristic of animals fed raw soybeans.

Other Legumes

Although the phytohemagglutinins appear to have little significance as far as the soybean is concerned, the situation with respect to some other legumes is quite different. The common bean, *Phaseolus vulgaris,* constitutes an important source of dietary protein for large segments of the world's population, and numerous reports may be found in the literature concerning the toxic effects which have sometimes accompanied the ingestion of raw or inadequately cooked beans (Liener and Kakade 1969). In order to evaluate the possible nutritional significance of this phytohemagglutinin we undertook the task of isolating sufficient quantities of this material from *Phaseolus vulgaris* in order to feed it to rats at approximately the same level of activity as is found in the raw bean (Honavar *et al.* 1962). This was preceded by a study to ascertain the effect of heat on the nutritive value of several legumes which enjoy popular consumption in some of the underdeveloped countries. It is apparent from Table 14.7 that of the five legumes tested, only the black bean and kidney bean, both classified as *P. vulgaris,* were markedly improved by heat treatment. Table 14.8 shows that these same two beans were the only ones to display high levels of hemagglutinating activity. When the phytohemagglutinins from these two beans were purified to the point where the trypsin inhibitor activity was elimi-

TABLE 14.8

HEMAGGLUTINATING AND ANTITRYPTIC ACTIVITIES OF
CRUDE EXTRACTS OF RAW LEGUMES

Legume	Hemagglutinating Activity (units/gm)	Antitryptic Activity (units/gm)
Phaseolus vulgaris		
Black bean	2450	2050
Kidney bean	3560	1552
Cicer arietinum	0	220
Cajanus cajan	0	418
Phaseolus aureus	0	260

Source: Honavar *et al.* (1962).

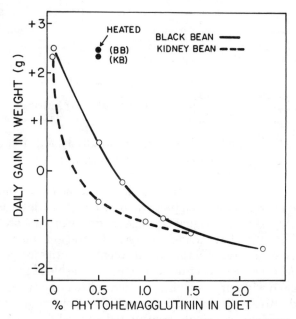

Taken from Hanovar et al. (1962)

FIG. 14.7.   THE EFFECT OF BLACK BEAN (BB) AND KIDNEY BEAN (KB) HEMAGGLUTININS ON THE GROWTH OF RATS

nated, their growth inhibitory effect and toxicity to rats became readily apparent (Fig. 14.7). Levels as low as 0.5% of the diet caused a definite inhibition of growth, and higher levels of the phytohemagglutinin hastened the onset of death. Similar effects were subsequently reported with chicks as the experimental animal (Wagh *et al.* 1965).

One of the complicating factors involved in relating hemagglutinating

TABLE 14.9

CORRELATION OF SPECIFIC HEMAGGLUTINATING ACTIVITY WITH THE
INTRAPERITONEAL TOXICITY IN RATS OF EXTRACTS OF
DIFFERENT VARIETIES OR CULTIVARS OF *P. VULGARIS*

Variety	Rabbit Blood	Trypsinated Cow Blood	Toxicity (No. of Injected Rats/no. of Dead Rats)
Valin de Albenga	+	+	5/4
Merida	+	+	9/9
Negro Nicoya	+	+	5/4
Saxa	+	+	5/5
Peruvita	+	−	5/0
Palleritos	+	−	6/0
Juli	+	−	5/0
Cubagua	+	−	5/0
Porillo	−	+	5/5
Negra No. 584	−	+	5/3
Varnica Saavegra	−	+	10/6
Hallado	−	−	5/0
Madrileno	−	−	5/0
Alabaster	−	−	5/0
Triguito	−	−	6/0

Source: Jaffé and Brücher (1972).
− = hemagglutinating activity absent; + = hemagglutinating activity present.

activity to toxicity is the fact that there are hundreds of different strains and cultivars of *Phaseolus vulgaris*. The hemagglutinins present in their seeds are known to exhibit different degrees of specificity, depending on the species of animal from which the red blood cells have been derived and whether or not the cells have been pretreated with proteolytic enzymes such as trypsin. Jaffé and his colleagues (Brücher *et al.* 1969; Jaffé and Brücher 1972; Jaffé *et al.* 1972) have made a systematic study of the hemagglutinating activity of a large number of different varieties or cultivars of *Phaseolus vulgaris* with respect to their action on the blood from different animals, with and without trypsinization, and the toxicity of their extracts when injected into rats. They made the significant observation that only those extracts which agglutinate trypsinated cow cells were toxic when injected into rats (Table 14.9). Feeding tests confirmed the fact that those varieties which exhibited agglutinating activity toward trypsinated cow cells were also toxic and supported very poor growth when fed to rats (Jaffé and Brücher, 1972; Jaffé and Vega Lette, 1968). Those varieties which were nonagglutinating or agglutinated only rabbit cells were nontoxic when fed. These results serve to emphasize the importance of testing the hemagglutinating activity of seed extracts against several species of blood cells before one is justified in concluding that a particular bean is toxic or not. The use of trypsinated cow cells would appear to be the most useful system for detecting potentially toxic beans.

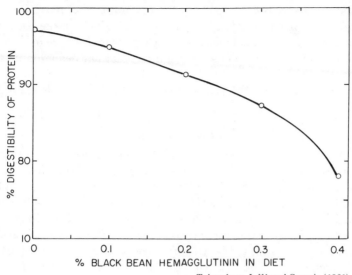

Taken from Jaffé and Camejo (1961)

FIG. 14.8. THE EFFECT OF BLACK BEAN HEMAGGLUTININ ON PRO-
TEIN DIGESTIBILITY AS MEASURED WITH RATS

As to the mechanism whereby phytohemagglutinins inhibit growth, Jaffé and Camejo (1961) have shown that the addition of the purified phytohemagglutinin from the black bean markedly reduced the digestibility of the protein (casein) component of the diet (Fig. 14.8). *In vitro* experiments with isolated intestinal loops, taken from rats fed the black bean hemagglutinin, revealed a 50% decrease in the rate of absorption of glucose across the intestinal wall compared to controls. Jaffé (1960) postulated that the action of the hemagglutinin was to combine with cells lining the intestinal wall, thus causing a nonspecific interference with the absorption of nutrients. This effect of course will be reflected in the extent to which the protein is apparently digested.

Although the toxic effects of the hemagglutinins present in plant foodstuffs can be generally eliminated by proper heat treatment, it should be recognized that conditions may prevail whereby complete destruction of the phytohemagglutinins may not always be achieved. For example, Korte (1973A) has recently observed that in mixtures of ground beans and ground cereal prepared under the field conditions prevailing in Africa, the hemagglutinin was not always destroyed, and the cooked product produced diarrhea and severe vomitting. Low concentrations of hemagglutinins may also affect the utilization of some amino acids as demonstrated by a reduced excretion of sulfur in the urine after the ingestion of insufficiently heated beans (Korte 1973B). A reduction in the boiling point of water in mountainous regions could also result in incomplete elimination of toxicity. An outbreak of massive poisoning after the consumption of partially cooked bean flakes has been reported by Griebel (1950). The marked resistance of phytohemagglutinins to inactivation by dry heat (De Muelenaere 1964) deserves special emphasis. Thus, the addition of kidney bean flour to wheat flour for the manufacture of bread (Anon. 1948) and the use of bean flour for making baked goods (Marcos and Boctor 1959) should be viewed with caution.

CONCLUSIONS

It should be apparent that, although there are numerous examples of so-called toxic constituents in legumes, they have nevertheless provided man with a valuable source of protein over the centuries. This can be attributed to the fact that man has learned how to detoxify them by suitable preparative measures. The varied nature of our diet also minimizes the contribution of a toxicant from any one foodstuff. Nevertheless, there is the ever present possibility that the prolonged consumption of a particular legume which may be improperly processed could bring to the surface toxic effects which would otherwise not be apparent. As the shortage of protein becomes more acute, it is not unlikely that much of the population of the world will, in the future, be faced with a more limited selection of protein foods, most of which will be of plant origin and hence potential carriers of toxic constituents. The nutritionist, food scientist and plant breeder should all be at least cognizant of such a possibility and be prepared to apply their knowledge and skill to meeting this challenge.

BIBLIOGRAPHY

ALUMOT, E., and NITSAN, Z. 1961. The influence of soybean antitrypsin on the intestinal proteolysis of the chick. J. Nutr. 73, 71.

ANON. 1948. Augmenting wheat flour supplies. Chem. Ind. Eng. News 26, 2516.

APPLEGARTH, A., FURUTA, F., and LEPKOVSKY, S. 1964. Response of the chicken pancreas to raw soybeans. Morphologic responses, gross and microscopic, of the pancreas of chickens on raw and heated soybean diets. Poultry Sci. 43, 733.

BESSLER, W., and GOLDSTEIN, I. J. 1973. Phytohemagglutinin purification: A general method involving affinity and gel chromatography. FEBS Letters 34, 58.

BOOTH, A. N., ROBBINS, D. J., RIBELIN, W. E., and DE EDS, F. 1960. Effect of raw soybean meal and amino acids on pancreatic hypertrophy in rats. Proc. Soc. Exptl. Biol. Med. 104, 681.

BORCHERS, R., and ACKERSON, C. W. 1950. The nutritive value of legume seeds. X. Effect of autoclaving and the trypsin inhibitor test for 17 species. J. Nutr. 44, 339.

BRESSANI, R., VITERI, F., ELIAS, L. G., DE ZAGHI, S., ALVARADO, J. and ODELL, A. D. 1967. Protein quality of a soybean protein textured in experimental animals and children. J. Nutr. 93, 349.

BRÜCHER, O., WECKSLER, M., LEVY, A., PALLOZZO, A., and JAFFÉ, W. G. 1969. Comparison of phytohemagglutinin in beans Phaseolus aborigineus and in common beans Phaseolus vulgaris and their inheritance. Phytochemistry 8, 1739.

CHERNICK, S. S., LEPKOVSKY, S., and CHAIKOFF, I. L. 1948. A dietary factor regulating the enzyme content of the pancreas. Changes induced in size and proteolytic activity of the chick pancreas by ingestion of raw soybean meal. Am. J. Physiol. 155, 33.

COAN, M. H., and TRAVIS, J. 1971. Interaction of human pancreatic proteinases with naturally occurring proteinase inhibitors. *In* Proceedings of the International Research Conference on Proteinase Inhibitors, H. Fritz, and H. Tschesche (Editors). Walter de Gruyter, Berlin.

DEAN, R. F. A. 1958. The use of processed plant proteins as human food. *In* Processed Plant Protein Foodstuffs, A. M. Altschul (Editor). Academic Press, New York.

DE MUELENAERE, H. J. H. 1964. Effect of heat treatment on the haemagglutinating activity of legumes. Nature *201*, 1029.

DESIKACHAR, H. S. R., and DE, S. S. 1947. Role of inhibitors in soybeans. Science *106*, 421.

EVANS, R. J., and MCGINNIS, J. 1948. Cystine and methionine metabolism by chicks receiving raw or autoclaved soybean oil meal. J. Nutr. *35*, 477.

FEENEY, R. E., MEANS, G. E., and BIGLER, J. C. 1969. Inhibition of human trypsin, plasmin and thrombin by naturally occurring inhibitors of proteolytic enzymes. J. Biol. Chem. *244*, 1957.

FIGARELLA, C., CLEMENTE, F., and GUY, O. 1969. On zymogens of human pancreatic juice. F.E.B.S. Letters *3*, 351.

FIGARELLA, C., NEGRI, G. A., and GUY, O. 1975. The two human trypsinogens. Inhibition spectra of the two human trypsins derived from their purified zymogens. European J. Biochem. *53*, 457.

GREEN, G. M., and LYMAN, R. L. 1972. Feedback regulation of pancreatic enzyme secretion as a mechanism for trypsin inhibitor-induced hypersecretion in rats. Proc. Soc. Exptl. Biol. Med. *140*, 6.

GRIEBEL, C. 1950. Erkrankungen durch bohnenflocken *Phaseolus vulgaris* L. und platterbsen *Lathyrus tingitanus* L. Z. Lebensm. Untersuch.-Forsch *90*, 191.

HABEEB, A. F. S. A. 1966. Determination of free amino groups in proteins by trinitrobenzene sulfonic acid. Anal. Biochem. *14*, 328.

HAM, W. E., SANSTEDT, R. M., and MUSSEHL, F. E. 1965. The proteolytic inhibitory substance in the extract from unheated soybean meal and its effects upon growth in chicks. J. Biol. Chem. *161*, 635.

HAYWARD, J. W., and HAFNER, F. H. 1941. The supplementary effect of cystine and methionine upon the protein of raw and cooked soybeans as determined with chicks and rats. Poultry Sci. *20*, 139.

HONAVAR, P. M., SHIH, C.-V., and LIENER, I. E. 1962. Inhibition of growth of rats by purified hemagglutinin fractions isolated from *Phaseolus vulgaris*. J. Nutr. *77*, 109.

JAFFÉ, W. G. 1960. Uber phytotoxine ans bohnen. Arzneimittel-Forsch. *12*, 1012.

JAFFÉ, W. G., and BRÜCHER, O. 1972. Toxicity and purification of the different phytohemagglutinins of beans *Phaseolus vulgaris*. Arch. Latinoam. Nutr. *22*, 267.

JAFFÉ, W. G., BRÜCHER, O., and PALOZZO, A. 1972. Detection of four types of specific phytohemagglutinins in different lines of beans *Phaseolus vulgaris*. Z. Immunitaetsforsch. Allerg. Klin. Immunol. *142*, 439.

JAFFÉ, W. G., and CAMEJO, G. 1961. La accion de una proteina toxica aislada de caroatas negras *Phaseolus vulgaris* sobre la absorcion intestinal en ratas. Acta Cient. Venezuela *12*, 59.

JAFFÉ, W. G., and VEGA LETTE, C. L. 1968. Heat-labile growth inhibiting factors in beans, *Phaseolus vulgaris*. J. Nutr. *94*, 203.

KAKADE, M. L., ARNOLD, R. L., LIENER, I. E., and WAIBEL, P. E. 1969. Unavailability of cystine from trypsin inhibitor as a factor contributing to the poor nutritive value of navy beans. J. Nutr. *99*, 34.

KAKADE, M. L., HOFFA, D., and LIENER, I. E. 1973. Contribution of trypsin inhibitors to the deleterious effects of unheated soybeans fed to rats. J. Nutr. *103*, 1772.

KAKADE, M. L., SIMONS, N., and LIENER, I. E., 1969. An evaluation of natural vs. synthetic substrates for measuring the antitryptic activity of soybean samples. Cereal Chem. *46*, 518.

KAKADE, M. L., SIMONS, N. R., LIENER, I. E., and LAMBERT, J. W. 1972. Biochemical and nutritional assessment of different varieties of soybeans. J. Agr. Food Chem. *20*, 87.

KHAYAMBASHI, H., and LYMAN, R. L. 1966. Growth depression and pancreatic and intestinal changes in rats force-fed amino acid diets containing soybean trypsin inhibitor. J. Nutr. *89*, 455.

KLOSE, A. A., HILL, B., and FEVOLD, H. L. 1946. Presence of a growth inhibiting substance in raw soybean. Proc. Soc. Exptl. Biol. Med. *62*, 10.

KONIJN, A. M., and GUGGENHEIM, K. 1967. Effect of raw soybean flour on the composition of rat pancreas. Proc. Soc. Exptl. Biol. Med. *126*, 65.

KORTE, R. 1973A. Heat resistance of phytohemagglutinins in weaning food mixtures containing beans, *Phaseolus vulgaris.* Ecol. Food Nutr. *1*, 303.

KORTE, R. 1973B. Weanling food nutrition. Paper presented at IVth Intern. Congr. Nutr., Mexico City.

KUNITZ, M. 1945. Crystalization of a trypsin inhibitor from soybeans. Science *101*, 668.

KWONG, E., BARNES, R. H., and FIALA, G. J. 1962. Intestinal absorption of nitrogen and methionine from processed soybeans in the rat. J. Nutr. *77*, 312.

LEWIS, J. H., and TAYLOR, F. H. L. 1947. Comparative utilization of raw and autoclaved soybean protein by the human. Proc. Soc. Exptl. Biol. Med. *64*, 85.

LIENER, I. E. 1973. Toxic factors associated with legume proteins. Ind. J. Nutr. Dietet. *10*, 303.

LIENER, I. E. 1974. Phytohemagglutinins: Their nutritional significance. Agr. Food Chem. *22*, 17.

LIENER, I. E., and KAKADE, M. L. 1969. Protease inhibitors. *In* Toxic Constituents of Plant Foodstuffs, I. E. Liener (Editor). Academic Press, New York.

LYMAN, R. L., and LEPKOVSKY, S. 1957. The effect of raw soybean meal and trypsin inhibitor diets on pancreatic enzyme secretion in the rat. J. Nutr. *62*, 269.

MALLORY, P. A., and TRAVIS, J. 1973. Human pancreatic enzymes. Characterization of anionic human trypsin. Biochem. *12*, 2847.

MARCOS, S. K., and BOCTOR, A. M. 1959. The use of *Dolichos lablab* and *Lathyrus sativus* in the making of taamiah (bean cakes) in Egypt. Brit. J. Nutr. *13*, 163.

MELNICK, D., OSER, B. L., and WEISS, S. 1946. Rate of enzymic digestion of proteins as a factor in nutrition. Science *103*, 326.

NESHEIM, M. C., GARLICH, J. D., and HOPKINS, D. T. 1962. Studies on the effect of raw soybean meal on fat absorption in young chicks. J. Nutr. *78*, 89.

NIESS, E., IVY, C. A., and NESHEIM, M. C. 1972. Stimulation of gall bladder emptying and pancreatic secretion in chicks by soybean whey protein. Proc. Soc. Exptl. Biol. Med. *140*, 291.

OSBORNE, T. B., and MENDEL, L. B. 1917. The use of soybean as food. J. Biol. Chem. *32*, 369.

PIAN, J. H. C. 1930. Biological value of the proteins of mung beans, peanut and bean curd. Chinese J. Physiol. *4*, 431.

RACKIS, J. J. 1965. Physiological properties of soybean trypsin inhibitors and their relationship to pancreatic hypertrophy and growth inhibition of rats. Federation Proc. *24*, 1488.

RACKIS, J. J., MCGHEE, J. E., and BOOTH, A. N. 1975. Biological threshold levels of soybean trypsin inhibitors by rat bioassay. Cereal Chem. *52*, 85.

SALMAN, A. J., DAL BORGO, G., PUBOLS, M. H., and MCGINNIS, J. 1967. Changes in pancreatic enzymes as a function of diet in the chick. Proc. Soc. Exptl. Biol. Med. *126*, 694.

SHURPALEKAR, S. R., CHANDRASEKHARA, M. R., SWAMINATHAN, M., and SUBRAHMANYAN, V. 1961. Chemical composition and nutritive value of soybean and soybean products. Food Sci. (Mysore) *11*, 52.

SMITH, A. K., RACKIS, J. J., HESSELTINE, C. W., SMITH, M., ROBBINS, D. J., and BOOTH, A. A. 1964. Tempeh: Nutritive value in relation to processing. Cereal Chem. *41*, 173.

STANDAL, B. R. 1963. Nutritive value of proteins of oriental soybean foods. J. Nutr. *81*, 279.

TRAVIS, J., and ROBERTS, R. C. 1969. Human trypsin isolation and physical-chemical characterization. Biochem. *8*, 2884.

TURNER, R. H., and LIENER, I. E. 1975. The effect of the selective removal of hemagglutinins on the nutritive value of soybeans. J. Agr. Food Chem. 23, 484.

VAN VEEN, A. G., and SCHAEFFER, G. 1950. The influence of the tempeh fungus on the soya bean. Doc. Neerl, Ondones. Morbis Trop. 2, 270.

WAGH, P. V., KLAUSTERMEIR, D. F., WAIBEL, P. E., and LIENER, I. E. 1965. Nutritive value of red kidney beans, Phaseolus vulgaris. J. Nutr. 80, 191.

WESTFALL, R. J., and HAUGE, S. M. 1948. The nutritive quality and the trypsin inhibitor content of soybean flour heated at various temperatures. J. Nutr. 35, 374.

CHAPTER 15

W. H. Martinez | Other Antinutritional Factors of Practical Importance

Antinutritional factors associated with edible proteins can be resolved into two classes, (1) factors which in themselves are physiologically deliterious, and (2) factors which induce a physiological deficiency, e.g., those which affect the availability of vitamins or minerals in the diet. Factors in the first class can be further subdivided into (a) those which are phytologically indigenous, such as gossypol, glucosinolates and the protease inhibitors, (b) those which are environmentally introduced, such as selenium and mercury, and (c) those which are concentrated to unacceptable levels by processing, such as fluoride or nucleic acids.

The factors selected for this discussion were chosen on the basis of the generally accepted potential of the proteinaceous materials in which they are found for contribution to world protein resources. Since the protease inhibitors are reviewed in Chapter 14, this discussion will be limited to a current review of the problems of gossypol in cottonseed and glucosinolates in rapeseed as examples of Class 1 factors, and a review of the phytates in plant proteins as an example of Class 2 factors. In two relatively recent books (Natl. Acad. Sci.–Natl. Res. Council 1973; Liener 1969), much of the information on the physiological response of these factors is reviewed. The emphasis of this discussion, therefore, will center on methods for elimination and research needs.

GOSSYPOL

The limiting factor in the use of cottonseed protein for man and animals has been the presence of the highly colored, highly reactive, phenolic pigment called gossypol (Berardi and Goldblatt 1969). Gossypol is a polyhydroxyl, binapthyl dialdehyde which is localized in specific extracellular glands within the seed kernel of the cotton plant (Leahy 1948; Boatner 1948; Moore and Rollins 1961). It is also found in specific glands in the stem, leaf and boll of the plant, and in the free form in the root tissue (Smith 1961) and the vascular system (Bell et al. 1975) of the plant. Various proposals on the function of gossypol and its precursors in the plant have been made. All suggest some host-plant resistance or phytoalexin mechanism (Bell and Presley 1969; Stipanovic et al. 1975; Sadykov et al. 1974). The premise that the glands in the seed merely serve as a storage site for the gossypol is supported by the facts that all of the gossypol in the seed is located within the glands and no differences have been found in the oil or protein characteristics of the glanded and glandless cottonseed (Thaung *et al.* 1961).

The pigment glands of the cottonseed can be spherical or ovoid, range from 100–400 μ on the long axis, comprise from 2.4–4.8% of the kernel weight and consist internally of a multiplicity of spherules containing a variety of gossypol pigments associated with lipid, phosphorus and some nitrogenous constituents. The exact distribution and type of pigments are determined by genetic factors and the climatic conditions during maturation of the seed, as well as by length of storage and environmental conditions during storage. Isolated and purified gossypol pigments are water insoluble, but the glandular contents of the cottonseed are very readily dispersed in water. This difference in dispersibility suggests that the pigments occur naturally in a complexed form.

Superimposed upon the complexity of this natural occurrence are (*1*) the induced effects of processing which affects both the pigments and the protein, (*2*) the necessity to distinguish between *in vitro* and *in vivo* reactions of purified gossypol pigments versus naturally occurring complexes, and (*3*) the need for accurate quantitative procedures for the physiologically active forms of the gossypol pigments. The physiological action of gossypol (and each of the other antinutritional factors in this discussion) is an extremely complex problem which in many instances cannot be easily or precisely separated from the total response obtained in feeding the proteins, carbohydrates and other nutrients with which the factor occurs.

Physiological Effects

The physiological effects of gossypol vary with the species. Ruminants are not adversely affected by gossypol and the acute oral toxicity for non-ruminants is relatively low. However, the biological effects of physiologically active "free" gossypol in nonruminants are cumulative (Smith and Clawson 1970; Albrecht *et al.* 1971) producing the general symptoms of depressed appetite and subsequent loss in weight. Studies by Abou-Donia *et al.* (1970, 1974) *in vitro* suggested that gossypol may exert its toxic effect by uncoupling respiratory chain-linked phosphorylation. The major *in vivo* observations in swine, however, suggest interaction with iron metabolism. A series of studies (Albrecht *et al.* 1971; Skutches *et al.* 1973, 1974) indicate that the primary pathway of gossypol excretion is via the biliary system as iron complexes. These studies also suggest that the initial effect of gossypol *in vivo* is to chelate iron which results in a reduced hematocrit and inhibition of the normal utilization of iron for the synthesis of hemoglobin and respiratory enzymes. Braham and Bressani (1975) obtained similar results with rats and, at high levels of "free" gossypol intake, noted increased blood serum and decreased liver transaminase activity. These findings support the well-accepted feeding practice of inhibiting the physiological activity of "free" gossypol in swine and poultry by the addition of ferrous sulfate to cottonseed meal rations (Phelps 1966). The existence or the precise site of the interaction between iron and gossypol in the diet or in the digestive tract has not been demonstrated or determined except in terms of the enhanced growth of the animal.

Gossypol Complexes

Commercially the application of heat, moisture and pressure at various points in the defatting operation is used to rupture the pigment glands. Under these conditions, the released gossypol pigments react with other cellular constituents.

The exact nature of the gossypol complexes with the cellular constituents has never been elucidated. *In vitro* evidence suggests the formation of a Shiff base between the aldehyde groups of gossypol and the epsilon amino group of lysine (Conkerton and Frampton 1959). In model-system studies of the reaction between pepsinogen and gossypol (Wong *et al.* 1972; Finlay *et al.* 1973) the formation of intra- and intermolecular cross linkages were indicated and confirmed by the isolation of one gossypol linked peptide and the product from borohydride reduction of the Shiff base. However, no direct evidence of the gossypol-lysine interaction in cottonseed has been obtained. It has been demonstrated that the level of epsilon-free lysine in cottonseed can be reduced in the absence as well as the presence of gossypol (Martinez *et al.* 1967).

Effects of Inactivation On Protein Quality

Cottonseed protein products for human consumption must, in accord with U.S. Food and Drug Administration regulations (Federal Register 1974), contain no more than 0.045% "free" gossypol. No limitation was placed on the total gossypol content. Total gossypol is that quantity which can be measured after acid hydrolysis. "Free" gossypol is that portion of the pigment which can be freely extracted with 70% aqueous acetone (Berardi and Goldblatt 1969). Since the total gossypol contents of defatted cottonseed products will range from 0.5–1.2%, the degree of processing required to inactivate or bind this quantity of gossypol is intensive and normally results in decreased lysine availability and reduced protein quality (Martinez *et al.* 1961; Eagle and Davis 1957). The processing of cottonseed seed is, therefore, a delicate compromise between gossypol inactivation and maintenance of protein quality. The duality of this problem also complicates the interpretation of the physiological effects of the processed materials.

Eliminating the "Gossypol Problem"

The most satisfactory solution to the gossypol problem would be total elimination. Presently, there are two approaches to this solution; one is genetic, the other is mechanical removal of the intact pigment gland using the liquid cyclone process (Gardner *et al.* 1973). In the latter process, the dehulled kernels are dried to a moisture content (1–3%) which will permit the use of impact milling to rupture the cells of the seed tissue without rupture of the pigment glands. The glands and coarse cell fragments are then separated from the subcellular particulates by differential centrifugation of a hexane slurry of the milled seed kernels in a liquid cyclone. The gland-free fine particles are separated from the oil-rich hexane on a rotary drum filter under vacuum and desolventized to produce a defatted cottonseed flour. This flour is low in both free and total gossypol and has a protein quality near that of casein (Martinez and Hopkins 1975). Commercial production of this flour, containing 65% protein and less than 0.045% "free" gossypol, is presently in the shakedown phases of the operation.

Glandless varieties of cotton are available from most of the commercial breeders. However, slow acceptance by the farmer due to lack of any economic incentive and questions of lint yield and insect resistance have limited the acreage to only contract production. With clearance from FDA, use of the dehulled kernels as condiment nuts is anticipated. Properly defatted glandless cottonseed is an excellent source of a variety of protein products (Martinez *et al.* 1970).

GLUCOSINOLATES

The seeds from two species of the mustard family (Cruciferae), rape (*Brassica napus*) and turnip rape (*Brassica campestris*), are known commonly as rapeseed. The toxicological problems associated with this major oilseed and potential world protein resource are equally as complex as gossypol. The major problem results from the presence of glucosinolates which, under the influence of moisture and the enzyme thioglucosidase, can be reduced to glucose, $KHSO_4$, isothiocyanate, nitriles and thiocyanates (Van Etten and Wolff 1973).

Like gossypol, the concentration of glucosinolates is influenced by variety, climatic environment, nutrition of the soil and maturity (Josefsson 1970; Kondra and Downey 1969; Finlayson 1971). It is also influenced by the pod position on the plants (Kondra and Downey 1970). The ultrastructure of the seed (Hofsten 1972) is typical of the oilseeds. Cells are densely packed with lipid droplets, aleurone grains and the globoid inclusions. Unlike gossypol, the exact location of the glucosinolates, intra- or extracellular, is not known. However, the inheritance of the glucosinolates has been determined (Kondra and Stefansson 1970).

Nitriles and Goitrins

The conditions of seed storage, treatment during the defatting operation and conditions during the time of enzymatic activity, if any, will determine the products formed from the glucosinolates. These can be predominantly either unsaturated nitriles or the isothiocyanates called progoitrins. The latter undergo cyclic rearrangements to form the compounds called goitrins because of their goitrogenic activity. The nitriles tend to have greater acute toxicity than the goitrins and can cause pathological kidney and liver lesions. The goitrins cause mild hyperplastic goiter with slight reduction in weight gain and mild liver enlargement (Oliver *et al.* 1971; Lo and Hill 1971A, 1972; Bell *et al.* 1972). Lanzani and Vacini (1971) and Lanzani *et al.* (1974A) have shown that a major goitrin of rapeseed, 5-vinyl-1,3-oxazolidin-2-thione, has an easily alterable structure and will polymerize with heat. Bjoerkman (1973) has shown that the isothiocyanates will react with the basic low molecular proteins during extraction at pH values greater than 6.

Detoxification

The methods proposed for inactivation or removal of the glucosinolates are numerous. Most consist of some variation of heat inactivation and/or aqueous extraction. Dahlen and Goude (1973) proposed a fluidized steam treatment. Lanzani *et al.* (1974B) suggested heating in the presence of $Na_2S_2O_3$. Others have used hydrogen peroxide (Anderson *et al.* 1975), and microbiological procedures (Poznanski *et al.* 1973; Staron 1974).

Proposals for aqueous extractions in many forms have been made: aqueous diffusion (Sosulski *et al.* 1972), aqueous ethanol (Ekmund *et al.* 1971; Lopez *et al.* 1973), hot water (Bergqvist *et al.* 1970), double water extraction (Ballester *et al.* 1970), salt extraction (Lo and Hill 1971B), water plus heat (Barros, 1968), and heat plus water (Eapen *et al.* 1969; Tape *et al.* 1970; Sims and Nunes 1970; Ohlson 1972).

Effects of Detoxification on Nutritive Value

All of the above treatments inactivated or reduced the glucosinolate contents to varying degrees and generally increased the favorable biological response as measured by animal growth. The amino acid profile of rapeseed cultivars suggests that the protein quality should be excellent. It is high in lysine, and the sulfur amino acids. Flours and concentrates with low glucosinolate contents reportedly were as good or better than casein. However, the total picture on the nutritive quality of defatted, detoxified rapeseed suffers from the complexity of the variables contributing to the growth response and again a lack of adequate methodology to determine the physiologically active levels of glucosinolates and their by-products.

Ogawa *et al.* (1971) has reported the presence of two groups of proteinase inhibitors which may account in part for the beneficial effects of moist heat in the presence of low glucosinolate concentrations.

Genetic Developments

Possibly the most important advance has been the genetic development of very low glucosinolate varieties. With the aid of a rapid analytical method for testing small samples of seed (Youngs and Wetter 1967), it has been possible to breed a variety of rapeseed, "Tower," low in glucosinolate (Stephansson 1975) and low in erucic acid, a long chain fatty acid which is also detrimental to animal and human health (Mattson 1973).

Preliminary evaluations of this new Tower variety have been favorable. Bowland (1975) reported the defatted, low-glucosinolate rapeseed meal was satisfactory as a complete replacement for soybeans in rations for growing pigs, and Jones (1975) showed that the protein efficiency of the flour was greater than casein. McLaughlan *et al.* (1975), however, have confirmed the detrimental effects, reported earlier by Eklund (1973), on pregnant rats. Jones (1975) and Shah *et al.* (1976), in turn, have demonstrated that the adverse effects of rapeseed meal on zinc metabolism can be overcome by proper supplementation of the diet with zinc.

PHYTATES

The chemical and antinutritional aspects of the presence of phytates in animal and human dietaries have been reviewed recently by Oberleas (1973) and Rackis (1974). The first is a general review of the problem; the second deals specifically with soybean protein products. The major aspects of concern are (1) the availability of phytate phosphorus and (2) the role of phytates in the availability of trace minerals and calcium.

Occurrence

Phytic acid and phytates are the common terms for myoinositol hexaphosphate and its salts. Inositol phosphates containing fewer than six phosphate groups commonly occur in the complex lipids of both animals and plants. The hexaphosphate, however, is only known to occur in plants, primarily seeds. Phytate concentration of the seed increases with maturation. Conflicting reports exist on the importance of phosphate fertilizer to the seed phytate concentration and the percentage of total seed phosphorus that it represents (Asada *et al.* 1969; Kazantseva 1971; Rutkowska and Tryebska-Jeske 1973). The effect of fertilizer probably varies with the soil phosphorus, the time of fertilization, type of fertilizer (N/P/K), and the type of seed.

Phytates are not generally distributed throughout the seed but are located in specific morphological components (O'Dell *et al.* 1972A; Kennedy and Schelstraete 1975). In the cereals they tend to be concentrated in the germ and aleurone layer of cells of the kernel, and in the bran or hull. Corn differs from most cereals in that almost 90% of the phytate occurs in the germ. Since the major morphological differences between normal and high lysine corn occur in the endosperm, the phytate distribution in high lysine corn is essentially the same as that of normal corn (O'Dell *et al.* 1972A). In the oilseeds, which generally contain little or no endosperm, the phytates are distributed throughout the kernel but rarely occur in the hull.

Cytological evidence continues to support the premise that the major portion of the phytates, in wheat and oilseeds, are located within the specific subcellular particulates called aleurone grains or protein bodies (Yatsu 1965; Lui and Altschul 1967; Dieckert and Dieckert 1972; Pomeranz 1973). The data of Pomeranz (1973) and Lui and Altschul (1967) indicate that phytate occurs as a potassium-magnesium salt rather than a calcium-magnesium salt as suggested in the early literature. The major portion of the calcium in seed, therefore, does not occur as calcium phytates. Iron phytates also are reported to occur in cereals (Kennedy and Schelstraete 1975; Morris and Ellis 1975).

Effects of Processing

The studies cited indicate that the location and concentration of phytates varies with the type of seed, the maturity of the seed and the portion of the seed consumed. Protein concentrates made from corn germ (O'Dell *et al.* 1972A; Blessin *et al.* 1974), abrasive milling of rice (Kennedy and Schelstraete 1975) or the by-products of flour milling (Ferrel *et al.* 1969) would all be relatively high in phytates. The phytate concentration and distribution in oilseed protein products will also depend upon the manner in which the seed is fractionated and processed (Vix *et al.* 1972). It must be recognized, however, that the phytate which occurs within aleurone grains or protein bodies is not generally distributed as a protein-phytate complex but is concentrated as a specific inclusion, 1–2 μ or less in diameter, within the protein matrix of the protein body which, in turn, is surrounded by a classical unit membrane. This aleurone grain in the unruptured cell is imbedded and surrounded by the cytoplasm of the cell and the cell wall. Access to these phytates—the phytates of the aleurone grains—is limited, therefore, by the permeability of a series of structures, by the degree to which these structures are disrupted during processing, by the solubility characteristics of the surrounding proteins, and by the solubility of the phytate salt itself.

In the preparation of protein isolates from undenatured, defatted cottonseed flakes by aqueous alkaline extraction at pH 10.5 (Berardi *et al.* 1969), the major portion of the seed phosphorus, which is phytin phosphorus (Martinez *et al.* 1961), remained in the residue. The fact that phytin is coextracted and precipitated with oilseed proteins such as soybean also is well documented (Smith and Rackis 1957; Wolf 1972). These statements are not meant to be contradictory but rather illustrative of the complexity of the problem and the need for specific quantitative analytical methodology. The major portion of the proteins of the undenatured soybean are water dispersible. That is, the aleurone grains are ruptured and the proteins surrounding the phytate inclusions are dispersed, thereby increasing the availability of the phytates for extraction. The aleurone-grain proteins of the undenatured cottonseed are not water dispersible, and in low ionic strength solutions can only be extracted at relatively high pH values in which the major portion of the phosphorus is not extracted. The exact cationic composition of the phytic acid salt which exists in the inclusions of the aleurone grains in either of the oilseeds, the phytate solubility characteristics, and the ability of the nature phytates to interact with the polyvalent proteins above the isoelectric point are not known. All that has been determined is that a certain portion of the phosphorus of the seed coprecipitates with the proteins. This could equally be the result of protein-phosphoprotein, protein-phospholipid, protein-nucleoprotein, or protein-phytate interactions where the phytic acid salt differs in cellular location and cationic constituents. The coextraction or presence of calcium ions in the extraction medium also can affect the nature and type of phytin-protein association above the isoelectric point, and disassociation below the isoelectric point, pH 4.9, of the major soybean proteins (Okubo et al. 1974A, 1974B, 1975).

Much of the information and many of the conclusions in the literature are based on phosphorus, not phytate analysis, and on the results obtained with model systems utilizing phytic acid or sodium phytate, aqueous protein extracts and metal salts. Little of this information has been substantiated with in situ evaluation and analysis, particularly in terms of identification of the native forms, the effect of processing on their extraction and solubility characteristics, and most importantly, the relationship between the form in which they are consumed and their ability in this form to contribute to reactions described in model systems. The major difficulties preventing substantiation are (1) the complexity of the materials in which they are found, (2) the difficulties involved in extraction of the native form, and (3) the lack of appropriate and definitive methodology for the assay of phytates. Recent advances in coupling X-ray reflectance methodology for the determination of metals with scanning electron microscopy offers great potential for further elucidation of certain aspects of these problems.

Effect on Nutritional Availability of the Elements

Methodology problems also exist in the determination of the physiological action of phytates. Too often, the mere presence of phytates in the native unprocessed form of the material consumed is construed to be axiomatic proof of the physiological reactivity. Oberleas (1973) makes the unqualified statement that "phytate should not be considered a source of available phosphate for monogastric animals or man." This statement must be qualified in terms of the physiological system and the form in which the phytate-containing material is consumed. Ranhotra et al. (1974) reported an increase in available phosphorus during bread making caused by hydrolysis of all of the wheat phytate and more than 75% of the added soy flour phytate by phytases in the wheat and/or yeast. The phosphorus in cottonseed meal was reported to be 80% available to turkey poults by Andrews et al. (1972) and the absorption of phytin-phosphorus by swine has been reviewed by Schulz and Oslage (1972). Nelson et al. (1968, 1971) also found that the addition of a mold phytase preparation increased the availability of phytate phosphorus in a chick diet.

Heating is reported (Carlson 1967) to overcome the physiological effects of phytin particularly with respect to raw or unheated soybean meal. This suggests that the extractability characteristics of the protein and phytates in the material and consequently the dispersibility in the various segments of the digestive system have been favorably altered. Moist heating or autoclaving usually produces denaturation of the cytoplasmic components of the cell and can consequently reduce the extractability of the aleurone grain proteins and their phytate inclusions. Solubilization of the phytates could, therefore, be restricted to the intestinal tract where enzymatic hydrolysis of the proteins could permit effective release of the phytates to the action of the phytases of the intestinal microflora.

The problem of phytate phosphorus availability in animal feeds is often compounded by the addition of calcium carbonate to the diet. The effect of this salt on the solubility and extractability of the phytin in oats, wheat and wheat bran was examined in detail in a series of papers by Hill and Tyler (1954A, 1954B, 1954C). The results suggest that the phytic acid and calcium solubilized under the acid conditions in the stomach would rapidly precipitate on entering the alkaline medium of the intestine and subsequently would be rendered unavailable for hydrolysis and adsorption. As recognized by the authors, the results of these studies do not necessarily directly relate to the solubility characteristics of the phytates in heated or processed materials or in the digestive tract. Much of the data on the extraction characteristics of the phytates in the oilseeds also has been obtained with carefully prepared undenatured materials and will not directly relate to conditions in processed materials. Morris and Ellis (1975) have noted that demonstration of the biological availability of the iron in monoferric phytate isolated from wheat bran does not mean that the iron is readily available since it could be bound in an undigestible bran matrix.

The situation with respect to the effect of phytates and phytic acid on trace mineral availability has much of the same complexity. Oberleas (1973) has reviewed the formation of metal complexes of phytate and the synergistic effect of two or more cations such as zinc and calcium in increasing the precipitation of phytates. On the basis of these studies, he concluded that zinc will form an insoluble salt of phytate at pH values found in the upper small intestine resulting in decreased availability. O'Dell and Savage (1960) showed that zinc added to a soybean isolate diet would increase chick weight at four weeks and the addition of phytic acid would decrease weight at four weeks. Weight increase, which can be influenced by a great number of variables, is a relatively nondiscriminating criteria of mineral availability. The sharp decreases and increases in weight on the addition of zinc and phytic acid suggest changes in amino acid availability rather than zinc availability.

O'Dell *et al.* (1972B) have recently utilized both a chick assay and a rat assay to determine the percentage of zinc that is available in various foodstuffs. The percentage of zinc available in wheat, corn, rice and soybean meal was 59, 63, 62, and 67, respectively. In view of the relative wide variation in phytate contents among these materials, the availability or decrease therein cannot be attributed solely to phytates. Reinhold (1975) has recently set forth a phytate hypothesis based on his work with unleavened Iranian breads in explanation of observed zinc and mineral deficiences. An evaluation of the importance of the fiber content of the unleavened bread to the availability of zinc would seem appropriate.

BIBLIOGRAPHY

ABOU-DONIA, M. B., and DIECKERT, J. W. 1974. Gossypol: Uncoupling of respiratory chain and oxidative phosphorylation. Life Sci. *14*, 1955.

ABOU-DONIA, M. B., LYMAN, C. M., and DIECKERT, J. W. 1970. Metabolic fate of gossypol: The metabolism of 14-C gossypol in rats. Lipids *5*, 938.

ALBRECHT, J. E., CLAWSON, A. J., SMITH, F. H., and ALSMEYER, W. L. 1971. Effect of initial weight and days on feed on the accumulation of gossypol in pig livers. J. Anim. Sci. *32*, 96.

ANDERSON, G. H., LI, G. S., JONES, J. D., and BENDER, F. 1975. Effect of hydrogen peroxide treatment on the nutritional quality of rapeseed flour fed to weanling rats. J. Nutr. *105*, 317.

ANDREWS, T. L., DAMRON, B. L., and HARMS, R. H. 1972. Utilization of various sources of plant phosphorus by the turkey poult. Nutr. Rept. Intern. *6*, 251.

ANON. 1974. Modified cottonseed products. Federal Register *39*, No. 177, 32735.

ASADA, K., TANAKA, K., and KASAI, Z. 1969. Formation of phytic acid in cereal grains. Ann. N.Y. Acad. Sci. 165.

BALLESTER, D., RODRIGO, R., NAKOUZI, V., CHICHESTER, C. O., YANEZ, E., and MONCKEBERG, F. 1970. Rapeseed meal III-A simple method for detoxification. J. Sci. Food Agr. *21*, 143.

BARROS, F. M. 1968. Extraction of toxic substances from a presscake of *Brassica napus*. U.S. Pat. 3,615,648.

BELL, J. M., BENJAMIN, B. R., and GIOVANETTI, P. M. 1972. Histopathology of thyroids and livers of rats and mice fed diets containing *Brassica* glucosinolates. Can. J. Anim. Sci. *52*, 407.

BELL, A. A., and PRESLEY, J. T. 1969. Temperature effects upon resistance and phytoalexin synthesis in cotton inoculated with verticillium. Phytopathol. *59*, 1141.

BELL, A. A., STIPANOVIC, R. D., HOWELL, C. R., and FRYXELL, P. A. 1975. Antimicrobial terpenoids of gossypium, hemigossypol, 6-methoxyhemigossypol and 6-deoxyhemigossypol. Phytochem. *14*, 225.

BERARDI, L. C., and GOLDBLATT, L. A. 1969. Gossypol. *In* Toxic Constituents of Plant Foodstuffs, I. E. Liener (Editor). Academic Press, New York.

BERARDI, L. C., MARTINEZ, W. H., and FERNANDEZ, C. J. 1969. Cottonseed protein isolates: two step extraction procedure. Food Technol. *23*, 75.

BERGQVIST, A. E., GONZALES, D. N., CIDUDAD, B. C., and GUAJARDO, G. V. 1970. Extraction of the toxic principle from rapeseed meal with hot water and application of the meal in chicken feed. Agr. Tec. (Chile) *30*, 19.

BJOERKMAN, R. 1973. Interaction between proteins and glucosinolate isothiocyanates and oxazolidinethiones from *Brassica napus* seed. Phytochem. *12*, 1585.

BLESSIN, C. W., GARCIA, W. J., DEATHERAGE, W. L., and INGLETT, G. E. 1974. An edible defatted germ flour from a commercial dry-milled corn fraction. Cereal Sci. Today *19*, 224.

BOATNER, C. H. 1948. Pigments of cottonseed. *In* Cottonseed and Cottonseed Products, A. E. Bailey (Editor). John Wiley & Sons, New York.

BOWLAND, J. P. 1975. Evaluation of low glucosinolate-low erucic acid rapeseed meals as protein supplements for young growing pigs, including effects on blood serum constituents. Can. J. Anim. Sci. *55*, 409.

BRAHAM, J. E., and BRESSANI, R. 1975. Effect of different levels of gossypol on transaminase activity, on nonessential to essential amino acid ratio, and on iron and nitrogen retention in rats. J. Nutr. *105*, 348.

CARLSON, C. W. 1967. Iodine, vitamins, minerals and phytic acid as related to soybean protein. U.S. Dept. Agr., ARS-71-35, 81.

CONKERTON, E. J., and FRAMPTON, V. L. 1959. Reaction of gossypol with free ϵ-amino groups of lysine in proteins. Arch. Biochem. Biophys. *81*, 130.

DAHLEN, J., and GOUDE, A. 1973. Use of steam as a heating medium and fluidizing agent for the heat treatment of oilseeds. Swedish Pat. Appl. 357,658.

DIECKERT, J. W., and DIECKERT, M. C. 1972. The deposition of vacuolar proteins in oilseeds. *In* Symposium: Seed Proteins, G. E. Inglett (Editor). Avi Publishing Co., Westport, Conn.

EAGLE, E., and DAVIS, D. L. 1957. Feed value and protein-quality determination on cottonseed meals. J. Am. Oil Chem. Soc. *34*, 454.

EAPEN, K. G., TAPE, N. W., and SIMS, R. P. 1969. Recovery of seed meal from thioglucoside-containing oilseed. U.S. Pat. 3,732,108.

EKLUND, A. 1973. Influence of detoxified rapeseed protein on reproduction in the female rat. Nutr. Rept. Intern. *7*, 647.

EKLUND, A., AGREN, G., and LANGLER, T. 1971. Rapeseed protein fractions. I. Preparation of a detoxified lipid-protein concentrate from rapeseed (*Brassica napus L.*) by a water-ethanol extraction method. J. Sci. Food Agr. *22*, 650.

FERREL, R. E., WHEELER, E. L., and PENCE, J. W. 1969. Phytic acid in millfeed by-products. Cereal Sci. *14*, 110.

FINLAY, T. H., DHARMGRONGARTAMA, E. D., and PERLMANN, E. 1973. Mechanism of the gossypol inactivation of pepsinogen. J. Biol. Chem. *248*, 4827.

FINLAYSON, A. J. 1971. Changes in the amounts of seed components of rapeseed during growth. Cereal Sci. Today *16*, 293.

GARDNER, H. K. JR., HRON, R. J. SR., and VIX, H. L. E. 1973. Liquid cyclone process for edible cottonseed flour production. Oil Mill Gaz. *78*, 13.

HILL, R., and TYLER, C. 1954A. The effect of increasing acidity on the solubility of calcium, magnesium and phosphorus in certain cereals and pure salts. J. Agr. Sci. *44*, 293.

HILL, R., and TYLER, C. 1954B. The effect of decreasing acidity on the solubility of calcium, magnesium and phosphorus in bran and certain pure salt solutions. J. Agr. Sci. *44*, 311.

HILL, R., and TYLER, C. 1954C. The influence of time, temperature, pH and calcium carbonate on the activity of the phytase of certain cereals. J. Agr. Sci. *44*, 306.

HOFSTEN, A. V. 1972. Ultrastructure of protein rich rapeseeds. J. Ultrastruct. Res. *38*, 198.

JONES, J. D. 1975. Problems associated with substitution of plant proteins in human nutrition. Paper presented at 18th Annual Meeting,Canadian Federation of Biological Societies, June 24–27, 1975, Univ. of Manitoba, Winnipeg, Canada.

JOSEFFSON, E. 1970. Glucosinolate content and amino acid composition of rapeseed (*Brassica napus*) meal as affected by sulfur and nitrogen nutrition. J. Sci. Food Agr. *21*, 98.

KAZANTSEVA, O. F. 1971. Productivity and phosphate metabolism by seeds of several bean varieties under various conditions of phosphorus-potassium nutrition. Byul. Vses. Nauch. Issled. Inst. Udobr. Agropochvoved. *14*, 83.

KENNEDY, B. M., and SCHELSTRAETE, M. 1975. Chemical, physical and nutritional properties of high-protein flours and residual kernel from the overmilling of uncoated milled rice. III. Iron, calcium, magnesium, phosphorus, sodium, potassium and phytic acid. Cereal Chem. *52*, 173.

KONDRA, Z. P., and DOWNEY, R. K. 1969. Glucosinolate content of developing *Brassica napus* and *Brassica campestris* seed. Can. J. Plant Sci. *49*, 623.

KONDRA, Z. P., and DOWNEY, R. K. 1970. Glucosinolate content of rapeseed (*Brassica napus* and *B. Campestris*) meal as influenced by pod position on the plant. Crop Sci. *10*, 54.

KONDRA, Z. P., and STEFANSSON, B. R. 1970. Inheritance of the major glucosinolates of rapeseed (*Brassica napus*) meal. Can. J. Plant Sci. *50*, 643.

LANZANI, A., CARDELLO, M., and JACINI, G. 1974A. Sulfur containing substances of rapeseed, II. Riv. Ital. Sostanze Grasse *51*, 147.

LANZANI, A., PETRINI, M. C., and JACINI, G. 1974B. Antithyroid components of rapeseed in the light of protein isolate production. Riv. Ital. Sostanze Grasse *51*, 113.

LANZANI, A., and VACINI, G. 1971. Sulfur-containing substances of rapeseed, I. Riv. Ital. Sostanze Grasse *48*, 471.

LEAHY, J. 1948. Structure of the cottonseed. *In* Cottonseed and Cottonseed Products, A. E. Bailey (Editor). John Wiley & Sons, New York.

LIENER, I. E. 1969. Toxic Constituents of Plant Foodstuffs. Academic Press, New York.

LO, M. T., and HILL, D. C. 1971A. Effect of feeding a high level of rapeseed meal on weight gains and thyroid function of rats. Federation Proc. *30*, 641.

LO, M. T., and HILL, D. C. 1971B. Evaluation of protein concentrates prepared from rapeseed meal. J. Sci. Food Agr. *22*, 128.

LO, M. T., and HILL, D. C. 1972. Cyano compounds and goitrin in rapeseed meal. Can. J. Physiol. *50*, 373.

LOPEZ, V. L., MASSON, S. L., NASER, G., PENNACHIOTTI, I., and SANCHEZ, A. 1973. Determination of the critical variables for a protein detoxification and concentration process in rapeseed cakes or meals using water-alcohol extraction. Grassi. Deriv. *9*, 65.

LUI, N. S. T., and ALTSCHUL, A. M. 1967. Isolation of globoids from cottonseed aleurone grains. Arch. Biochem. Biophys. *121*, 678.

MARTINEZ, W. H., FRAMPTON, V. L., and CABELL, C. A. 1961. Effects of gossypol and raffinose on lysine content and nutritive quality of proteins in meals from glandless cottonseed. J. Agr. Food Chem. *9*, 64.

MARTINEZ, W. H., BERARDI, L. C., FRAMPTON, V. L., WILCKE, H. L., GREEN, D. E., and TEICHMAN, R. 1967. Importance of cellular constituents to cottonseed meal protein quality. J. Agr. Food Chem. *15*, 427.

MARTINEZ, W. H., BERARDI, L. C., and GOLDBLATT, L. A. 1970. Potential of cottonseed: products, composition and use. Proc. 3rd Intern. Congr. Food Sci. Technol. (SOS/70), 248, Institute of Food Technologists, Chicago, Ill.

MARTINEZ, W. H., and HOPKINS, D. T. 1975. Cottonseed protein products: variation in protein quality with product and process. *In* Protein Nutritional Quality of Foods and Feed. Part II. Quality Factors: Plant Breeding, Composition, Processing, and Anti-Nutrients, M. Friedman (Editor). Marcel Dekker, New York.

MATTSON, F. H. 1973. Potential toxicity of food lipids. *In* Toxicants Occurring Naturally in Foods, 2nd Edition. National Academy of Sciences, Washington, D.C.

MCLAUGHLAN, J. M., JONES, J. D., SHAH, B. G., and BEARE-ROGERS, J. L. 1975. Reproduction in rats fed protein concentrate from mustard or rapeseed. Nutr. Rept. Intern. *11*,

327.

MOORE, A. T., and ROLLINS, M. L. 1961. New information on the morphology of the gossypol pigment gland of cottonseed. J. Am. Oil Chemists' Soc. *38*, 156.

MORRIS, E. R., and ELLIS, R. 1975. Isolation of a soluble iron complex from wheat bran and its biological availability to the rat. Federation Proc. *34*, 923.

NATL. ACAD. SCI.-NATL. RES. COUNCIL. 1973. Toxicants Occurring Naturally in Food, 2nd Edition. National Academy of Sciences, Washington, D.C.

NELSON, T. S., SHIEH, T. R., WODZINSKI, R. J., and WARE, J. H. 1968. The availability of phytate phosphorus in soybean meal before and after treatment with a mold phytase. Poultry Sci. *47*, 1842.

NELSON, T. S., SHIEH, T. R., WODZINSKI, R. J., and WARE, J. H. 1971. Effect of supplemental phytase on the utilization of phytate phosphorus by chicks. J. Nutr. *101*, 1289.

OBERLEAS, D. 1973. Phytates. *In* Toxicants Occurring Naturally in Foods, 2nd Edition. National Academy of Sciences, Washington, D.C.

O'DELL, B. L., and SAVAGE, J. E. 1960. Effect of phytic acid on zinc availability. Proc. Soc. Exptl. Biol. Med. *103*, 304.

O'DELL, B. L., deBOLAND, A. R., and KOIRTYOHANN, S. R. 1972A. Distribution of phytate and nutritionally important elements among the morphological components of cereal grains. J. Agr. Food Chem. *20*, 718.

O'DELL, B. L., BURPO, C. E., and SAVAGE, J. E. 1972B. Evaluation of zinc availability in foodstuffs of plant and animal origin. J. Nutr. *102*, 653.

OHLSON, R. 1972. Projection and prospects for rapeseed and mustard seed. J. Am. Oil Chem. Soc. *49*, 522A.

OGAWA, T., HIGASA, T., and HASA, T. 1971. Proteinase inhibitors in plant seeds. V. Inhibitors in rape seeds. Mem. Res. Inst. Food Sci. Kyoto Univ. *32*, 1.

OKUBA, K., IACOBUCCI, G. A., and MEYERS, D. V. 1974A. Effect of divalent calcium ion on phytate binding to glycinin. Cereal Sci. Today *19*, 401.

OKUBA, K., MEYERS, D. V., and IACOBUCCI, G. A. 1974B. Binding of phytic acid to glycinin. Cereal Sci. Today *19*, 401.

OKUBA, K., WALDROP, A. B., IACOBUCCI, G. A., and MEYERS, D. V. 1975. Preparation of low phytate soybean protein isolate and concentrate by ultrafiltration. Cereal Chem. *52*, 263.

OLIVER, S. L., McDONALD, B. E., and OPUSZYNSKA, T. 1971. Weight gain, protein utilization, and liver histochemistry of rats fed low- and high-thioglucoside-content rapeseed meals. Can. J. Physiol. Pharmacol. *49*, 448.

PHELPS, R. A. 1966. Increasing the amount and performance of cottonseed protein concentrates in nonruminant rations. *In* Proc. Conf. Inactivation of Gossypol with Mineral Salts. National Cottonseed Products Assoc., Memphis, Tennessee.

POMERANZ, Y. 1973. Structure and mineral composition of cereal aleurone cells as shown by scanning electron microscopy. Cereal Chem. *50*, 504.

POZNANSKI, S., BEDNARSKI, W., JAKUBOWSKIM, J., and SAWICKI, Z. 1973. Microbiological removal of toxic substances from rapeseed meal. Przemysl. Ferment. Rolny. *17*, 27.

RACKIS, J. J. 1974. Biological and physiological factors in soybeans. J. Am. Oil Chemists' Soc. *51*, 161A.

RANHOTRA, G. S., LOEWE, R. J., and PUYAT, L. V. 1974. Phytic acid in soy and its hydrolysis during breadmaking. J. Food Sci. *39*, 1023.

REINHOLD, J. G. 1975. Zinc and mineral deficiencies of man: the phytate hypothesis. Proc. 9th Intern. Congr. Nutr. *1*, 115.

RUTKOWSKA, U., and TRYEBSKA-JESKE, I. 1973. Content of total and phytate phosphorus in wheat grains in relation to various levels of mineral fertilizers. Rocz. Panstrv. Zakl. Hiz. *24*, 707.

SADYKOV, A. S., METLITSKII, L. V., KARIMDZHANOV, A. K., ISMAILOV, A. I., MUKHAMEDOVA, R. A., AVAZKHODZHAEV, M. K. H., and KAMAEV, F. G. 1974. Isohemogossypol: a phytoalexin of cotton. Dokl. Akad. Nauk. SSR *218*, 1472.

SCHULZ, E., and OSLAGE, H. J. 1972. Intestinal hydrolysis of inositol phosphoric acid ester and the absorption of phytin phosphorus by swine. Research problems and analytical method. Z. Tierphysiol. Tierernaehr. Futtermittelk. *30*, 55.

SHAH, B. G., JONES, J. D., MCLAUGHLIN, J. M., and BEARE-ROGERS, J. L.   1976.   Beneficial effect of zinc supplementation in young rats fed protein concentrate from rapeseed or mustard.   Nutr. Rept. Intern. *13*, 1.

SIMS, R. P. A., and NUNES, A. C.   1970.   Rapeseed and sunflower protein.   Proc. 3rd Intern. Cong. Food Sci. Technol. (SOS/70), 262, Institute of Food Technologists, Chicago, Ill.

SKUTCHES, C. L., HERMAN, D. L., and SMITH, F. H.   1973.   Effect of intravenous gossypol injection on iron utilization in swine.   J. Nutr. *103*, 851.

SKUTCHES, C. L., HERMAN, D. L., and SMITH, F. H.   1974.   Effect of dietary free gossypol on blood components and tissue iron in swine and rats.   J. Nutr. *104*, 415.

SMITH, F. H.   1961.   Biosynthesis of gossypol by excised cotton roots.   Nature *192*, 888.

SMITH, F. H., and CLAWSON, A. V.   1970.   The effects of dietary gossypol on animals.   J. Am. Oil Chem. Soc. *47*, 443.

SMITH, A. K., and RACKIS, J. J.   1957.   Phytin elimination in soybean protein isolation.   J. Am. Chem. Soc. *79*, 633.

SOSULSKI, F. W., SOILMAN, F. S., and BHATTY, R. S.   1972.   Diffusion extraction of glucosinolates from rapeseed.   Can. Inst. Food Sci. Technol. J. *5*, 101.

STARON, T.   1974.   Detoxification of rapeseed cakes by a biological method.   Aliment Vie. *62*, 165.

STEFANSSON, B. R.   1975.   Tower summer rape.   Can. J. Plant Sci. *55*, 343.

STIPANOVIC, R. D., BELL, A. A., MACE, M. E., and HOWELL, C. R.   1975.   Antimicrobial terpenoids of gossypium cotton: 6-methoxy gossypol and 6,6'-dimethoxygossypol.   Phytochem. *14*, 1077.

TAPE, N. W., SABRY, Z. I., and EAPEN, K. E.   1970.   Production of rapeseed flour for human consumption.   J. Inst. Can. Technol. Aliment. *3*, 78.

THAUNG, U. K., GROS, A., and FEUGE, R. O.   1961.   Characterization of oils from low gland and glandless cottonseed.   J. Am. Oil Chemists' Soc. *38*, 220.

VAN ETTEN, C. H., and WOLFF, I. A.   1973.   Natural sulfur compounds. *In* Toxicants Occurring Naturally in Foods, 2nd Edition.   National Academy of Sciences, Washington, D.C.

VIX, H. L. E., GARDNER, H. K. JR., LAMBOU, M. G., and ROLLINS, M. L.   1972.   Ultrastructure related to cottonseed and peanut processing and products. *In* Symposium: Seed Proteins, G. E. Inglett (Editor).   Avi Publishing Co., Westport, Conn.

WOLF, W. J.   1972.   Purification and properties of the proteins. *In* Soybeans: Chemistry and Technology, Vol. 1, A. K. Smith, and S. J. Circle (Editors).   Avi Publishing Co. Inc. Westport, Connecticut.

WONG, R. C., NAKAGAWA, Y., and PERLMANN.   1972.   Studies on the nature of the inhibition by gossypol of the transformation of pepsinogen to pepsin.   J. Biol. Chem. *247*, 1625.

YATSU, L. Y.   1965.   The ultrastructure of cotyledonary tissue from *Gossypium hirsutum* L. seeds.   J. Cell. Biol. *25*, 193.

YOUNGS, C. G., and WETTER, L. R.   1967.   Microdetermination of the major individual isothiocyanates and oxazolidinethiones in rapeseed.   J. Am. Oil Chem. Soc. *44*, 551.

Index